"As someone with both chronic conditions and recurring cancer this book and approach is beyond essential. The lens, perspective, tips and insights are so accurate, powerful and important. The difference these could make to the whole person is more than I could put into words. Every professional should read this and use it as a guide and manifesto. Thank you to Dr Treisman for her work and for writing this unmissable book."

– Ellen Lake, patient and user of numerous health services

"Dr. Karen Treisman's extensive professional and personal experience of psychological trauma has resulted in a compendious exploration of the complexities in the provision and accessibility of healthcare. This academically robust yet accessible book makes trauma-informed healthcare everyone's business. At a time when healthcare professionals are facing unprecedented challenges, this hopeful book offers pragmatic and creative ways for us to return to our core values and ensure that patients are not just 'treated' but are compassionately cared for."

– Dr Carlotta Raby, Paediatric Clinical Psychologist/
Child and Adolescent Trauma Specialist

"Dr. Treisman has done it again – she has produced a book directed at anyone working in healthcare that grapples with the enormous complexity of working as a caregiver in these troubling times without overwhelming the reader. Peppered throughout the very accessible but comprehensive text are illustrations that make the material come alive. This should be a basic text in medical, nursing, public health and all allied health educational institutions."

– Sandra Bloom, M.D. Associate Professor, Health Management and
Policy, Dornsife School of Public Health, Drexel University

"Dr. Treisman's timely and enlightening book offers a transformative approach to patient care, blending relevant research with real-world examples. As a specialist, I can wholeheartedly recommend this as a must-read for all healthcare professionals committed to compassionate, holistic trauma-informed patient care."

– Dr. (Prof) Deepak Ravindran, NHS Pain Consultant
and author of The Pain Free Mindset

T0384448

Also by this author

A Treasure Box for Creating Trauma-Informed Organizations
A Ready-to-Use Resource for Trauma, Adversity, and Culturally
Informed, Infused and Responsive Systems
Dr Karen Treisman
ISBN 978 1 78775 312 9
eISBN 978 1 83997 188 4
Therapeutic Treasures Collection

**A Therapeutic Treasure Box for Working with Children
and Adolescents with Developmental Trauma**
Creative Techniques and Activities
Dr Karen Treisman
ISBN 978 1 78592 263 3
eISBN 978 1 78450 553 0
Therapeutic Treasures Collection

The Parenting Patchwork Treasure Deck
A Creative Tool for Assessments, Interventions, and Strengthening
Relationships with Parents, Carers, and Children
Dr Karen Treisman
Illustrated by Richy K. Chandler
ISBN 978 1 78775 308 2

Dr Treisman's Big Feelings Stories
Six-Book Collection
Dr Karen Treisman
Illustrated by Sarah Peacock
ISBN 978 1 83997 374 1

Dr Treisman's Therapeutic Activity Books
Six-Book Collection
Dr Karen Treisman
Illustrated by Sarah Peacock
ISBN 978 1 83997 375 8

Trauma-Informed Health Care

A Reflective Guide for Improving Care and Services

Dr. Karen Treisman

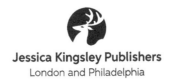

Jessica Kingsley Publishers
London and Philadelphia

First published in Great Britain in 2024 by Jessica Kingsley Publishers
An imprint of John Murray Press

2

A CIP catalogue record for this title is available from the
British Library and the Library of Congress

ISBN 978 1 83997 614 8
eISBN 978 1 83997 613 1

rinted and bound in the United States by Integrated Books International

Jessica Kingsley Publishers' policy is to use papers that are natural, renewable and recyclable
products and made from wood grown in sustainable forests. The logging and manufacturing
processes are expected to conform to the environmental regulations of the country of origin.

Jessica Kingsley Publishers
Carmelite House
50 Victoria Embankment
London EC4Y 0DZ

www.jkp.com

John Murray Press
Part of Hodder & Stoughton Limited
An Hachette UK Company

Contents

CHAPTER 1

Traumas, Adversities, and Stressors

There are many different types of traumas, adversities, and stressors. These have far-reaching diverse impacts, which can affect one's body, sensory world, and health.

It is beyond the scope of this book to provide a fully comprehensive deep dive into the many different forms of trauma. Similarly, this book will not describe therapeutic interventions for trauma.

What I aim to provide you with is a broad foundational knowledge to enable you to understand the relevance of trauma in health settings – for individual practice and trauma-informed teamwork and services – and just how prevalent trauma, stress, and adversity are within the "patient" population.

1.1. What will be covered in this chapter

- Defining trauma and adversity

- Trauma as widespread and common

- Trauma as unseen, less visible, often camouflaged

- A wider frame than the post-traumatic stress disorder (PTSD) classification

- Different types of traumas

- Some reflective questions on the different types of traumas which have been covered

1.2. Defining trauma and adversity

There are so many different definitions of trauma and adversity, and just as many opinions about these definitions. Use of the word trauma may differ depending on the context in which it is used. There are also many types: complex trauma, single-event trauma, community trauma, cultural trauma, and so on. This chapter will expand on the different forms and nuances.

To avoid getting caught up in a definitional maze, I offer a definition which is commonly used: *trauma is an event, series of events, or set of circumstances that is experienced as physically or emotionally harmful or life-threatening, overwhelms someone's ability to cope, and has lasting adverse effects on a person's mental, physical, social, emotional, or spiritual wellbeing.*

Interestingly, the word 'trauma' originates from the Greek word 'traumata', which means an injury, a wound, or to pierce. This resonates with the way that experiences of trauma can pierce or wound individuals, families, organizations, and communities.

A broader, related term is 'adversity', which will be used throughout this book. Adversity is a term commonly used to describe a range of challenging life experiences. The noun 'adversity' originally comes from the Latin word 'adversus', meaning 'turned against', and figuratively 'hostile or unfavourable': when things seem against you, you are facing adversity.

Adversity is an important additional perspective to keep in mind as we go on to consider different types of trauma. We need to be mindful that trauma does not occur within a vacuum. It is influenced by multiple systemic, relational, cultural, political, and wider contextual elements. Specific adversities might include social exclusion, social dislocation, discrimination, poverty, addiction, abuse, and so on.

As a result, trauma will necessarily mean different things to different people and different communities at different times.

My approach in writing this book is also to avoid positioning or viewing trauma as a reductive label or concept, and instead to keep the focus on the unique person within their unique context. We will have created our own sense and meaning from the experience which we have lived through, or are continuing to navigate.

You should by now be getting the idea that the impact and consequences of trauma vary – they can be broad, complex, and multi-layered.

Whether an event is 'traumatic' depends not just on the nature of the event itself, but on our experience and meaning-making of the trauma, as well as a range of other wider contextual factors.

As Gabor Maté has said in his talks, 'Trauma is not what happens to you but what happens inside you.'

Manifestations of how trauma impacts individuals are extraordinarily idio-syncratic and present on a spectrum (McDonald, 2020).

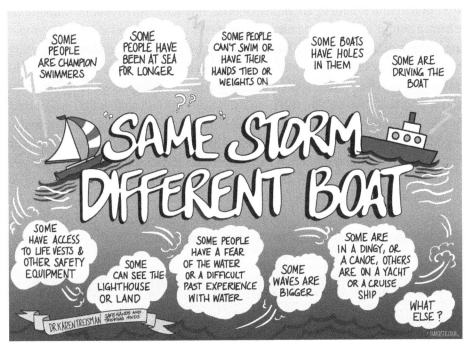

1.1. SAME STORM, DIFFERENT BOAT

Think about the common saying 'same storm, different boat' and take a look at image 1.1. To consider this saying in relation to trauma, I would suggest that it is a different storm but is also certainly a different boat. Some people don't have a boat. Others have a raft, a canoe, or a kayak. Others are on a fully staffed super yacht. Some people love the water and are amazing swimmers. Others don't know how to swim and have a fear of the water. They may have had a previous experience of almost drowning, or have weights on their legs.

Some people are alone, others have crewmates. Some have access to life jackets and food and can see the lighthouse, others are sailing without a map. Some have been at sea for longer, or the waves they are navigating through are taller and bigger.

When we talk about something like sexual abuse, we might know it as a western socially constructed term or legal category. However, it is a case of same/different storm and different boat. There is not a checklist or a one-size-fits-all. There might be ten different people who have experienced sexual abuse. They might not view it as sexual abuse or use or recognize this term; they might not share or disclose it either.

Just because I might know this term or that someone has experienced sexual abuse doesn't mean it will present the same or that it will impact people in the same or even similar ways. I don't have an emotional or life x-ray, and people are not machines. People are multi-layered, nuanced, and dynamic individuals within a unique context and culture. Each person will have different sense-making, beliefs, attributions, and feelings about the sexual abuse. Each person will have a different cultural, family, societal, and educational context, which will influence how the sexual abuse is conceptualized, interpreted, responded to, and supported. Each person will be at a different age and stage when it occurred or when they are processing it – not just chronologically but more importantly socially, emotionally, and developmentally. Each person will have a different relationship with the person who abused them, and there will be different key factors, such as was the person believed, what support was put in place, how the abuse interplays with other buffering and risk factors, and so much more.

The image below captures some of these interplaying and influencing factors (this is by no means an exhaustive or prescriptive list).

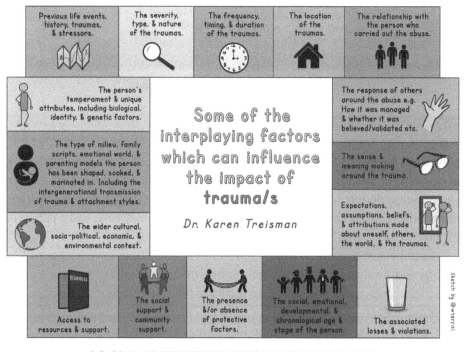

1.2. SOME OF THE INTERPLAYING FACTORS WHICH CAN
INFLUENCE THE IMPACT OF TRAUMA

★ Take some time to reflect on the above factors and what they mean, what they might look like, and how they might apply to you, and to those you support.

★ Which others would you like to add, reword, or change?

People can view or describe trauma in different ways and use different terms. The infographic below captures some of the meaning-making, words, and explanations that over 100 people shared when asked.

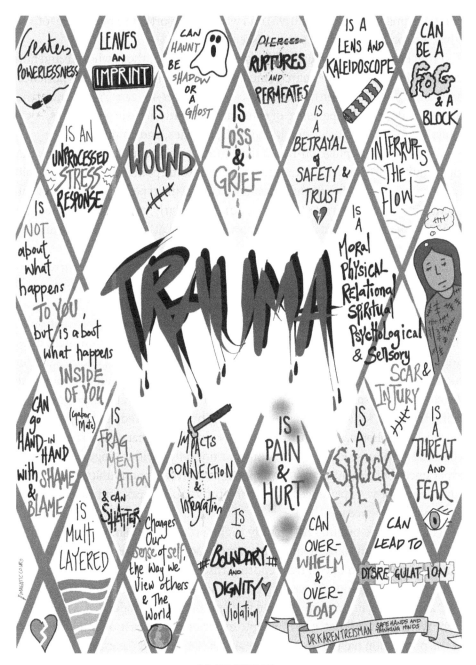

1.3. TRAUMA IS...

1.3. Trauma as widespread and common

Before we go on to explore some of the different types of trauma and adversity, it's important to highlight how pervasive and widespread trauma and adversity can be. This is one of the key reasons why services and systems need to become more adversity, culturally, and trauma-informed and responsive (or as a starting point, trauma aware and sensitive) and why it is important to be mindful of, and advocate for, a universal approach (see Chapter 7).

From evaluations, professional reports, accounts of those who use and have used services, and from research (including the adverse childhood experiences ACE and Dunedin longitudinal studies (Poulton *et al.*, 2015)), we know that there is widespread experience of trauma, dissociation, toxic stress, loss, social injustice, and adversity among individuals, families, and communities.

For example, population-based data from various countries indicates that most adults will experience a traumatic event at some point in their lives, despite cross-national variation in the prevalence of specific types of traumatic events (Benjet *et al.*, 2016; Burri & Maercker, 2014). Similarly, one study revealed that almost 90% of nearly 3000 respondents reported at least one exposure to a traumatic event in their lifetimes, with multiple exposures within the range of normal experience (Kilpatrick *et al.*, 2013). This widespread occurrence of trauma has been echoed in numerous prevalence studies, such as ones using the (ACE) measure (critiques and limitations of the ACE study and scoring are shared in Chapter 2). Such studies are likely to reflect an underestimation, as they are based on self-report, retrospective data, and the ten-item ACE questionnaire, which discounts possible key experiences that are not enquired about, such as being in war, being bullied, and negative experiences outside the home, in schools, in hospitals, or other environments. There are also aspects such as being in foster, kinship, or residential care, being adopted, and experiencing racism, homophobia, and other forms of discrimination that need to be included. For a full picture, studies need to consider not only a wider range of childhood experiences but also adverse adult experiences, adverse community experiences, adverse collective experiences, adverse cultural experiences, and adverse organizational experiences.

That said, the original ACE study (Felitti *et al.*, 1998) showed that almost two-thirds of study participants (just over 17,000 people) reported at least one ACE, and more than one in five reported three or more ACEs. And in one ACE study in the USA, approximately 60% of the sample experienced at least one ACE and more than 10% experienced five or more ACEs (Anda, *et al.* 2006). Data from Wales showed that 47% of people experienced at least one ACE, with 9% of the population having four or more ACEs (De Bellis & Zisk, 2014). In Brazil, looking at an adolescent cohort, 85% of teens reported experiencing at least one ACE, with females experiencing more adverse events (Soares *et al.*, 2016).

In addition to ACE and other studies showing a widespread occurrence of trauma and adversities, we see higher prevalences in certain populations. Research has shown that people who are homeless are more likely to have experienced higher incidences of adverse childhood experiences and some form of trauma (Buhrich *et al.*, 2000; Sundin & Baguley, 2015), and this was echoed in a report which found that 85% of those in touch with criminal justice, substance use, and homelessness services had experienced trauma as children (Bramley *et al.*, 2015). Similarly, in a study by Kushel *et al.* (2003), it was found that homeless and marginally housed adults in San Francisco experienced much higher rates of physical and sexual assault than people in the general population. And within this, people who were homeless were also more likely to experience injuries or accidents.

Moreover, we know that there is a strong relationship between trauma and the use of drugs or alcohol. For example, in the National Survey of Adolescents in the USA, teenagers who had experienced physical or sexual abuse/assault were three times more likely to report past or current substance use than those without a history of trauma (Kilpatrick *et al.*, 2003). In surveys of adolescents receiving treatment for substance use, more than 70% of patients disclosed that they had a history of trauma exposure (Funk *et al.*, 2003). This is consistent with numerous other studies that show high levels of childhood trauma in those who use drugs (Anda *et al.*, 2006; Wu *et al.*, 2010).

Additionally, research indicates that people abused as children are nearly ten times more likely to develop psychosis (Janssen *et al.*, 2004). For people who have endured three kinds of abuse – sexual abuse, bullying, and physical abuse – their risk of psychosis increases 18-fold, and those experiencing five types of abuse are 193 times more likely to experience psychosis (Shevlin *et al.*, 2007). And yet so often in these areas, trauma is not considered; in some cases, services unintentionally add to and reinforce the trauma.

This is a public health issue that warrants our attention; it is not an 'us or them' debate. Trauma and adversity are umbrella terms, and, within them, there are so many different types of trauma and adversity-related experiences and events, ranging from interpersonal, attachment, social, and relational, through to cultural and community, to historical and intergenerational, to health, medical, birth, and disability trauma. We need to think beyond the focus on ACEs to widen our understanding and create services that acknowledge and integrate adverse adult, community, cultural, social, political, economic, and organizational experiences. This includes wider factors which need to be considered, such as poverty, racism, sexism, exclusion, social dislocation and rejection, social oppression, and many more.

These experiences do not only occur at an interpersonal and individual level or happen within a vacuum. Rather, they can occur at a socio-political, community, societal, and collective level. Due to the complex nature of trauma, toxic stress, and adversity, the impact can be pervasive, cumulative, intergenerational, long term, and widespread. There may be a multi-layered impact on behaviours, emotions, cognitions, beliefs, attitudes, and relationships, on the body, on one's sensory world, including regulation, and on the brain – at an individual, family, system, organizational, and societal level. Therefore, practitioners and organizations need to be more equipped to understand and proactively respond, otherwise they will miss so many of the core causes and needs, and potentially add more harm through trauma-inducing or re-traumatizing practices.

1.4. Trauma as unseen, less visible, often camouflaged

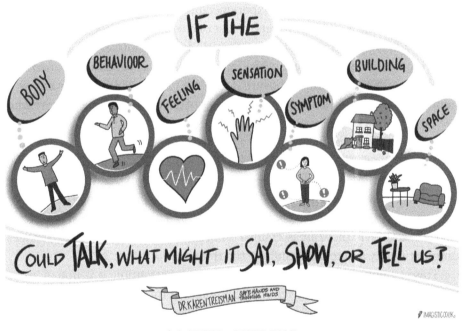

1.4. IF THE...COULD TALK

Trauma is often ignored, hidden, misunderstood, invalidated, silenced, disenfranchised, and minimized. Often, we don't know who has experienced trauma, stress, or adversity, because it isn't within our role or because trauma can be unseen, marinated in secrecy and shame, and it is multi-layered and varied. It can come in many different forms, so it doesn't fit into a neat box or a checklist.

Additionally, due to ill-equipped individual, system, and societal responses, including blaming, shaming, denying, avoiding, and criticizing, it can be difficult to name or disclose, and is often understandably not shared. People can be marinated in dismissive, blaming, and shaming discourses such as 'You asked for it/You wanted it', 'It is in your head', 'It isn't a big deal/Get over it', 'It's our little secret/No one will believe you', 'It will toughen you up', 'What goes on behind closed doors stays behind closed doors', 'Don't air your dirty laundry', 'Keep your head down', 'Others have it much worse', 'It was a lifetime ago, don't hold on to it, move on', and 'You're overreacting, making a mountain out of a molehill'.

Moreover, experiences of trauma are often positioned as a deficit about the person and they are labelled as 'badly behaved', 'difficult', 'hard-to-reach', 'resistant', 'attention-seeking', and so on. Services can themselves be trauma avoidant, with practices such as not asking about life experiences, having male staff on one-to-one observations with women who have been sexually abused by men, and focusing on the diagnosis or presenting difficulties such as self-harm or an eating disorder, without viewing the person within the context of their experiences.

Trauma might have occurred during the in-utero experience or when a child was pre-verbal, and/or the person may not choose to label it as 'trauma' or may not conceptualise or view it as such. Also, trauma and emotional pain are often less visible, so it can be hard to empathize with some people. For example, when someone has a diagnosis of Downs Syndrome or when someone is in a wheelchair, this is more visible (which can come with its own complexities and doesn't mean we know what it is like for that unique individual).

For these reasons and many others, trauma and adversity can be more easily missed, mislabelled, or avoided. This will be discussed further within the context of a trauma-informed approach in Chapter 7.

1.5. A wider frame than the post-traumatic stress disorder (PTSD) classification

Throughout this book, although it is based on trauma, I do not use the term PTSD, unless the study I am referring to specifically uses it. I take the position that while the diagnostic classification of PTSD and the associated evidence base can be useful, it often doesn't fully do justice to the multifaceted nature of what we see in real-world clinical settings where people have experienced trauma, adversity, and hardships, particularly children who have experienced cumulative and complex relational and developmental trauma. This view is echoed by a body of professionals who continue to advocate for 'developmental trauma' to be seen as a new diagnostic category, or for a revision of existing categories within the PTSD classification (Van der Kolk, 2005).

This is also based around notions that PTSD was initially conceptualized in the western world from an adult perspective and was mainly focused on single-event traumas and often on veteran studies. Therefore, it is posited that the understanding of PTSD does not consider the chronic and cumulative nature of attachment and relational trauma from a child development perspective. For example, there are several unique characteristics of trauma which occur during a child's critical sensitive developmental trajectory that are not fully considered in the PTSD inclusion criteria. These include complex disruptions in affect, sensory, and physiological regulation, changes in attachment patterns and styles, interferences in developmental competencies and skills, and feelings such as ineffectiveness, shame, and self-blame (Cook *et al.*, 2005). In addition, the term PTSD does not consider areas which we know can have an important impact, such as moral injury, iatrogenic harm (harm caused by medical treatment), and insidious trauma.

Furthermore, researchers suggest that many stressful experiences are not included in PTSD Criterion A (Exposure to traumatic event), such as caregiver separation, verbal abuse, bullying, chronic sibling discord, multiple home or foster moves, and living with a caregiver with mental health difficulties (D'Andrea *et al.*, 2012). The term PTSD also neglects other important multi-layered aspects of other types of traumas and the intersectionality between them, such as intergenerational, historical, cultural, community, organizational, and institutional trauma, betrayal, poverty, social exclusion, rejection, and dislocation, which warrant acknowledgement and, if needed, support. This negates the wider socio-political, cultural, and economic climate and context.

Thus, PTSD has often focused on the individual-event dyad, as opposed to group, collective, or relational dyads, which do not encompass the complex relational changes and impact of the traumas, or consider fundamental factors such as caregiver involvement, social support, whether the person was believed, and their response to the trauma.

In its very name, PTSD is positioned around a time frame of 'post', which does not adequately capture children and adults whose trauma remains ongoing, is cumulative, or started during the in-utero period. It doesn't extend to those who experience insidious trauma and are living in a traumatic or toxic stress environment or an emotional battlefield, such as those with daily experiences of racism, discrimination, injustice, poverty, and stigma.

In addition, many clinicians and academics have become increasingly critical of the universal applicability of a narrow biomedical model, based on western notions of trauma (Papadopoulos, 2007; Quosh & Gergen, 2008; Summerfield, 2004). This is not to deny that trauma can't be usefully conceptualized in biological and psychological terms, but that an over-emphasis on symptomology can result in the divorcing of the mind from the body, the individual from the community, and the community from the environment. It is essential to consider the cultural, historical, familial, political, and individual meaning of the symptoms and signals. For example, nightmares are designated as a symptom of PTSD in the *Diagnostic and Statistical Manual of Mental Disorders* (DSM), yet whether they are reported will depend on whether an individual/society regards them as problematic. In some cultures, nightmares are viewed as conveying ancestors' messages, or as indicators of the person's spiritual status. This can also negate wider crucial impact, where socio-political forces can perpetuate oppression and political violence.

PTSD is referred to as a 'disorder', which can medicalize and pathologize human distress and experience, and positions the difficulty within the person, rather than considering the wider contextual and cultural factors. Such views are also linked to 'deficit models' of trauma and its impacts (Burstow, 2005) within which individuals' attempts to cope with trauma and to survive are described as 'dysfunctional' or 'disordered'.

Additionally, many people who have experienced trauma often are 'misdiagnosed' or the intervention focuses on the behaviour, rather than the root cause – for example, substance use or self-harming. This fits with the notion of 'What is wrong with you?', as opposed to the trauma-informed approach of 'What has happened to you? Why has it happened? Who was with you when it happened? What is the behaviour telling us? What matters to you?'

Alternatively, many people do not meet the criteria for a PTSD diagnosis, as their experiences do not fit in this box or the categories within it, so they cannot access support or resources but might still importantly be experiencing trauma and therefore want and need support.

Therefore, this book advocates for considering and respecting existing diagnostic criteria, while attending to the wider trauma and adversity framework and conceptual lens. This broadening framework aims to see the whole person and context rather than just the diagnosis – in essence re-contextualizing trauma and adversity.

1.6. Different types of traumas

There are numerous different types of traumas, stressors, and adversities, some of which are illustrated in image 1.5; however, it is by no means an exhaustive or prescriptive list. This image is also important as there are a lot of people and organizations who claim (with the best intentions) that they are trauma-informed, but who actually mean that they have learned about one type of trauma, or that they have had some training in one of these areas – or that they use certain measures or assessment tools designed to assess trauma, but which often only focus on a sub-section of trauma. Therefore, this image is intended to give the reader a broader sense of what the different types of traumas might be. It is also important to show the different types of traumas, as often certain aspects of trauma are prioritized or spoken about, while others are unacknowledged or silenced. At other times, there are hierarchical claims made about which trauma is 'worse', such as sexual abuse is worse than neglect.

Each of these types of traumas could be the subject of multiple books in their own right, so they are just briefly shared here to raise awareness of them. They are represented as a patchwork as many can be interlinked with each other, adding to the intersectionality and complexity. I will not go into the details of the academic differences between these different types of traumas, but rather offer a brief introduction to them, and give some examples as to what sorts of experiences these might include. Please refer to my resource *The Trauma Treasure Deck of Cards: A Creative Tool for Assessments* (Treisman, 2021) for individual illustrations of these types of traumas.

★ How might these be interlinked with each other?

★ Which others might you add?

★ Which are you familiar or less familiar with? For you as a practitioner and within your service, which are considered/screened for/targeted/assessed/acknowledged? Which do you have training on?

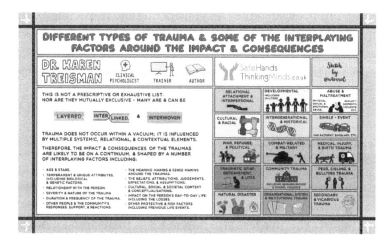

1.5. DIFFERENT TYPES OF TRAUMAS: WHAT IS IT LIKE SEEING
SOME OF THE DIFFERENT TYPES OF TRAUMAS?

1.6.1. Single-event trauma

This is where there has been a one-off traumatic experience or single event, such as a burglary, an assault, or a car accident. Of course, they do not occur within a vacuum and can be interwoven with other experiences, such as those described in image 1.3.

1.6.2. Medical, health, injury, and birth trauma

This is a wide area which refers to some of the trauma related to our health, including medical and birth-related elements. This includes the potential trauma of a diagnosis of a particular illness; the trauma following a heart attack, a stroke, or a serious accident; female genital mutilation, or having a traumatic fertility, IVF, birth, or pregnancy experience; having a child with health or learning needs; having a visible difference, such as a facial scar, burn, or cleft lip; having a still-born baby or a miscarriage; having speech and language difficulties; experiencing pain or having a traumatic time during or after a procedure, treatment, medical experience, or operation; or having a serious injury, such as an amputated leg, or going blind. This might also relate to some of the traumas and stressors that can occur due to mass public health situations, such as the recent cases of Ebola, SARS, and Covid-19. Of course, these can be layered with other types of traumas, such as the injuries sustained from sexual violence, a car accident, or the impact of racism on possible health outcomes.

In the context of medical trauma, people might have experienced fear, overwhelm, loss and grief, helplessness, and disbelief. They may have felt inca-pacitated, trapped in intense, toxic, immobilizing shock, with the pain or fear being inescapable. They may have been faced with the fear of dying, being in pain, or being different, or feel dread for what the future holds or what is coming next, including their condition deteriorating, or their illness progressing or reoccurring. People can also be faced with their own vulnerability, fragility, and fallibility. Many may relive memories, experiences, or sensations (in flashbacks, nightmares, images).

These experiences understandably contribute to added distress and stress, and can increase barriers to screening, check-ups, ongoing monitoring, adherence to or uptake of treatment, and much more. As described in the Enduring Somatic Event model (Edmondson, 2014), this can also be additionally distressing as the threat and fear can be ongoing and more frequent, with many people requiring ongoing medical treatment, tests, and hospital appointments. And people often have to continue to monitor symptoms and be more aware of their bodies and symptoms. This model also discusses how the threat can be real and present, for example the cyclical impact of change in heart rate, blood pressure, sleep, and so on.

Often, people are so focused on the health and medical side – the symptom management, the treatment required, and so on – that the psychological and social side of what the person is experiencing, including the possible medical trauma, can be overlooked or sidelined. Therefore, people may feel misunderstood, and left alone with the ripples of the trauma. This is likely to be even more the case in medical settings where emotions can be timetabled out and not attended to, and where the physical symptoms can be overshadowing. This may have implications for a person's:

- identity or sense of self and belonging, including their self-esteem, confidence, and body image

- spirituality and belief systems – they may question, 'Why me?'

- quality of life, including impacting on their daily activities and hobbies, or ability to carry out tasks and their job

- financial situation – loss or change of job, additional bills to pay, equipment needed, adjustments to home or transport arrangements, treatments, medication costs, insurance, change of home

- friendships, relationships, and parenting (see Chapter 2 for a section on this)

- memories, nightmares, flashbacks, and re-experiencing of the illness or treatment

- future fears, worries, and uncertainties.

The potential impact can far extend beyond the days, weeks, or months in the hospital or when the symptoms occur, or when the diagnosis is given. For example, someone can experience a burn and have it treated and healed but the psychological impact and memories can linger for far longer; or someone with a diagnosis of cancer can find that the changes and impact can last far beyond the operation, chemotherapy, or radiotherapy.

Consider the potential impact on a baby and their family after being in the neonatal intensive care unit (NICU). In a study of parents who had a baby in the NICU, 35% of mothers and 24% of fathers met the criteria for acute stress and 15% of mothers and 8% of fathers of PTSD (Lefkowitz *et al.*, 2010). There is also the possible impact on attachment, connection, and bonding to take into account, as well as uncertainty over the baby's health, ongoing medical treatment and check-ups, parental fears about work and finances, and implications for future pregnancies.

Receiving an HIV diagnosis for some people itself can be seen as traumatic

(Garrido-Hernansaiz *et al.*, 2017). There are possible fears around or actual experiences of increased trauma, such as intimate partner violence, family separation, discrimination, social exclusion, rejection, stigma, or being fired or mistreated at work. There are also the possible side effects of medication, nuanced around disclosure and one's sex life, and possible additional measures around pregnancy and breastfeeding. These among other factors may be a barrier to disclosure of HIV status, accessing HIV care, and adherence to medication (Kouyoumdjian *et al.*, 2013; Leserman, 2008).

More quotes and stories about difficult health experiences that can contribute to trauma can be found in Chapters 3 and 4.

1.6.3. Disability trauma (a spotlight on intellectual/learning disabilities)

There is huge variety within this group of people and it is important to acknowledge that this explanation offers only a snapshot of the whole picture. It focuses on the areas of trauma and some of the associated difficulties, and there is also an emphasis here on intellectual/learning disabilities. However, many can be applied and adapted to physical disabilities (as well as other specific considerations added), as well as within a neurodiverse context.

People with intellectual disabilities can face a range of complexities, stressors, oppressive practices, and traumas. These can be cumulative and insidious in nature and can include:

- stigma and discrimination
- social and societal isolation, dislocation, rejection, and exclusion
- being separated from loved ones when going into care or hospitals
- living or receiving care in non-trauma-informed settings or receiving trauma-inducing care
- facing a lack of choice, voice, and agency
- being treated with a lack of dignity and integrity
- being silenced, ignored, underestimated, or negatively treated
- being seen or positioned as a burden or as an embarrassment
- being physically restrained or secluded
- not being communicated with, and feeling and being 'done to', not 'with'

- having additional health and medical needs

- experiencing services, systems, environments, and wider society as less accessible and inclusive and more restrictive, overwhelming, and hostile

- being teased, humiliated, and bullied

- feeling different and left out

- being patronized or infantilized

- being in cultures or families where having a disability is associated with further stigma and discrimination.

There are many others – what would you add to this list?

People with intellectual disabilities are at a significantly increased risk of experiencing all forms of abuse – believed to be three to four times more likely to be abused than those without a disability (Jones *et al.*, 2012; Kvam, 2004; Lightfoot *et al.*, 2011; Sullivan & Knutson, 2000). For example, people who are deaf report nearly twice the rates of intimate partner violence and sexual assault (Anderson *et al.*, 2011; Porter & Williams, 2011) and may experience more than six unique types of traumas across their lifespan, as well as stressors or experiences unique to being deaf (Mastrocinque *et al.*, 2015; Schild & Dalenberg, 2012).

Here are some reasons why people with disabilities are at risk of trauma:

- A tendency for the diagnosis to overshadow everything else, so people see the disability first and not the needs of the person, or can see signs of distress and misinterpret or attribute them as being part of the disability rather than a signal of distress or something additional such as trauma.

- An inability to communicate or verbally disclose or articulate the abuse.

- Higher exposure to multiple different people and environments.

- The need for personal care increasing vulnerability and access. For example, children with disabilities may have a limited ability to protect themselves or to understand what abuse is or whether they are experiencing it (Lightfoot, 2014).

- Increased caregiver stress and tension, due to the level of complexity and behaviours. This can also mean that there may be more likelihood for people to react or retaliate.

- In an intellectual disability context, less education, openness, focus, and discussion about sex, abuse, and consent.

- An increased wish to make friends, to be liked, or to trust others (particularly for people with intellectual disabilities).

- Some systems tolerating a lower standard of care for people with intellectual disabilities.

- Reluctance or avoidance for people to believe or think about someone with an intellectual disability being abused or being seen in a sexual way.

- Abuse being ignored, hidden, or missed. This includes people often separating abuse and disability in services; for example in the UK, where social services often have separate teams for those with disabilities to those in child protection, with some teams having little interface. Or there being 'mainstream' residential homes and disability residential homes, with little communication between them. In many training programmes, trauma and disabilities are not discussed. Moreover, many staff in trauma-specific services are not trained or equipped to work with those with an intellectual disability.

- Some people with intellectual disabilities having different processing speeds, and different concepts of time, and so the trauma may show itself at different times, or with a delay in time.

- Incorrect assumptions that people with intellectual disabilities don't understand or feel things in the same way that people without intellectual disabilities do, and therefore the impact can be minimized (e.g. 'They won't remember', 'They don't understand', 'They are always happy').

- People with intellectual disabilities being told to 'calm down' and to be 'settled', and so communications of distress might be suppressed or unheard.

What else would you add to this list?

There are many reports and studies of disparities in service provision for those with a learning/intellectual disability (discussed further in Chapter 6). For example, when studies have looked at those with a learning/intellectual disability accessing mainstream services for their physical health, a range of barriers have been highlighted, including communication difficulties, resulting in individuals with intellectual disability being excluded from consultations (Ward et al., 2010; Wullink et al., 2009). This also included general practitioners (GPs) not conducting certain blood tests and investigations, as well as there being a lack of health promotion and screening (Broughton & Thomson, 2000), and a lack of transport and accessible buildings. Studies have also shown an inadequate knowledge of doctors about the health needs of people with an intellectual disability (Fisher *et al.*, 2005; Minnes & Steiner, 2009), which has contributed to diagnostic overshadowing. Other studies have found that some health professionals exhibited more negative attitudes and behaviour towards individuals with an intellectual disability (Dinsmore, 2012; Webber *et al.*, 2010). Thiara *et al.* (2011) shared that unless women who were disabled made explicit disclosures of abuse, social workers and other professionals were unlikely to recognize signs of partner abuse because they tended to focus on the disability.

1.6.4. Traumatic grief, bereavement, and loss

This includes bereavement, as well as aspects such as murder, manslaughter, death, a stillborn baby, and suicide. However, importantly, and often less discussed, there is *disenfranchised loss and grief*. This is grief and loss that can be socially minimized, hidden, or not acknowledged. This is where grief that isn't as common or understood is not given the same regard as other forms of grief – for example, the huge loss for a mother, father, or relative when their child is removed by social services. In death there is usually empathy, compassion, support, and ways to mourn and process the loss. Whereas, for the parents of a child removed by social services, their grief and loss are not socially acknowledged and they can be met with discrimination, blaming, shaming, social exclusion, and rejection. Often, they must contend with a lack of services put in place to support them, ongoing system and institutional trauma, physical reminders such as breast milk coming through or pain from their caesarean scar, people asking if they have children, or getting letters reminding them to bring their child for their health check-up, and so much more.

Similarly, grief following an abortion can be disenfranchised as it can be socially unacknowledged and not given the same response that other forms of loss might be. Other examples of disenfranchised grief might include miscarriages, infertility, death of an ex-partner, or death of a pet.

Loss and grief should be viewed through a much wider lens. It can also include the loss of things which often occur because of the trauma, such as, in the context of sexual abuse, the loss of trust, safety, connection, virginity, boundaries, security, hope, integrity, dignity, confidence, and childhood. Someone who can't have children but longs for them may mourn this loss; someone who has had an amputation may mourn for their limb and for their health; a parent may grieve the loss of the healthy child they longed for on finding out that their child has a serious medical condition; someone may mourn the loss of their eyesight when they go blind. Traumatic loss might also include the loss of someone's home, their role in their community, their sense of belonging and identity, or their language (if they have had to flee their country). There can be multi-layered multi-sensory losses and changes experienced by a child moving into foster care or being adopted. Traumatic loss can also include *collective grief* and mourning mass losses, such as those that occur in war or through community trauma.

There is also the loss of someone as you knew them or the relationship or life you had together or the role they played, following a diagnosis of dementia, a stroke, multiple sclerosis, or other progressive or terminal illnesses which can affect a person's personality and interactions. This sometimes can be referred to as *anticipatory loss or grief*, where there is mourning in the anticipation of the loss.

Ambiguous and unresolved grief and loss can result when there is a lack of emotional closure or clear understanding – for example, someone goes missing in a war and is not found; a child's parent has abandoned them, or is estranged; someone dies before the person they abused can confront or report them; someone has never known the identity of their father.

1.6.5. Cultural and identity trauma

This refers to trauma that can occur around someone's identity and culture; for example, racial trauma, antisemitism, islamophobia, sexism, homophobia, ageism, and discrimination against those with a disability and those who identify as refugees or asylum-seekers. These are in themselves wide and multi-layered areas; for instance, racial trauma may include direct experiences of racial harassment, such as threats of harm, injury, and humiliation, witnessing racial violence towards others, and experiencing discrimination and institutional racism. This can also include being avoided or ignored because of one's race, and experiencing collective disrespect and devaluing, and blocked opportunities, as well as experiencing 'microaggressions', putdowns, and dismissals (brief, everyday verbal or behavioural exchanges that intentionally or unintentionally communicate hostile, derogatory, or negative racial messages) (Bryant-Davis & Ocampo, 2005; Carter, 2007; Sue, 2010).

This type of trauma can also include more subtle aspects such as a look, moving away, a question such as 'Where are you really from?', or a statement such as 'Wow, you speak so well'. Within this, there is also the notion of 'insidious trauma' which has also been used to describe the reality of trauma experienced by individuals who live under constant oppressive conditions, such as those who experience daily racism (Brown, 1994), or those who may be discriminated against because of their disability, their sexuality, their expressed gender, or something like a stammer, etc. It is around the chipping away, weathering, and ongoing nature of trauma that can occur.

There is also the theory around minority stress, which discusses the impact of chronic psychosocial stress such as discrimination, prejudice, and stigma. This includes considering distal and external stressors (e.g. actual experiences of discrimination, violence, rejection) and internal or proximal stressors (e.g. expectations of rejection and discrimination, chronic vigilance). Much research has looked at this theory in relation to groups such as the anti-lesbian, gay, bisexual, transgender, queer or questioning, intersex (LGBTQI) experience. This is likely to be compounded and influenced by other threads of identity, such as older people who identify as gay who might also have experienced high levels of intolerance, exclusion, shame, and othering.

Trauma can also occur around areas of identity, such as when someone shares or expresses their sexual or gender identity or preference with their family and receives negative responses, or the stigma, harassment, and discrimination someone might face due to their cultural identity or expression. Of course, this varies, but for some people can also lead to internalized stigma, as well as vacant esteem (believing oneself to have little worth, exacerbated by the group and social pronouncement of inferiority).

All the above can be embedded within the policies and practices of services and systems, showing them as institutionally racist, sexist, ageist, and so on. There can also be a lack of cultural humility and responsiveness (see Chapter 6). This extends to considering how there can be culturally specific ways of processing and expressing distress and trauma, as well as coping and healing, and cultural idioms of distress, including those related to trauma (see Chapter 6).

This cultural and identity trauma can also go hand-in-hand with collective and community trauma, such as when people are persecuted against and oppressed due to aspects of their identity (as occurred in the Holocaust and in the Rwandan Genocide, for example), or are subjected to honour-based violence, forced marriage, female genital mutilation, and so on.

We also know that trauma in a broader sense can often impact and influence one's sense of self. The experience of trauma can require:

- a transition and adaptation to a new identity

- processing of other parts of one's identity

- making sense of mixed and conflicting parts of one's identity

- mourning the loss of an aspect of one's identity

- re-connecting with one's identity or different parts of one's identity

- searching for one's identity, and, in the context of trauma, possibly developing a more fragile and incoherent sense of identity.

Within this, trauma can also lead to people questioning their core belief systems, and the things which make them who they are. For example, they may ask them-selves key questions such as 'Who am I now?' and 'Why me?'

1.6.6. Intergenerational, multigenerational, transgenerational, historical, and inherited trauma

These often refer to several different elements, including the patterns, links, repetitions, coping mechanisms, and cycles of trauma and adversity which can be passed down through relationships, parenting, and generations. This includes the social, emotional, and psychological chains of pain, the ghosts of the past (Fraiberg et al., 1975), unresolved trauma and loss, and relationship patterns.

This also can extend to how beliefs around others and the world – such as a conspiracy of silence (Yael Danieli), fear, grief, guilt, blame, shame, pain, mistrust, violence, dysregulation, powerlessness, danger, injustice, hopelessness, and avoidance – can travel through families and generations. Certain behaviours or experiences, such as substance use, domestic abuse, and behaviour of a crim-inal nature, can reoccur and shape multiple people through the generations. Trauma that is not transformed can be transferred.

The trauma of past generations, including wider contextual themes and experiences such as poverty, oppression, discrimination, and systemic inequalities, can continue to impact people and communities. Trauma can travel, it can pierce layers and create moral, social, and psychological wounds. For example, historical trauma has been defined by Yellow Horse Brave Heart et al. (2011) as 'cumulative emotional and psychological wounding across generations, including the lifespan, which emanates from massive group trauma'. Historical, collective, and cumu-lative trauma includes aspects such as colonization, racism, oppression, slavery, famine, genocide, segregation, a state-sanctioned policy of extermination, forced abandonment of religious and cultural practices, forced removal of children, stolen lands, and so on. These have sometimes been referred to as soul wounds.

In addition to possible psychological and social themes and experiences that can be passed through generations – the chain of pain – there are biologi-cal aspects passed down, for example through epigenetics (a set of potentially heritable changes in the genome that can be induced by environmental events). Studies have looked at some of the epigenetic changes in second- and third-gen-eration survivors of things like the Dutch famine, the Rwandan Genocide, the Troubles in Northern Ireland, and the Holocaust. These changes occur across a range of aspects from health, such as digestive systems and inflammation markers, through to patterns of things like depression and anxiety. (Google the work around epigenetics by Dr Rachel Yehuda, Dr Szyf, Dr Kundakovic, and Dr Champagne for more on this.)

1.6.7. Community and collective trauma (social suffering)

This is often interlinked with some of the previously mentioned types of traumas. When trauma has occurred at a community, large group, and collective level, it can widely impact societies and communities. The ripples can often be felt for generations, especially in societies which have been marinated in trauma and adversity. In these situations, the moral, social, political, economic, and psychological fabric of a society and community can be permeated and pierced, and these events and experiences can impact the collective memory of a community or a large group of people. As Michael Kober termed it, trauma can move from society to cell (Schmidt *et al.*, 2021).

These experiences might also influence the collective meaning-making, such as the narrative and stories that are told or untold, the traditions and rituals which derive from the trauma or additionally are or were threatened by it, as well as the different survival and coping mechanisms that have developed and continue to be filtered into other areas of the community. This can also filter into subsequent social comparisons of other groups, and through the reconstruction of memories and narratives of what happened. This collective and community trauma can have an impact on many aspects, such as cohesion and unity, or the division and splitting of and within a community. These events can also create a sense of disconnection and discontinuity, as well as fear, mistrust, heightened vigilance, insecurity, pain, othering, oppression, and so on.

This was captured powerfully by Erikson in 1976 (pp.153–154):

> ...by collective trauma, I mean a blow to the basic tissues of social life that damages the bonds attaching people together and impairs the prevailing sense of communality. The collective trauma works its way slowly and even insidiously into the awareness of those who suffer from it, so it...[is] a gradual realization that the community no longer exists as an effective source of support and that an important part of the self has disappeared... 'We' no longer exist as a connected pair or as linked cells in a larger communal body.

Kleinman *et al.* (1997) describe this as social suffering and Honwana (1997) as social pollution.

As with many of the broad categories of trauma, collective and community trauma can also be overlapping and linked with other types of traumas, such as cultural, generational, and political trauma. Examples may include (of course there are a range of factors within these and they are multi-layered) things like war, genocide, poverty, segregation, a culture of youth violence, events such as the Grenfell fire, bombings, terrorism, school shootings, famine, Brexit, and certain political regimes. This can also include community grief and mourning mass losses, as well as violence on a large scale, stolen lands, forced removal of children, and much more. There are so many layers and intersectionality within this, and these are explored more in Chapter 6, which focuses on cultural humility and responsiveness.

1.6.8. War, genocide, political, and refugee trauma

This refers to the trauma that can occur during genocide or war and the trauma of certain political regimes, the oppression and violence which people can experience because of their political beliefs, and the trauma experienced by those who are forced to be child soldiers, those subjected to sexual violence and other forms of torture, and those who are trafficked. This also includes the trauma associated with the asylum-seeking and refugee experience, including before, during, and after migration – for example, being in refugee and detention centres, arduous journeys, hostile environments, oppressive legal and immigration systems, discrimination, stigma, language barriers, poverty, housing difficulties, cultural dislocation and bereavement, separation from loved ones, loss and change of role, sense of belonging, and identity.

1.6.9. Abuse, violence, and maltreatment

This type of trauma refers to financial, physical, relational, emotional, online/cyber, organizational/system, cultural and sexual abuse, neglect, violence, and maltreatment, which can happen across and throughout a person's life, including adulthood. This also overlaps with other areas of trauma, such as sexual, criminal, and financial exploitation, trafficking, slavery, honour-based violence, and child labour.

1.6.10. Military, veteran, and combat-related trauma

This refers to the combat-related trauma which can occur for military personnel and war veterans, as well as some experiences which can be relevant to other occupations, such as the police and security personnel. There are many studies showing that some people who join these professions are more likely to have experienced childhood trauma.

This type of trauma includes memories and experiences of war, death, injury, and illness, separation from loved ones, navigating and re-adjusting to civilian life, having mixed feelings about the reasons why they are there, or the decisions being made (moral injury and wounding), and possible survivor guilt.

1.6.11. Peer, sibling, and bullying trauma

This includes a wide spectrum of trauma which can occur within peer and sibling relationships. This might be difficult relationships between siblings, abuse between siblings, one sibling receiving preferential treatment to another, trauma re-enactment, being separated from one's sibling/s, complex and conflictual sibling relationships, and so on. It also includes trauma through bullying and harassment at school, at home, in the community, in the workplace, and online through social media and cyber bullying.

1.6.12. Natural disaster trauma

This is trauma which can occur because of a natural disaster, such as an earthquake, a volcanic eruption, fire, flooding, tsunami, hurricane, and landslide.

1.6.13. Secondary and vicarious trauma (compassion fatigue, emotional saturation, and burnout)

People can experience symptoms of trauma when working with those who have experienced trauma, when hearing or seeing stories of trauma, when bearing witness or being exposed to other people's trauma, and when living with, caring for, or parenting those who have experienced trauma. Secondary and vicarious trauma, compassion fatigue, and burnout are so crucial to the focus of this book that they are explored in much more detail in Chapter 5.

1.6.14. Organizational, institutional, and system trauma (see Chapter 5)

Similarly, as trauma within organizations, institutions, and systems is so important in this book, instead of going into detail here it is described in much more depth in its own chapter (Chapter 5). Just a brief outline will be shared here.

Institutional trauma refers to the trauma and the abuse that can occur within an institution, such as the abuse within residential and nursing homes, from religious organizations and figures, within schools, hospitals, and medical facilities, within the military, and within prisons. This includes failure to prevent, acknowledge, or respond supportively to these abuses. It comes with a host of additional considerations, such as the violation of expectations, safety, trust, and protection, and the abuse of power and authority. Where people are oppressed, silenced, or not acknowledged or believed, this can also go hand-in-hand with institutional injustice.

System trauma generally refers to trauma that can be created and reinforced by the systems themselves, for example for a survivor of rape, whose trauma might be exacerbated by the trauma-inducing victim-blaming police and court systems. Re-traumatizing experiences through restraint, seclusion, or institutional racism, or through health care situations adding to or worsening the symptoms or presenting diagnosis (see Chapters 3 and 4 for some examples), are further examples of this. This can also include iatrogenic harm (where the intervention or treatment itself can cause harm).

Organizational trauma often refers to how an organization, system, or team can become unhealthy and traumatized, and how an organization itself can create trauma for the people who work there and the people it serves, through organizational adverse experiences.

1.6.15. Developmental trauma

This is trauma and toxic stress that occurs during someone's developmental trajectory which is likely to impact some of the areas of their development (brain/neurological/cognitive, sensory integration and processing, speech, communication, and language, social/relational, emotional/psychological, identity, moral, sexual, physical development/health). It can be induced by experiencing neglect (including relational and emotional poverty), domestic abuse, sexual abuse, and/or physical abuse during a person's critical sensitive periods of development. This includes the in-utero experience (a baby's first classroom, and their first lesson and introduction to life and relationships). This type of trauma impacts on the neurobiology of attachment. There are many variations and different degrees of severity, impacted by an array of factors.

This trauma may be seen in developmental delays in certain areas or domains, such as in speech and language or sensory processing, regulation, and integration, or it might be seen in a child or adult presenting, particularly at times of need and distress, at a different emotional, social, and developmental age and stage from their chronological age or stage, as they did not have those skills taught, mastered, or developed fully at the time. This is expanded on in my books and cards *Working with Relational and Developmental Trauma in Children and Adults* (2016), *A Therapeutic Treasure Box for Working with Children and Adolescents with Developmental Trauma* (2017a), and *The Parenting Patchwork Treasure Deck* (2020); and various training courses on childhood trauma.[1]

---

1   See www.safehandsthinkingminds.co.uk.

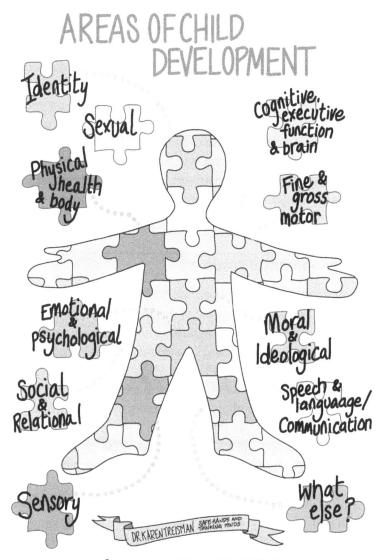

AREAS OF CHILD DEVELOPMENT

Identity

Sexual

Physical health & body

Cognitive, executive function & brain

Fine & gross motor

Emotional & psychological

Moral & Ideological

Social & Relational

Speech & language/ Communication

Sensory

What else?

DR KAREN TREISMAN   SAFE HANDS AND THINKING MINDS

1.6. AREAS OF CHILD DEVELOPMENT

1.6.16. Relational, interpersonal, and attachment trauma

This often refers to trauma which occurs within someone's relationships and is likely to impact how people are in relationships and what people might expect from relationships. This includes how people are interconnected and relational beings and so serve and return interactions, particularly from primary and early caregivers. Our way of being held, treated, and responded to can contribute to the formation of our guiding beliefs and narratives around themes such as 'I am lovable and worthy, or unlovable and unworthy', 'Relationships/people/

others are predictable, reliable, caring, or painful, scary, unpredictable', and 'The world is a safe and secure place, or the world is dangerous and unsafe'. These can inevitably shape, influence, and colour people's relational maps. As child psychotherapist and adult psychoanalyst Valerie Sinason says, 'We can pattern the world from the shapes that we have seen'; or as philosopher and writer Alan Watts says, 'We do not come into the world, we come out of it.'

This also can refer to the trauma which can occur around someone's attachment and early caregiving experiences, and might include things like sexual abuse, physical abuse, domestic abuse, and relational poverty, if taken place within a child's relationships. See more about this in my books and cards highlighted in the previous section (1.6.15).

1.6.17. Traumatic fog and oxygen

It is important to mention that while some people may not be directly hurt or harmed through physical contact, they may be marinated in a traumatic fog, energy, or emotional battlefield, one of hostility, friction, tension, stress, fear, panic, aggression, oppression, emptiness, disconnection, and so on. This may be at a family, system, community, or global level and can have an impact or leave an imprint, especially as feelings can be contagious and can travel through other people. This traumatic fog can understandably impact the overall feel, climate, and energy. We pick up clues and messages and feelings from our environment.

Please note that there is a spotlight on poverty and racial trauma in Chapter 2 and a separate chapter on secondary and organizational trauma (Chapter 5), and how these traumas can impact someone's health and sensory world (Chapters 2 and 3).

1.7. Some reflective questions on the different types of traumas which have been covered

★ This chapter provides a brief introduction to some of the different types of traumas. Which are you most familiar with? Which are you least familiar with? Are there others you would like to add?

★ Of course, there is not a them and us - many people reading might also have experienced one or multiples of these forms of trauma, or ones not listed. However, think about a family or individual whom you support - what types of trauma might they have experienced, and how do we consider the intersectionality of these? What about in the context and communities you work in?

★ Which types of trauma are at the forefront of your organization? Which are visible and acknowledged? Which might be less acknowledged or less visible?

★ Which of these types of trauma are covered in the training offered by your organization or in your initial professional training? Which might you like to expand on and learn more about? Also, remember that the interventions and what is needed will differ depending on these different types of traumas and the settings.

★ How can you consider a person's lived experiences of these traumas, rather than getting overly caught up in a category? (They are so much more than a category, a tick box, or a word.)

CHAPTER 2

The Impact of Trauma, Stress, and Adversity on the Body, Health, and Sensory World

Having explored some of the different types of traumas and the interplaying factors around experiencing these in Chapter 1, we will now build on this by exploring the potential influence and impact of trauma, stressors, and adversities on the body, on our sensory worlds, and on our overall health. Chapter 3 will go further into the detail of possible body-based and sensory 'triggers' and hotspots that are key to understand when supporting people.

Of course, this is a brief introduction and it is not intended to be a comprehensive systematic review but rather give the reader a baseline knowledge and a starting platform from which to further explore and inform their practice.

2.1. What will be covered in this chapter

- Pregnancy and the in-utero experience period
- Other possible impacts of childhood trauma on later health outcomes
- Other impacts of stress on the body
- Trauma and the brain
- Some other areas where trauma can impact the body
- Health inequalities and social injustice
- Connections between areas of poverty and health
- The impact of racism and other forms of discrimination on health

2.2. Pregnancy and the in-utero period

2.2.1. The in-utero period

This section is a snapshot, and it is acknowledged that there is huge variety and diversity within the pregnancy experience and the possible consequences on the developing baby. This section doesn't go into detail on various important areas such as prenatal attachment and bonding, nutrition, neurodiversity, or the numerous different types and levels of trauma and stress exposure. However, it highlights the importance of the pregnancy

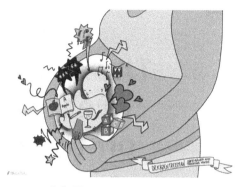

2.1. THE IN-UTERO PERIOD

period, some of the potential factors to hold in mind, and how the pregnancy experience can impact the developing baby. The in-utero experience is a vital time for the developing baby, as the womb can be likened to a baby's first classroom, an introduction to the world, and their first lesson of what it is like to be in a relationship and to be connected to another person.

2.2.2. The womb as a war zone

While the pregnancy period for some women has been documented as a protective and positive experience, for others it can be a very stressful time (and for some, a blend of both). For instance, some women during pregnancy and labour can feel out of control, powerless, in pain, and as if their body is being taken over or invaded, which can be reminiscent of some of the feelings and sensations they might

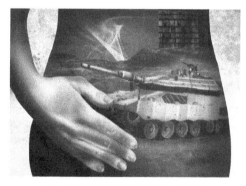

2.2. THE WOMB AS A WAR ZONE

have felt during previous experiences of abuse. For many, becoming a parent can understandably stir up memories, sensations, and associations from their own childhood and parenting experiences. There might also be a lot of medical appointments and examinations, which can leave some women feeling exposed, judged, and violated, among other feelings.

The pregnancy period can also bring to the fore wider societal and health opinions around aspects such as breastfeeding, child rearing, and parenting styles. These possible resurfacing experiences and 'triggers' will be discussed more in Chapters 3 and 4. Pregnant women are more likely to experience trauma and re-experience past traumas and abuse during the prenatal, delivery, and postpartum periods (Gelaye *et al.*, 2016), and are at an increased risk for violence and abuse (Kendall-Tackett, 2009). In the context of ongoing violence or fear, the baby too might be marinated in high levels of stress, fear, and cortisol or, as Bruce Perry (1997) says, incubated in terror.

Moreover, pregnancy can also be a time of possible transition, identity change, and role adjustment and can impact people's self-esteem, body image, relationship to sex and sexuality, relationships, purpose and meaning within life and society, and their overall sense of identity. It has commonly been characterized as a time for increased rumination and worry, and many women who experience emotional difficulties may find that these resurface or are exacerbated during their pregnancy, with increased anxiety about their health and about the baby's health, financial concerns, others' opinions about the baby, the impact on their relationships, and so on. Pregnancy can also require a change of medication or intervention which someone has previously been on, for example a change of anti-psychotics or anti-depressants.

This can all be further complicated by the intersectionality of experiences (what follows is by no means an exhaustive or prescriptive list nor do these necessarily lead to a particular consequence as people are unique within unique contexts):

- Having experienced previous difficulties with fertility, miscarriages, stillbirths, perinatal loss, or child loss.

- Having experienced previous birth, health, or medical trauma.

- Having current or previous post-natal depression, and/or finding it difficult to bond or connect with the new baby or previous babies.

- Being in an unsupportive, violent, or abusive relationship.

- Experiencing sexual, physical, domestic, financial, or emotional abuse during pregnancy.

- Being pregnant as a result of being raped.

- Being socially isolated, alone, or excluded.

- Living in poverty or financial difficulties. This might include being homeless, or living in a war zone, fleeing for one's safety, or living somewhere hostile, unsafe, or surrounded by toxic stress.

- Undergoing a parenting assessment and/or being known to social services; previously having children removed by social services.

- Having been in care oneself, or adopted.

- Having a disability or physical health condition, and/or finding out that the baby has additional health or learning needs. This might include concerns or news around hereditary and genetic conditions.

- Being HIV-positive and having associated recommendations, such as those around breastfeeding and caesarean section.

- Using substances, withdrawing from drugs, or being on certain medications.

- Going through the asylum-seeking process or living in a detention centre or refugee camp; or being in prison or in a psychiatric hospital while pregnant or postpartum.

- Having new or exacerbated emotional distress difficulties such as depression, anxiety, and hearing voices.

- Identifying as transgender, with the additional experiences that someone might experience around this, including stigma, discrimination, and lack of awareness.

- Experiencing a traumatic event or the bereavement of a loved one during pregnancy.

- Being discriminated or mistreated at work.

Are there any others you could add?

2.2.3. Effects of stress and dysregulation on the developing baby

Pregnancy is a crucial time, as studies have demonstrated how the neural connectivity between the brainstem, limbic, and cortical brain regions undergoes rapid development and growth during pregnancy. Therefore, this time is particularly important as the foetal immune system is very vulnerable to disruptions caused by environmental factors, such as toxins, substance use, malnutrition, over-nutrition, poor prenatal care, trauma, and stress. The environment in which the baby is developing and being contained may shape and influence the baby. They will be evolving and adapting in response to that environment. Studies have demonstrated that foetuses can respond to maternal stress, and that maternal mood such as anxiety, including elevated cortisol levels, can cross the placenta (Monk *et al.*, 2012; Sarkar *et al.*, 2006). This is in line with the 'foetal-origins hypothesis' (Kinsella & Monk, 2009), which argues that stress directly affects foetal development. The baby can be the receiver of the mother's stress, mood, and other aspects, and so their prenatal life might have been shaped by those stressed or heightened foundations.

For example, women who were pregnant and were present at the September 11 attacks in New York, and later showed PTSD symptoms, were more likely to have babies who also had altered stress responses and elevated cortisol levels (Yehuda *et al.*, 2005). Similarly, Field *et al.* (2006) found that babies who were born to mothers who were categorized as being depressed and withdrawn were more likely to display flattened moods and had lower dopamine and serotonin levels. While there is a huge amount of variability and inconsistency in study findings, and they need to be interpreted with caution, exposure to and experiences of toxic stress and trauma in the in-utero period can be associated with negative affect, poorer motor and cognitive development, increased behavioural difficulties, problem-solving difficulties, and increased anxiety disorders in children. There are also other potential difficulties in foetal development, blood flow, placental size, brain growth, motor development, premature birth, and low birth weight (Baibazarova *et al.*, 2013; Belkacemi *et al.*, 2010; Buss *et al.*, 2012; Lazinski *et al.*, 2008; Talge *et al.*, 2007).

Additionally, prolonged childhood abuse has been directly linked to neuroendocrine alterations, such as cortisol and oxytocin dysregulation in the mother (Bublitz & Stroud, 2012; Carpenter, 2007; De Bellis & Zisk, 2014). For example, in the context of relational and developmental trauma, such as domestic abuse, sexual abuse, and physical abuse, developing babies in the womb are often marinated in a sea of emotional, sensorial, and physiological waves, with their stress systems being frequently activated. They are on a steady diet of fear. Therefore, when they are born, they can understandably be used to an adrenaline buzz and sometimes have a lower window of tolerance (Siegel, 2012) and a higher reaction intensity.

Moreover, when babies are flooded with high levels of cortisol and have had chronic and/or ongoing exposure to stress hormones or unregulated toxic stress, this can suppress and weaken their developing immune system in multiple different ways, for example making them more prone to colds, gastroenteritis, and other viral respiratory infections (Karlen *et al.*, 2015), hypersensitivity (such as allergies, eczema, and asthma), and autoimmune disease such as Graves (Baldwin *et al.*, 2018; Burke Harris, 2018; Fujimura *et al.*, 2016; Gensollen *et al.*, 2016).

2.2.4. Foetal memory

There are numerous studies that shed light on foetal memory and babies being able to hear or be influenced by external stimuli such as sounds while they are in-utero. For example, Hepper (1991) conducted a study where women heard the TV show *Neighbours* theme tune approximately 360 times during their pregnancy. Two to four days after the baby's birth, on hearing the music from the *Neighbours* theme tune, the newborn babies became more alert, stopped moving, and exhibited lower heart rates. The same babies showed no similar reaction when other unfamiliar songs were played. Similarly, DeCasper and Fifer (1980) provided evidence that babies can recognize their mothers' voices shortly after birth. Using a non-nutritive nipple attached to a sensing apparatus, the newborns would suck more when listening to a tape of their mother's voice compared to a tape of a stranger's voice. Because they were newborns, it was hypothesized that the babies must have become familiar with the mother's voice while still in the womb. In a follow-up study, DeCasper and Spence (1986) had 16 pregnant mothers read a three-minute-long passage from the Dr Seuss book *The Cat in the Hat* to their foetuses twice a day for the last six and a half weeks of pregnancy. The mothers were also recorded reading three-minute excerpts from two other stories. By the time the babies were born, the researchers calculated they had heard *The Cat in the Hat* for about five hours in total. DeCasper and Spence used the sucking test again. The babies sucked more when listening to *The Cat in the Hat*.

2.2.5. Alcohol and cocaine use the in-utero experience

Building on the above, there are also the added layers of exposure to substance use during the in-utero period. However, it is important to say that some research shows that women are more likely to be poly-drug users, meaning that there is a higher likelihood that children have been exposed to the impact of multiple substances interacting with each other, each with their own unique properties and effects, and this makes researching the unique impact more difficult. Additionally, some of this knowledge is based on self-report, and this can understandably be impacted by the lack of awareness, misinformation, and feelings of shame, blame, and guilt which might impact how much people share or disclose. In foster care, where developmental histories might be unknown, there also can be a lack of information about exposure during the in-utero experience.

While it is beyond the remit of this book to go into this issue in detail, new studies are constantly emerging and it is an important area of research.

Taking alcohol as an example, prenatal exposure to alcohol occurs when alcohol crosses the placenta and increases the level of alcohol in the blood of the foetus. Foetal alcohol spectrum disorder (FASD) is believed to be one of the most common, non-genetic causes of learning disability in the UK (British Medical Association, 2016). International research proposes that between 2% and 5% of the population may be affected by FASD (May *et al.*, 2018), with this worryingly increasing. The most recent research in the UK (McCarthy *et al.*, 2021) highlighted that for planning and commissioning purposes we should be considering a prevalence rate of 3–4%. FASD is the umbrella term for the whole spectrum of those who may be affected by foetal alcohol exposure, including partial foetal alcohol syndrome (pFAS), alcohol-related neurodevelopmental defects (ARND), neurobehavioural disorder associated with prenatal alcohol exposure (ND-PAE), alcohol-related birth defects (ARBD), and foetal alcohol syndrome (FAS).

Importantly, experts believe FASD remains hugely under- and misdiagnosed, as children often present with an alphabet soup of symptoms. What is crucial is that this condition is preventable if there is no prenatal alcohol exposure, so early intervention, a public health approach, and education are key. There are also some studies which show that the extent of the disability can worsen for each subsequent child born to that mother. So, if a mother continues drinking the same amount, we might see the third child with a more significant impact than the second, and the fourth with more than the third, and so on. This is another reason for early intervention and prevention.

There are numerous variations in how alcohol exposure can impact the child, and these are influenced by a range of factors, including the developmental timing of the exposure, and the mother's and baby's metabolic systems. Of course, no two children are the same and there are a variety of interweaving factors. And because alcohol can be soaked into the whole of a child's brain, we can see a plethora of difficulties and symptoms in multiple areas. There is a large body of evidence on the relationship between exposure to alcohol prenatally, and later cognitive and executive function difficulties, including selective inhibition, verbal and non-verbal fluency, abstract reasoning, working memory and processing difficulties, speech and language, particularly receptive difficulties, arousal, attention, and concentration, hyperactivity, problem-solving, and planning (Green *et al.*, 2009; Rasmussen & Bisanz, 2009). Moreover, within this population of children, there are observations of regulation difficulties, and the ability to manage internal, sensory, emotional, behavioural, and bodily states. There can also be associated difficulties with vision and hearing, including sensory sensitivities. Some children (not the most serious but the most recognizable) may also present with facial feature differences such as a smooth philtrum, thin upper lip, and small palpebral fissures. Other associated features may include an upturned nose, underdeveloped ears, flat nasal bridge and midface, epicanthal folds, and small head circumference.

Cocaine use is another example of substance abuse during the in-utero period. As with alcohol, there is huge variance and multiple interplaying factors, but in babies prenatally exposed to cocaine, studies show higher incidences of amniotic sac ruptures and placentas separating from uteruses (Addis *et al.*, 2001). Moreover, cocaine can produce a high by blocking the reuptake of dopamine into the proximal nerve endings, while methamphetamine 'triggers' a high by stimulating excess release of dopamine. This excess of dopamine can interfere with blood flow across the placenta from the mother to the baby, leading to possible increased heart rate, poor growth, and sometimes contractions of the uterus producing premature labour. There have also been found to be some associations with changes in the cortical structure, and the physical and neurocognitive development of the baby. Singer *et al.* (2008) used the Brazelton Neonatal Assessment Scale and found that babies exposed to cocaine in-utero showed more difficulties in sensory asymmetry, orientation, habituation, regulation, autonomic stability, reflexes, muscle tone, motor performance, mood, and alertness.

Additionally, chronic exposure to cocaine or methamphetamine can result in the down-regulation of the neurotransmitter receptors, which can impact the central nervous system, behavioural regulation, and muscle tone. This can lead to consequences such as arching, trembling, feeding difficulties, and issues with coordinating the muscles involved in sucking and swallowing, as well as difficulties such as bowel or cardiac infarction. There have also been difficulties with the child's ability to process and respond to sound and visual stimulation, including, for some, being more easily startled or overstimulated. There can be increased difficulty with regulating behaviours, which one might expect if a baby is crying more, is harder to soothe, sleeps less, and is more dysregulated; this can understandably impact how they are parented or responded to by others such as childcare providers, which can then lead to a cycle of difficulties (Chasnoff, 2011). Likewise, longitudinal studies of prenatally cocaine-exposed four- to seven-year-olds found the children performing at below standard norms on sustained and selective attention tests (Bandstra *et al.*, 2010). Bennett *et al.* (2007) found that boys aged ten with histories of prenatal cocaine exposure were more likely to display high-risk traits, including aggression, hyperactivity, and disregard for safety. (Please see Chasnoff's (2011) *The Mystery of Risk* for a review of the impact of various substances.)

2.2.6. A brief spotlight on epigenetics

Another key part of pregnancy are the biological aspects which can be passed through the generations, for example through epigenetics ('epigenetics' refers to a set of potentially heritable changes in the genome that can be induced by environmental events; 'epi' refers to the things which can attach or be on top of the genes – it is not what is carried but what gets expressed). Studies have shown that changes in gene expression can occur in response to environmental factors (i.e. trauma and stress), and that these can be transmitted intergenerationally, leaving children with a gene expression that has been uniquely influenced by their parents' experiences. These are nuanced and of course other numerous factors create unique differences within people, so while new studies are emerging all the time, these need to be interpreted with caution.

However, some of these epigenetic influences have been demonstrated in a variety of contexts, including during the Dutch famine (Lumey *et al.*, 1995), the Chinese famine (Shen, 2019), and in the offspring of Holocaust survivors (Kellerman, 2013). Another example is provided by a longitudinal assessment of the children of women who were pregnant during Hurricane Sandy in 2012. These children showed elevated cortisol levels, measured in hair samples when they were three to four years old, which were accompanied by increased anxiety. These were linked to broad placental mRNA changes, including with genes associated with endocrine and immune processes that may have influenced the later biological and behavioural changes observed (Nomura *et al.*, 2021). Moreover, in some babies aged three months, they found that increased methylation of the genes for glucocorticoid receptors, along with increased cortisol stress responses, was apparent if mothers had been anxious/depressed (broad category or terms) during the third trimester of pregnancy (Oberlander *et al.*, 2008).

These studies reveal a whole new arena of possibilities around not just how gene sequences can be passed from parents to children, but also how and why gene expression and regulation can vary from parent to child. For example, during the Holocaust, people's bodies adapted to overwhelming chronic stress, including prolonged starvation and malnourishment, but these changes or adaptations were less helpful or needed or came out in a different way when they were in different contexts and environments, and for the following generations. For a more thorough discussion look online at the work of Dr Rachel Yehuda, Dr Stephanie Parade, Dr Kundakovic, and Dr Champagne.

Having briefly explored some of the possible health impacts of trauma experienced during pregnancy, let's look at other possible impacts of early life adversity and trauma.

2.3. Other possible impacts of childhood trauma on later health outcomes

As discussed in Chapter 1, experiences of trauma, stress, and adversity are unfortunately widespread. Data from adverse childhood experiences studies is key, especially as the effects of trauma can continue throughout the lifespan. Links between a range of physical health and autoimmune disorders, and childhood abuse and neglect, have been repeatedly shown in longitudinal research (Dube et al., 2009; Felitti et al., 1998). For instance, the Dunedin longitudinal studies in New Zealand show that, 20 years after people were abused in childhood, four different markers of inflammation in the body were higher than those who hadn't been maltreated. In the sections below, the role of stress on the hypothalamic-pituitary-adrenal axis, on the C-reactive protein, and on a person's ability to regulate and their window of tolerance will be briefly shared.

For example, studies (the original and numerous other replications of the ACE study) showed a close response relationship between ACEs and poor health outcomes, meaning that the higher a person's ACE score is, the greater risk there is for their physical and emotional health, including lower life expectancies and early mortality (Liming & Grube, 2018). Someone with four or more ACEs in the studies was found to be three-and-a-half times more likely to develop chronic obstructive pulmonary disease; they were also more likely to be obese, and have cardiac disease, sleep difficulties, migraines, fibromyalgia, reflux, chronic obstructive pulmonary disease, chronic bronchitis, stomach ulcers, or auto-immune disease (such as rheumatoid arthritis, lupus, type 1 diabetes, stroke, coeliac disease, Graves disease). Those with multiple ACEs have also been found to be more likely to smoke both cigarettes and cannabis, and struggle with difficulties with alcohol and other drugs, and have increased rates of psychosis, schizophrenia, anxiety, depression, suicidal ideation, and suicide (De Bellis et al., 2013; Dube et al., 2009; Huang et al., 2015; Hughes et al., 2017; Morris et al., 2020; Quinn et al., 2019; Zarse et al., 2019). As shared in Chapter 1, some research indicates that people abused as children are over nine times more likely to develop psychosis (Janssen et al., 2004) and that people who have endured three kinds of abuse – sexual abuse, bullying, and physical – are at an 18-fold higher risk of psychosis. Those experiencing five types of abuse are 193 times more likely to experience psychosis (Shevlin et al., 2007).

Nadine Burke Harris (2018), inspired by the original ACE study, did a similar evaluation of 702 patients accessing her clinic (however, unlike the original study, they were children not adults). Dr Burke Harris found not only similar results but also, among other findings, that those children with four or more ACEs were 32.6 times more likely to have been diagnosed with one or more learning and behavioural difficulties. In another large study from the UK (Chandan *et al.*, 2020), patients who experienced childhood trauma had a statistically significant adjusted incidence rate ratio for hypertension of 1.42. The same study showed an adjusted incidence rate ratio of 2.15 for strokes or transient ischaemic attacks. Numerous studies have shown the possible link between experiences of toxic stress during childhood and things like hypertension and diabetes.

Interestingly, while not providing evidence that adverse childhood experiences can increase the likelihood of developing autoimmune diseases, there have been studies showing that ACEs may affect their severity and trajectory. For example, Dube *et al.* (2009) found that those with an ACE score of 2 or more had twice the odds of being hospitalized for their autoimmune condition compared to those who had no ACEs. This indicates that those who had experienced childhood trauma even years later as adults had an increased likelihood of hospitalization with a diagnosed autoimmune disease. And similarly, a study using data from the California Lupus Epidemiology Study examined the relationship between adverse childhood experiences and systemic lupus erythematosus (SLE) in adults. They found that there was an association between higher ACE scores and higher levels of patient-reported SLE activity (DeQuattro *et al.*, 2020). This activity ranged from depression and health status to disease symptoms. Moreover, a cohort study (Almuwaqqat *et al.*, 2020) following 300 patients aged 18–60 showed that those with a high childhood adversity score and a documented prior myocardial infarction were twice as likely to have worse outcomes with more recurrent myocardial infarctions, strokes, heart failure, hospitalizations, and cardiovascular deaths over a median three-year follow-up than those without childhood adversity. Similarly, there have been numerous studies suggesting that life stressors can exacerbate symptoms and flare-ups in people with a diagnosis of multiple sclerosis (Mohr *et al.*, 2004). Moreover, some studies indicate that the risk for new diagnoses of coronary artery disease and mortality related to this was increased by more than 25% among individuals who reported high levels of distress.

There is also some evidence that exposure to trauma may also negatively affect immune function, leading to possible faster HIV disease progression, and that experiences of trauma were associated with lower rates of treatment adherence and increased viral load and virologic failure among people living with HIV. Depression and anxiety are often linked to poorer adherence, increased viral load, and decreased CD4 counts (Jewkes *et al.*, 2015; Kouyoumdjian *et al.*, 2013; LeGrand *et al.*, 2016; Machtinger *et al.*, 2012).

> Box 2.1.
>
> ## Caution around the ACE study and data
>
> Studies of adverse childhood experiences have been crucial in highlighting the widespread and prevalent nature of traumas and adversities (even more so as the original study by Felitti *et al.* (1998) was done in a predominantly white middle-class population and so is believed to not be representative of other communities). They show how trauma, adversity, and the body and health are interlinked, giving further weight to the importance of early intervention and prevention and presenting issues around childhood trauma and adversity as a public health responsibility. However, while the original ACE study can be incredibly helpful and illuminating, it is also important to mention that this study and all areas of similar research need to be interpreted with caution and viewed critically and within wider contexts. Here are just some of the limitations to consider around the ACE study (Felitti *et al.* 1998):
>
> - There are huge variations in reported numbers, which might be explained by the type of ACE studied, different characteristics of the sample studied, and variations in the definition of ACEs.
>
> - This was a self-report measure often completed by adults, and is about sensitive and personal information, so it is based on people sharing, naming, remembering, and disclosing. And, of course, the results vary depending on what terms and words people used or recognized or attributed to their experience. For example, what one person saw or labelled as physical abuse may differ from another person and may be viewed differently in different families and cultural contexts (see Chapter 1).
>
> - There were only ten items selected in the original ACE study, which of course is not an inclusive list, and importantly discounts possible key experiences that were not enquired about, such as being in war, being bullied, or having negative experiences outside the home, in school or hospitals, or within other environments. It also excludes being in foster, kinship, or residential care or being adopted, or experiencing racism,

homophobia, antisemitism, xenophobia, and other forms of discrimination (e.g. towards those who are neurodiverse). We also know that the adversities faced vary depending on the context and which are more common, which are highlighted, and which are culturally acknowledged. So often the measure is not as transferable, relevant, or applicable.

- The ten-item scale focused on adverse childhood experiences but it isn't just childhood experiences that are possibly impactful. We also need to consider adverse adult, adverse community, adverse collective, adverse cultural, and adverse organizational experiences.

- This measure focused on adverse experiences and therefore is one-sided and does not acknowledge protective, positive, and buffering factors which can inevitably have a huge impact. It is not helpful to discount or ignore these.

- This measure asked for a yes or no answer and we know that there is limited information about other crucial factors. For example, it is not just about saying yes or no to questions on sexual abuse, as there are so many other key factors which have been shown repeatedly in the literature. Trauma doesn't happen in a vacuum but is influenced by a plethora of additional factors within a wider context, such as the age and stage of the child, not just chronologically but socially, emotionally, and developmentally, their explanations and sense-making of the abuse, the support put in place and other buffering and protective factors, the frequency of the abuse, their relationship with the person, whether they were believed, their cultural and family context around the abuse, and so many other interplaying factors. A number does not describe or shed light on the lived and living experience and the nuance of what someone experienced.

- One item on the measure is about divorce. We know that there are multiple interplaying factors which will inevitably shape or influence how impactful a divorce can be, and yet divorce would be given the same score as sexual abuse.

- People are far more multi-layered than a score and should not be reduced to or described as a number. For example, we know someone might have a score of 1 but the impact might be profound, whereas someone else might have a score of 10 but be doing very well.

- This was a population epidemiological tool, not designed or intended to be used as a clinical or diagnostic tool, therefore care should be taken in where, how, when, and if it should be used, shared, and disseminated. People should not be asked to complete a measure which can be activating, personal, shocking, and sensitive without a clear rationale as to why, what will be done, and how they will be supported.

- Paying attention to ACEs and using the ACE tool does not in itself constitute a trauma-informed approach.

2.4. Other impacts of stress on the body

This section continues to explore some of the possible impacts of trauma on the body. As we have seen, chronic or ongoing exposure to stress hormones or unregulated toxic stress can suppress and weaken the immune system in many different ways. Karlen *et al.* (2015) found that children who were exposed to early stress showed increased cortisol levels and were more likely to be affected by colds, gastroenteritis, and other viral infections. We also know that dysregulation of the stress response can lead to increased inflammation, hypersensitivity (such as allergies, eczema, and asthma), and autoimmune diseases such as Graves (Anisman & Kusnecov, 2022; Burke, 2018). Other studies have shown that stress can have an impact on the length and health of telomeres (regions of repetitive DNA sequences that protect the end of chromosomes from becoming frayed or tangled) (Blackburn & Epel, 2012).

Moreover, some studies have also shown that trauma and stress experiences can impact cortisol levels and key regulatory processes (Cicchetti *et al.*, 2010; Heim *et al.*, 2008; Thayer & Lane, 2009). These can include the executive systems for emotion and information processing, the reward/motivation systems (e.g. dopamine), the sympathetic nervous system (i.e. survival responses, maintaining homeostasis, equilibrium, regulation), the serotonin system (i.e. regulating functions including mood, sleep, appetite, bowel function, and weight), the endocrine system, and the distress-tolerance system, such as the limbic-hypothalamic-pituitary-adrenal (HPA) axis. These can have significant implications, for example the HPA axis plays a fundamental role in the response to external and internal stimuli, including psychological stressors. Changes in the HPA axis, such as over-activity, have been linked to a range of difficulties including panic disorder and anorexia; and under-activity, to conditions such as depression and chronic fatigue (Afifi *et al.*, 2016; Neigh *et al.*, 2009; Schwaiger *et al.*, 2016). This happens for a range of reasons, including how chronic hyperarousal can lead to dysregulation of the physiologic stress system and the development of stress-related conditions.

In line with the above, Danese and McEwen (2012) found that chronic increased inflammation, in turn, is a dysregulation of the immune system and can lead to impaired cell-mediated acquired immunity. They illustrated the physiological connection between chronic stress and disease, showing, for example, that chronic increased inflammation is related to cardiovascular disease and atherosclerosis. C-reactive protein (CRP) is considered to be one of the most reliable indicators of inflammation.

In a longitudinal, prospective study, a birth cohort of 1037 participants was followed for 32 years (Danese *et al.*, 2007). Childhood maltreatment was investigated in the first decade of life and CRP levels were measured at age 32 years. Children with two or more indicators of maltreatment (9.8%) were 1.8 times more likely to have elevated CRP levels in adulthood compared to those children with no indicators of abuse; children with one indicator of abuse (26.7%) were 1.18 times more likely. Children in this study who were abused were also significantly more likely to experience co-occurring early life risks, including low birth weight, socioeconomic status, and intelligence scores. However, even when controlling for early life risks, the relation between childhood maltreatment and elevated adult CRP maintained significance (relative risk = 1.58). These results were also supported by a recent meta-analysis of 18 studies which found significantly elevated levels of CRP among adults with a history of childhood trauma (Baumeister *et al.*, 2016). This was further echoed in a meta-analysis of 20 studies which concluded that childhood maltreatment was associated with increased levels of C-reactive protein, fibrinogen, and proinflammatory cytokines (Coelho *et al.*, 2014). A study looking at 67, 516 women found that the experience of physical and emotional abuse in childhood was associated with 2.57 times greater risk of lupus erythematosus (Feldman *et al.*, 2019).

The above studies, in combination with other factors, also shed some light as to why people who have experienced abuse, toxic stress, and neglect (relational, sensory, and emotional poverty) often demonstrate behavioural and sensory changes in the way in which they regulate their stress systems, with their systems either being chronically elevated and up-regulated, or chronically suppressed and under-regulated (Gunnar & Fisher, 2006), or fluctuating between the two. (Of course, this can also be seen and influenced in other contexts – it is nuanced and we cannot just attribute all regulation difficulties to trauma.)

Some children who have been marinated in uncertainty and inconsistency are left feeling powerless, unsafe, and out of control. Their stress, threat, and fear responses and systems have been needed and activated repeatedly. They have been in persistent fear states, on an ongoing diet of stress, where their survival and protective responses have been continually over-used, like a well-exercised muscle taken to the fear and stress gym frequently. This offers an explanation as to why some of these children (and later adults) can have overly sensitive defence systems, be more hypervigilant, and understandably preoccupied with detecting, expecting, and surviving threats. Their defence systems can be likened to constantly beeping burglar alarms, which means they are often more vigilant for threats and signs of danger, like a constantly scanning danger detecting magnet, or a highly active threat radar.

This sense of fear and feeling unsafe and having to be at a higher arousal/alert level can sadly for some become their norm, their internalized sense of being. Therefore, this fear and sense of unsafety, like a trauma jacket, can follow them into different environments, such as a medical setting during a health check-up. The world around them can often feel too loud, too big, too bright. Some people experience regular hijacking of their fear/emotional/limbic systems, and one drop of an emotion can feel like a vast all-consuming ocean which can override their inhibitory systems.

This fits with Stephen Porges' polyvagal theory, in which the process of automatically and continually scanning our environment for features of danger or safety is called neuroception. In neuroception, our defence systems can be heightened or dampened down (or fluctuate between the two), and our social engagement system comes online (Porges, 2007). However, in the context of trauma, people might have had regularly activated systems of fear and danger. It is almost as if the wound or injury of trauma can be imprinted on our nervous, regulation, and arousal systems. Porges calls this neural expectancy. Peter Levine (founder of somatic experiencing and author of many books) shares that when an event elicits a high emotional charge where the body is unable to metabolize in the moment, the body might have to adapt to such overwhelm to the system in a way that protects the person when they are directly under threat. This emotional charge can become programmed in the nervous system, which is protective when under threat but can be distressing and disorienting in everyday life.

This also sheds some light on why some children (and adults) can often be more easily 'triggered' (even by what seems like a 'small trigger' or level of distress), can have a lower window of tolerance (Ogden & Fisher, 2014; Siegel, 2012), and have an out-of-sync emotional, sensory, physical, and behavioural homeostasis and equilibrium. This means that some people can often have a lower threshold for high-intensity emotions and can be slower to return to what is often a heightened baseline. They can be more habituated to an adrenaline buzz and more programmed to respond in ways to survive and protect themselves. These chronic and long-lasting stressors can put an excessive and heavy load on critical systems, which can result in allostatic overload and vulnerability to a variety of health issues (McEwen & Akil, 2020).

Moreover, those who have experienced ongoing and cumulative toxic stress, for example in the context of sexual, physical, and domestic abuse, can also often present with a poorer ability to regulate, process, and modulate affect and sensory stimuli (Warner & Koomar, 2009). This can show itself in a variety of different ways, including impacting sleep, concentration, attention, and focus. Of course, sleep is a vast area and there are numerous aspects within it (and many people with no trauma or adversity history have difficulty sleeping); however, we do know that sleep difficulties including insomnia, sleepwalking, night terrors, nightmares, wetting the bed during the night, struggling to fall or stay asleep, having more sleep disturbances, and feeling exhausted and fatigued are more common in those who have experienced trauma and adversity (Brown *et al.*, 2022; Fuligni *et al.*, 2021; Wu *et al.*, 2022). Trauma experiences can understandably increase threats of harm or unpredictability, resulting in increased vigilance and hyperarousal that are not conducive to sleep and thus might lead to more sleep disturbances (Noll *et al.*, 2006). Moreover, the trauma might have occurred in the dark, in their bedroom, or at night-time and thus they may feel more alone and vulnerable, and have more time to think or reflect. And if a child struggles to down-regulate, it can be harder to get into a 'calmer' state to be able to sleep.

Many people have had to survive and protect themselves by psychologically 'running away' (dissociating), blocking out their feelings, cutting off their mind from their body, and numbing themselves. In the face of inescapable fear and stress, children often cannot run or fight; therefore dissociating is their way of surviving and shielding themselves. For some, their fantasy world or place where their mind goes to is far more tolerable than their reality. Others may have to retreat into themselves, clam up, or put up a protective bubble to keep out the 'bad', but this can also stop the 'good' coming in. Those for whom dissociation has become their habituated way of being might be more likely to have systems that are chronically suppressed and down-regulated. This is also echoed in some studies of chronic neglect, showing increased dorsal vagal tones, diminished brain activity, and decreased heart rates (Marshall & Fox, 2004; Schore, 2009a, 2009b).

2.5. Trauma and the brain

Many studies have explored the possible impact or influence of trauma on brain development, particularly in the context of childhood trauma. However, it is important when talking about brain development to hold in mind that our knowledge of the brain is changing daily, and there is a lot we still do not know, and studies that are contradictory. The brain, like trauma and the various inter-playing factors, is complex and nuanced. Therefore, information about the brain needs to be interpreted and shared with caution. So, while we can hypothesize or use some of the information here to inform ourselves, it is not helpful to regard it in a reductionist, assumptive, or deterministic way. We also know that there may be some children and adults who have experienced trauma whose brains have been significantly impacted and influenced, and others on the other side of the spectrum for whom the trauma has had very little impact. There is much variety and many other influencing factors that can impact a person, and we need to consider the bigger picture including protective, positive, and buffering factors, learning disabilities, physical health conditions, neurodiversity, nutri-tion, head injuries, medications, poverty, exposure to substances, and so on. Moreover, there are various definitions of what trauma is and how it is defined or reported; most people won't have brain scans or be experts in neuroscience, so a lot is based on possible scenarios.

This said, because a child's developing brain is in a state of neural plasticity, this makes them particularly sensitive to the effects of trauma and toxic stress. Therefore, complex trauma has been shown in some studies to impact a child's psychobiology at multiple levels, from neurohormonal to neuroanatomical (Teicher et al., 2016). These biologic traumas can affect several developmental processes, such as synaptic overproduction, pruning, and myelination (Glaser, 2000), and, in some cases, influence the architecture, structure, and function of the developing brain. Most consistently evidenced in the child trauma litera-ture is the effect on the ventromedial and orbitofrontal-limbic regions, and the networks of affect control (e.g. the sensory integration, emotional regulation, and decision-making/reward-processing functions). There is also emerging evidence for discrepancies in the lateral fronto-striatal and parietal-temporal regions, which mediate a range of functions, including executive functioning (e.g. inhibition, attention, concentration, and working memory).

Interestingly, there have also been studies documenting decreased cerebral volumes (Schore, 2009a, 2009b; Teicher et al., 2016), larger lateral ventricles and frontal lobe cerebrospinal fluid volumes (Carrion et al., 2009), and an over-activity of the amygdala (Tottenham et al., 2010). This is pertinent, as the amygdala plays an important role in fear conditioning, survival, and protective responses, and assigning emotional significance to stimuli. The amygdala is the brain's fear centre, and helps to identify and react to threats. So, if the amygdala has been repeatedly 'triggered', it makes sense that this might have a variety of consequences.

In some studies, changes have also been found in the corpus callosum (CC) volume and white matter integrity (Jackowski *et al.*, 2008), which is significant, as the CC is a main connection point, like a bridge, between the left and right cerebral hemispheres of the brain and is also key in facilitating interhemispheric communication for both emotion and higher cognitive abilities. Studies looking at the severe neglect experienced by institutionalized Romanian orphans resulted in some (not all) of the children showing developmental delays, impacted executive functioning, increased 'autistic-like' behaviours, and elevated salivary cortisol levels (Gunnar & Fisher, 2001; Rutter *et al.*, 2004).

This is just a tiny flavour of the large body of brain literature that exists, but it is important to remember that while within the context of neuroplasticity (synaptic and cellular plasticity) some parts of the brain might be negatively shaped, it can also be positively shaped and supported through enriched environments and buffering and reparative relationships. This is demonstrated in the well-known work by Meaney with rat pups (Meaney & Szyf, 2005). Meaney looked at two groups of rat mothers and rat pups and observed that, after the pups were handled by the researchers, the rat mothers would soothe their pups by licking and grooming them. However, some rat mothers exhibited high levels of licking and others exhibited lower levels of licking. Researchers observed the rat pups' response to stress and found that the pups with the higher licking mothers had lower levels of stress hormones, including corticosterone, when they were handled by the researchers or had something stress-inducing done to them. The more licking they received, the lower their stress response was. The pups receiving lower licking not only had higher spikes of corticosterone in response to a stressor, but also had a harder time shutting off or regulating their stress response. This continued throughout their lifetime. They also found that for some these changes were passed on to the next generation, because female pups who had high-licking mothers were more likely to be high lickers themselves.

2.6. Some other areas where trauma can impact the body

There isn't space here to discuss all areas of the body potentially affected by trauma, and it is hoped that the reader will undertake research in relation to their specific area of interest. However, to give a flavour, some areas of possible interest have been selected.

In relation to urology and gynaecology practice, Felitti *et al.* (1998) observed that adults who experienced childhood trauma (a vague and broad category) and who had higher ACEs reported an increased number of sexual partners and sexually transmitted diseases. There have also been other studies which have looked at higher levels of chronic pelvic pain in women who experienced childhood abuse (As-Sanie *et al.*, 2014; Sachs-Ericsson *et al.*, 2007; Schrepf *et al.*, 2018).

Interestingly, Harris *et al.* (2018) found that among the 60,595 pre-menopausal women in the Nurses' Health Study II cohort after 24 years of follow-up, there were 3394 cases of laparoscopically confirmed endometriosis. Compared to those reporting no physical or sexual abuse, the risk of endometriosis was greater among those who experienced severe physical abuse (rate ratios = 1.20; 95% confidence intervals = 1.06, 1.37) or severe sexual abuse (rate ratios = 1.49; 95% confidence intervals = 1.24, 1.79). There was a 79% increased risk of laparoscopically confirmed endometriosis for women reporting severe chronic abuse of multiple types (95% confidence intervals = 1.44, 2.22). There are so many wider and interesting avenues within the trauma umbrella to be explored, for example women who have been abused and who are going through menopause, or those with HIV.

With respect to chronic pain, so much more research is needed. A retrospective population-based open cohort study (Chandan *et al.*, 2020) using the UK primary care database studied 80,657 adult patients who had experienced childhood trauma, who were matched to 161,314 unexposed patients by age and sex. Among people who had experienced childhood trauma (this is a vast area and an umbrella term, so it is hard to distinguish between types), there was an increased risk of developing fibromyalgia, chronic fatigue syndrome, chronic lower back pain, restless leg syndrome, and irritable bowel syndrome when compared to the unexposed group. Moreover, in a series of meta-analyses, relations were found between the experience of chronic pain in adulthood and retrospective reports of childhood sexual abuse, physical abuse, and neglect (Davis, 2005).

It has also been shared that childhood traumas can have a long-term effect on cortisol secretion patterns and this mediates symptom demonstration in chronic pain syndromes such as fibromyalgia (Yavne *et al.*, 2018). Several studies have found that people with fibromyalgia have a higher incidence of sexual or physical abuse than a control group, with a frequency varying between 34% and 88% (Bayram & Erol, 2014; Combas *et al.*, 2022; Miró *et al.*, 2020; Näring & Van Lankveld, 2007; Nijenhuis *et al.*, 2003; Semiz *et al.*, 2014). Moreover, a meta-analysis study of patients with fibromyalgia found that individuals were 2.52 times more likely to develop fibromyalgia after exposure to trauma (Afari *et al.*, 2014).

There have also been several studies which have discussed some of the associations found between headaches and childhood trauma (Juang & Yang, 2014). For example, in a large, multicentre study of migraine patients, Tietjen *et al.* (2010) found that childhood trauma was reported by 58% of the study population. This higher level and association with headaches and migraines was also found in a Canadian study of 23,395 people (Afifi *et al.*, 2016).

Other interesting studies found that stomach problems, nausea, heartburn, and ulcers have been found to occur with significantly greater frequency in those with abuse or neglect histories (Goodwin *et al.*, 2003; Heitkemper *et al.*, 2011; Randolph & Reddy, 2006; Ross, 2005). For example, a meta-analysis of 28 irritable bowel syndrome studies revealed that reported trauma exposure increased the likelihood of irritable bowel syndrome development by 2.22 times (Afari *et al.*, 2014).

2.7. Health inequalities and social injustice

We know wider system and structural inequalities such as poverty, austerity, social hardship, social injustice, discrimination, and emotional distress can be intertwined with poorer health. There is a growing body of evidence which shows that population health is determined to a great extent by social, environmental, economic, political, and cultural factors (the social determinants of health), and that an unequal distribution of these factors drives inequalities in physical and mental health. This includes the way that varying social identities, such as ethnicity and gender, can influence and interact with these factors and how different levels of power, prestige, and access to resources between groups in society can affect health outcomes (Commission on Social Determinants of Health, 2008; Marmot, 2010; World Health Organization, 2013). We also know that higher social position, whether measured by education, income, or occupational status, is associated with better health and longevity.

It is clear that we need to influence and proactively address the causes of these disparities themselves. As Bishop Desmond Tutu aptly said, 'There comes a point where we need to stop just pulling people out of the river, and we need to go upstream to find out why they are falling in.' This is about being proactive, intentional, and preventative rather than reactive and crisis-driven. If we want to make needed intergenerational changes, we need to not just focus on 'quick fixes'. Einstein said that only a fool keeps on doing the same thing over and over again and expects different results. Do we want to be saying the same thing or seeing worse in a year, five years, 20 years, 100 years? This is echoed in the Marmot review (Marmot, 2010) which advocates putting wellbeing, not just economic growth, at the heart of policy. It also makes the powerful statement that 'social injustice is killing people on a grand scale'.

2.8. Connections between areas of poverty and health (see also Chapter 6)

There are numerous links between poverty and health discussed in the extant literature base and within practice, and it is beyond the scope of this book to explore this area in depth. However, it is important to acknowledge some of the key points in this crucial area. Poverty trauma is often referred to as a neurotoxin and, as with other forms of discrimination, the experience can be ongoing and cumulative, chipping away at a person.

Of course, as with other areas discussed in this chapter, there is huge variation in the experience of poverty, and in the definitions that people and research studies use around poverty, and we must also consider any possible buffering and protective factors.

Poverty and some of the associated outcomes can inevitably be linked with areas such as housing and neighbourhood quality. Some of the most extensively studied examples of institutional racism and residential segregation are associated with significant differences in neighbourhood quality, living conditions, and access to opportunities that undermine health through multiple pathways (Bailey et al., 2017; Schulz et al., 2002; Williams & Collins, 2001). Numerous studies show that neighbourhood conditions and resources, such as access to adequate early childhood programmes, libraries, schools, health facilities, and green spaces, influence children's development and long-term outcomes (Acevedo-Garcia et al., 2020). Between a few roads and neighbourhoods, there is a postcode lottery where mortality and health outcomes as well as access to health care can be vastly different.

The Royal College of Paediatrics and Child Health (2022) produced a paper on child health inequalities driven by child poverty in the UK and the key findings are detailed below, interwoven with some international and other studies.

- Children living in poverty are significantly more likely to suffer from acute and long-term illness. They are significantly more likely to require hospital admission (Kyle et al., 2011) and are 72% more likely than other children to be diagnosed with a long-term illness (Spencer et al., 2015).

- Children raised in poverty are more likely to develop a variety of chronic health conditions including obesity (Kakinami *et al.*, 2014; Lee *et al.*, 2014), asthma (Commodore *et al.*, 2021; Mendes *et al.*, 2011), and chronic kidney disease (Friedman & Luyckx, 2019).

- Rates of obesity and severe obesity in children living in the most income-deprived areas are rising, while the rates are decreasing in the least income-deprived areas in England (NHS Digital, 2021). Similar rates are found in other parts of the UK.

- Children living in poverty are more likely to be at risk of tooth decay. In England, children from the most income-deprived areas have more than twice the level of decay compared with those from the least income-deprived areas (Public Health England, 2018).

- Air pollution exposure is highest in the most income-deprived areas (Brunt *et al.*, 2016), and children are disproportionally exposed to the highest levels of pollution (Barnes & Chatterton, 2016; Commodore *et al.*, 2021; Mullen *et al.*, 2020). They are also more likely to be exposed to noise pollution (Collins *et al.*, 2019) and lead poisoning (Baek *et al.*, 2021; Egendorf *et al.*, 2021). Children are most likely to be exposed to these toxins in their homes (Manduca & Sampson, 2019; Wheeler *et al.*, 2019) and schools (Collins & Grineski, 2018; Collins *et al.*, 2019), the two places where they spend the majority of their time. Air quality, in particular, has been linked with the prevalence and severity of childhood asthma, with higher levels of air pollution exacerbating asthmatic symptoms (Commodore *et al.*, 2021; Kranjac *et al.*, 2017). Black and Hispanic children are more likely to be exposed to higher levels of air pollution due to higher traffic levels in their neighbourhoods and have a higher prevalence of asthma/asthma-like symptoms than white and Asian children (Commodore *et al.*, 2021).

- Children in more income-deprived families are three times more likely to be exposed to second-hand smoke (Orton *et al.*, 2014).

- Children in income-deprived areas are more likely to live in housing with poor ventilation (Ferguson *et al.*, 2020) and other features of substandard housing.

- Poverty for some is associated with lower academic attainment, including school readiness, grades, and standardized test scores (Hair *et al.*, 2015; Morrissey *et al.*, 2014).

- Parents in poverty are less able to afford healthy foods and offer their children a healthy lifestyle. Healthy foods are nearly three times more expensive than less healthy foods per calorie, which means families may be more likely to eat food that is cheap but nutritionally poor, leading to obesity and malnutrition in children (The Food Foundation, 2021). This is likely to increase in the current cost of living situation.

- Living in a cold home has a negative impact on physical health, for example by exacerbating respiratory illnesses (Child Poverty Action Group & Royal College of Paediatrics and Child Health, 2017).

- Low-income families may be unable to afford basic hygiene products due to financial constraints. For example, period poverty is the lack of access to sanitary products and one in ten young people who menstruate are unable to afford period products, which can lead to missed school days or improvising menstrual products (Tingle & Vora, 2018).

- Depending on the country and setting, children in low-income families have less access to the medical care they need. Families have reported missing paediatric appointments because of the financial costs of attending one due to travel, parking, food, childcare costs, and potential loss in earnings.

- Low-income families may also be experiencing digital exclusion, where households may not have a smartphone or internet access and are unable to benefit from digital health technologies as a result.

There are many other related areas, such as possible experiences of discrimination, stigma, social exclusion/rejection, chronic loneliness, and social dislocation. Some longitudinal studies have found that childhood poverty is associated with increased risk of developing mental health difficulties (McLaughlin et al., 2011), type 2 diabetes (Maty et al., 2008), metabolic syndrome (Puolakka et al., 2016), and cancer (Vohra et al., 2016), as well as with less stable employment and lower earnings (Duncan & Magnuson, 2013) in adulthood. There is evidence from whole-population-linked data that even fleeting childhood poverty increases the risk of mortality in adulthood (Rod et al., 2020). One study (Hughes et al., 2015) of people who were unemployed found that they had higher markers of inflammation in their bodies, and that the longer the unemployment period lasted the greater the risk of inflammation.

Additionally, other examples of these inequalities were revealed in a survey carried out in 2015 which showed that men and women who were living in lower-income households were more likely to have received a psychiatric diagnosis than those living in higher-income households (Bridges, 2015). This and various other aspects were echoed in the powerful book *The Spirit Level: Why Equality is Better for Everyone* (Wilkinson & Pickett, 2010), which showed that there was a strong correlation at a national level between income inequality (i.e. the difference between the richest and poorest in society) and World Health Organization mental health surveys. Countries such as the UK or USA, with the highest levels of income inequality, had higher levels of mental health difficulties, whereas others such as Japan or Belgium, with more equality of income, had lower levels of distress.

Moreover, in a Joseph Rowntree Foundation Report (2020), it was reported that, in 2017/18, 31% of the 13 million people with disabilities in the UK lived in poverty, which is around four million people. It also stated that an additional three million non-disabled people in poverty live in a household where someone is disabled, meaning that, overall, nearly half of the 14 million people in poverty are affected by disability. Aspects like this are further compounded by policy restrictions, such as employment barriers, access to benefits, and carers' rights. The report also found that there were nearly four and a half million informal adult carers in the UK in 2017/18, around 7% of the population, and nearly a quarter (more than a million people) were living in poverty. More than half of these carers were women and three-quarters were of working age. Working-age carers had a higher rate of poverty than those with no caring responsibilities, with over a quarter of the group being in poverty compared with around one in five non-carers. Women of working age who were carers had the greatest risk of all. Younger carers (aged under 35) had higher rates of poverty than older carers.

For those who are homeless, poverty is not necessarily the cause, as there are also numerous systemic, family, and individual aspects to this. However, those living on the streets have been found to have higher rates of illness, including hypertension, asthma, diabetes, and HIV. Some studies indicate homelessness has an impact on lowering life expectancy, and there are also likely to be further related health concerns such as exposure to communicable diseases, harmful weather conditions, malnutrition, drug use, and violence.

2.9. The impact of racism and other forms of discrimination on health (see also Chapter 6)

Of course, this is a flavour and by no means an exhaustive review and there are so many nuances within this data but this section is intended as food for thought. And people will have differing experiences of discrimination, and there are multiple layers, such as being a woman, and Black, and in a wheelchair , and so forth.

Minoritized and marginalized populations may experience 'weathering', a physiological response to chronic stress that increases allostatic load, accelerated epigenetic ageing, and adverse health outcomes (Brody *et al.*, 2014; Geronimus *et al.*, 2010). The experience of discrimination can be ongoing and chip away at a person but also people can be marinated in these experiences from an early age. This is also sometimes referred to as insidious trauma (the daily and ongoing marginalization, objectification, exclusion, social rejection, dehumanization, and intimidation experienced by people or certain groups).

Interestingly, we know that some stressors can activate the stress-response systems – both the sympathetic-adrenal-medullary axis and the hypothalam-ic-pituitary-adrenal axis – and, when toxic stress is ongoing, can lead to dysreg-ulation or impact on these systems (Michopoulous *et al.*, 2017; Thames *et al.*, 2019). Therefore, it has been posited that ongoing race-based discrimination and other forms of discrimination could alter the physiological responses of people and contribute to increased inflammation.

Research has also indicated positive associations between reports of dis-crimination and adverse cardiovascular outcomes, body mass index (BMI), and incidence of obesity, hypertension, alcohol use, and poor sleep (Bernardo *et al.*, 2017; Dolezsar *et al.*, 2014; Gilbert & Zemore, 2016; Lewis & Van Dyke, 2018; Slopen *et al.*, 2016). Experiences of racism have been associated with a range of illnesses and symptoms, including higher levels of colds, diabetes, high blood pressure, memory and cognitive difficulties, asthma, and hypertension (Coogan *et al.*, 2020; Kapadia *et al.*, 2022; Lewis *et al.*, 2015; Pascoe & Smart Richman, 2009; van Daalen *et al.*, 2022). Moreover, in a study which compared the telomeres of Black and white women in the US, women who were Black were found on average over seven years to age more biologically than the white women (Geronimus *et al.*, 2010).

Building on the above, there have been links between self-reported racial discrimination and physical health outcomes, as documented in multiple recent reviews. For example, discrimination has been linked to amygdala activation, the formation of fear memories, and sympathetic engagement, leading to possible increases in blood pressure, core body temperature, heart rate, perspiration, respiration rate, startle reflex, and arousal levels, and disrupted regulation and immune responses. There have also been other links discussed, such as height-ened suicidal ideation, 'negative thinking', and increased alcohol consumption (Ben-Zeev *et al.*, 2005; Grasser & Jovanovic, 2022; Scanzano & Cosentino, 2015; Williams *et al.*, 2019).

Correspondingly, the brain regions and circuits that underlie emotional function, namely the amygdala, hippocampus, and prefrontal cortex, have been shown to be influenced by negative life experiences like stigmatization, racism, and discrimination (Grasser *et al.*, 2022). For example, Black adults who reported greater exposure to racial discrimination showed altered connectivity between the amygdala and the insula, known as the neural correlates of vigilance (Webber *et al.*, 2022). There has also been some discussion around experiences of racism and discrimination and how they can be linked with variation in white matter microstructure, which may indicate a mechanism through which such experiences enhance vulnerability to brain health problems (Fani *et al.*, 2021).

The Adolescent Brain Cognitive Development (ABCD) Study is a large longitudinal population-based study of brain development, with a sample of 11,857 nine- and ten-year-old children throughout the US (Karcher & Barch, 2021). Data from this cohort has indicated that Black and Hispanic/Latino young people in structural stigma contexts (based on analysis using indicators of attitudes related to racial prejudice, attitudes of immigrants and immigration policies, gender attitudes, and the Implicit Attitudes Test) have smaller hippocampal volumes compared to young people living in lower stigma contexts, and non-stigmatized youth did not show any difference between contexts (Hatzenbuehler *et al.*, 2021).

Moreover, a recent review of 30 studies focused on the effects of second-hand discrimination on children and young people (i.e. situations where the child was not the direct target) and reported significant impacts on a variety of socio-emotional outcomes, although it is worth mentioning that there was no standard definition of vicarious racism (Heard-Garris *et al.*, 2018). Additionally, a longitudinal study of 704 poor Black and Latina urban mothers who were also teenagers found that everyday discrimination reported during pregnancy predicted greater inhibition/separation difficulties and negative emotionality in their children at six months and at one year of age (Rosenthal *et al.*, 2018). And a longitudinal study of infants born in the UK found reports of discrimination experienced by Black and other minoritized mothers to be positively associated with child social and emotional problems six years later (Bécares *et al.*, 2015).

See Chapter 6 for more on health biases and disparities.

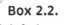

Box 2.2.

Recommended further reading on brain science and body-based approaches

Some books which might be of interest are listed below – this is just a small selection of the wide variety of books available:

- *The Health Gap* by Michael Marmot

- *The Death Gap* by David Ansell

- *The Spirit Level* by Kate Pickett

- *The Social Determinants of Health* by Kathryn Strother Ratcliff

- *Reproductive Injustice: Racism, Pregnancy, and Premature Birth* by Dana Ain-Davis

- *Medical Apartheid* by Harriet Washington

- *Just Medicine: A Cure for Racial Inequality* by Dayna Bowen Matthew

- *Black and Blue* by John Hoberman

- *Breathing Race into the Machine* by Lundy Braun

- *Infectious Fear* by Samuel Kelton Roberts

- *Killing the Black Body* by Dorothy Roberts

- *On Race and Medicine* by Richard Garcia

- *Unequal Treatment* by Brian Smedley

- *Transcultural Health Care* by Betty Paulanka

See also texts written by the following authors:

Hymie Anisman	Susan Aposhyan	Frances Champagne
Louis Cozolino	Antonio Damasio	Michael De Bellis
Alan Fogel	Marija Kundakovic	Joseph LeDoux
Peter Levine	Kimberley Matheson	Charles Nemeroff
Pat Ogden	Jaak Panksepp	Bruce Perry
Stephen Porges	Babette Rothschild	Robert Scaer
Allan Schore	Hannah Schreier	Daniel Siegel
Martin Teicher	Bessel Van der Kolk	Rachel Yehuda

The Impact of Trauma on the Body and Sensory World: 'Triggers', Hotspots, and Activating Experiences

3.1. What will be covered in this chapter

- The body as a physical and emotional container
- What might people's bodies have experienced in the context of trauma?
- Trauma-related body sensations and 'triggers'
- Ideas around sensory and body-based 'triggers', hotspots, and activating experiences

3.2. The body as a physical and emotional container

The body itself is fundamental in all stages of life, from conception and being contained within the womb, to travelling with us throughout every life stage, memory, and experience. Our body is also physically visible to the outside world, and acts as an actual physical and emotional container, and as a vehicle of expression and communication (e.g. scars, bruises, injuries, malnourishment). Think about where and what happens in your body when watching, witnessing, feeling, and experiencing something powerful, loving, emotive, or sickening.

This notion of trauma (from the Greek word traumata, meaning an injury, a wound, or to pierce) permeating and piercing through layers and really getting under one's skin has been aptly described as 'the body keeping the score' (Van der Kolk, 2014) and 'the body remembering' (Rothschild, 2000). As Frank

Gillette Burgess was known to have said, 'Our bodies are apt to be our autobiographies.' The multi-layered impact of trauma is also powerfully described by Gabor Maté who says, 'Trauma is not what happens to you, but what happens inside you.'

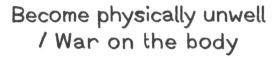

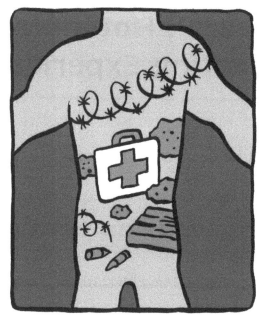

3.1. THE BODY AS A PHYSICAL AND EMOTIONAL CONTAINER

★ If your body could talk, what would it say? If your body could show you a map of the journey it has been through, what would you see and learn?

★ What do the concepts and quotes shared above mean to you and make you think about?

3.3. What might people's bodies have experienced in the context of trauma?

In the context of abuse and certain types of traumas, people might have experienced too much or too little touching, which is particularly important in the context of health settings where people are examined, prodded, touched, drugged, anesthetized, moved around, placed in machines, and so on. People's bodies have often been violated, neglected, hurt, and dehumanized. These experiences can be compounded by conflicting messages that people might have received during trauma; for example, in the context of sexual abuse, 'You got wet so you must have liked it', 'It is because you are so pretty'. This can impact people's relationship to their body, sensory world, feelings, sensations, and more, and also manifest in people being more sensory seeking and needing, or sensory avoidant, and many shades in between.

Images 3.2 and 3.3 give a flavour of some of the ways people's bodies may have been touched or treated in the context of trauma. This can be a helpful platform to then explore some sensory and body-based 'triggers' and hotspots.

★ Looking at these images, what thoughts, feelings, sensations, and associations come to mind?

★ Are there others you would add or change?

★ What possible impact might these have? How might these show themselves in someone's body, health, sensory experience, and relationship to touch?

★ How might these show themselves in health or medical settings and during appointments, procedures, and so on?

★ How might these experiences be 'triggered', resurfaced, and activated?

Each one of these experiences is written as words, almost as a list, but what might it feel like to experience them, the lived multi-sensory aspect of them? Consider, for example, that someone who has been sex trafficked, tortured, or sexually abused is likely to have experienced a multitude and entanglement of some of these. The next few sections will give an insight into how these experiences can be relived, resurfaced, 'triggered', and activated.

SOME OF THE EXPERIENCES, SENSATIONS, & WAYS THE BODY MIGHT HAVE BEEN TREATED IN THE CONTEXT OF TRAUMAS (NOT AN EXHAUSTIVE LIST)

- HAVING TOO MUCH OR TOO LITTLE TOUCHING
- BEING DRUGGED, POISONED, INJECTED OR MEDICATED
- BODY IMAGE INCLUDING SHAME / FEAR (EG WEIGHT, TEETH, SCARS)
- HAVING DIFFERENT EXPERIENCES OF TOILETING / WEANING, FEEDING / BRUSHING TEETH / BATHING, NAPPIES BEING CHANGED / TUMMY TIME / SLEEPING ETC
- BOUNDARIES BEING VIOLATED, INTRUDED & / OR INVADED
- EXPERIENCE OF HOW HURTS, PAIN, WOUNDS OR ILLNESS WERE NAMED, ACKNOWLEDGED & ATTENDED TO
- BEING USED AS A SHIELD / WEAPON / A TARGET / ATTACKED
- HAVING TO SURVIVE OR COPE BY CUTTING OFF, NUMBING OR DISSOCIATING FROM ONE'S BODY
- BEING NEGLECTED & ABUSED
- HAVING CONFLICTED BODY FEELINGS & SENSATIONS E.G THE BODY'S RESPONSE DURING SEXUAL ABUSE
- BEING EXPOSED, STRIPPED, HUMILIATED & OR OBJECTIFIED
- BEING OR FEELING TRAPPED, STUCK, PINNED DOWN, TIED OR RESTRICTED
- BEING IN PAIN, HURT, HARMED, BURNED, CHOKED & MORE

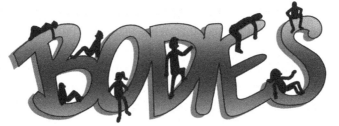

DR KAREN TREISMAN SAFE HANDS AND THINKING MINDS

IMAGISTIC.CO.UK

3.2. SOME OF THE EXPERIENCES, SENSATIONS, AND WAYS THE BODY MIGHT HAVE BEEN TREATED IN THE CONTEXT OF TRAUMAS – PART 1

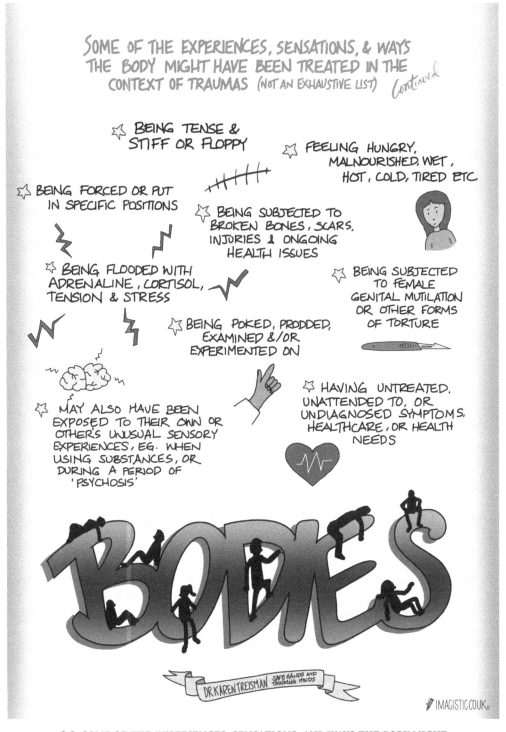

3.3. SOME OF THE EXPERIENCES, SENSATIONS, AND WAYS THE BODY MIGHT
HAVE BEEN TREATED IN THE CONTEXT OF TRAUMAS – PART 2

Some reflections and caution around the term and word 'trigger'

Throughout this book the word 'trigger' has been used with " intentionally; this is to acknowledge that this term for some can be unhelpful, unclear, and/or activating. This links to the power of language and of finding words which mean something and resonate for the unique person and their context. Some thoughts and alternatives to this term are shared in the below image. Following this, some reflective exercises, and examples of these will be shared to expand on this concept.

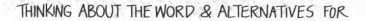
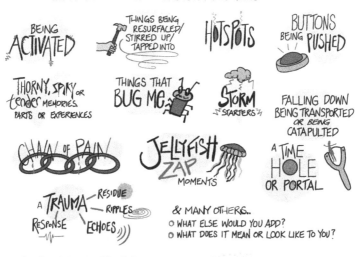

3.4. BEING MINDFUL ABOUT USE OF THE WORD 'TRIGGER'

3.4. Trauma-related body sensations and 'triggers'

Research has shown that when trauma or highly charged emotional experiences occur, they are often embedded in the limbic system, in the right brain, as sensory, somatic, and emotional memories (Van der Kolk, 2014). Therefore, due to these information-processing systems, trauma often shows itself in vivid images, fragments, memories, and sensations which are unintegrated, unprocessed, and lack a verbal narrative or context (e.g. nightmares, flashbacks, hotspots, activation experiences, trauma 'triggers'). This can make autobiographical memory, logic, reason, and the ability to put internal experience into words more difficult (Levine & Kline, 2007; Perry, 2009; Van der Kolk, 2014). This is particularly the case for children who are often pre-verbal at the time of the trauma, or during the in-utero period, and who naturally function more in the right brain hemisphere (feeling and sensing hemisphere). According to Van der Kolk (2014), 'Trauma can come back not as a memory, but as a reaction or response.'

Consequently, trauma is more likely to be embedded in the body, and to be re-experienced or re-lived through bodily sensations. In essence, the body may remember what the mind wants to forget. This may result in increased sensitization to subtle affective and sensory reminders of the traumatic event, which may easily set off false alarms (Fisher, 2006). The following exercise aims to demonstrate some of the ways trauma can impact and influence the body and sensory worlds and create sensory and body-based 'triggers' and hotspots, causing a person to fall down a memory time hole (Hobday, 2001).

Flashbacks / Re-experiencing signals and triggers

(Falling down a memory time-hole, a time machine or a chain of pain)

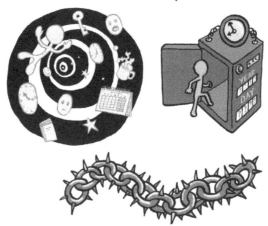

3.5. FLASHBACKS AND RE-EXPERIENCING SIGNALS AND 'TRIGGERS'

Box 3.1.

Reflection exercise – a multi-sensory experience of trauma

This is a powerful and potentially emotive but important exercise, so please make sure if you do this that you are in a safe, grounded, and regulated place and take care and time. I recommend making time for a grounding and regulating exercise afterwards. The rationale for doing this exercise is to be able to empathize, connect with the experience, and truly understand how trauma can be a multi-sensory experience which can have a multi-sensory impact. The exercise highlights the importance of multi-sensory awareness and inter-ventions and seeks to bring this alive far more than words or just reading an explanation or saying it cognitively can do.

Think about a trauma scenario, such as a child/adult experiencing domestic abuse, sexual abuse, neglect, or war.

Draw an outline of a child on a piece of paper or on a flip chart and write your answers to the following questions around the outline of the child. So, for example, think about the experience of domestic abuse from the eyes of a child. Think about it from a multi-sensory perspective (e.g. visual, auditory, olfactory, taste).

- What can/might the child see with their eyes in the context of domestic abuse within their home? What can they look at? What items, faces, colours, body positions, actions, images might they see in the context of domestic abuse? What might they zoom in on? (This includes the spectrum, so a child might see a lot, including the violence itself, or nothing as they are not there, or they might see something from hiding under a bed, or from inside a cupboard, or they might be blind. They might see facial expressions, colours, broken items, blood, bruises, spots on the wall that they focus on, the violence itself, certain body positioning, weapons, shadows, darkness, big bodies, flashing blue lights, things on the TV.)

- What noises and sounds might they hear with their ears (auditory) in the context of domestic abuse and in general within their home? (Of course, a child might be deaf or have headphones on. This might include footsteps, doors opening/locking/banging, the clock on the wall, the TV or music, cries, begging, pleading, or whispering. They might hear their own heartbeat or breathing, keys jangling, cars parking, belts being unbuckled, bottles being opened, sirens, silence, certain words, accents, shouting, swearing, items breaking.)

- What smells and aromas might they smell in their house and in the context of domestic abuse? (This might vary from things in the house like cooking smells, candles, pets, shampoo, or fabric conditioner, through to things like bleach, poo, wee, disinfectant, fear, alcohol, or blood, work smells, or breath and body odour, through to flowers and chocolates in the aftermath.)

- What can they or might they taste? (This might include saliva, vomit, certain foods, drinks, a metallic taste, certain textures.)

- What body sensations might they feel? (This might include shaking, trembling, headaches, pain, butterflies in tummy, nausea, muscle tension, hot, cold, wet, tired, sleepy, hungry, nothingness, frozen.) If their body could talk, what might it say?

- What body positions might they get into? (This might be things like shielding, hiding, foetal position, making themselves bigger, running away, joining in.)

- What emotions might they be feeling? (This could include anything from floods of emotions to numbness.)

- What thoughts might they be having? If the walls could talk, what might they say?

After writing these on the body outline, take a moment to look at the image.

- What do you notice? See? Feel? What words capture the image or your feelings from looking at the image? (For example, chaos, overwhelming, trapped, lost, sensory overload, drowning, sad, lost.)

- Reflect on what might it be like going to school or work with that experience. Or having a lovely family day and then going back into that, as it is likely there are multiple changes of sensory input. Imagine parenting in that experience, or parenting in that experience when you might have also had that experience when you were a child.

- What might it be like for someone's sensory integration and processing system to be developed and marinated in this?

- What might it be like for someone's body, nervous system, and immune system to be developed and marinated in this?

- What might it be like for someone's arousal and regulation systems to be developed and marinated in this?

- What insight does this give into why a child or adult might be consciously or unconsciously 'triggered' or activated when there is a sensory experience? (For example, it might be something like feeling hungry, feeling powerless or angry, hearing raised voices, or seeing certain types of facial expressions, hearing keys opening a door, feeling trapped in a machine, hearing footsteps, smelling a perfume.)

- What might this look like from a worker's perspective? (For example, a health professional who experiences these different feelings and behaviours at work and goes from person to person being marinated in different emotional and sensory experiences.)

This gives some insight into why trauma, stress, and adversity can have a multi-sensory impact, and why we need multi-sensory awareness, approaches, and interventions. Take some time to process and digest, as this can understandably be an emotive, 'triggering', and overwhelming activity to do.

3.5. Ideas around sensory and body-based 'triggers', hotspots, and activating experiences

Following the exercise above, we can now look at some examples of body-based and sensory 'triggers'. These are crucial to share as they shed further light on the multi-sensory impact of trauma and how treatment, the environment, facial expressions, tone of voice, language, touch, and other interventions can be activating and 'triggering', and why words are not enough (including explanations, letters, brochures, and interactions). These may be difficult to read and connect with, so please be mindful. They are anonymized and represent a composite of experiences.

There are certain experiences, sensations, and feelings which people can experience in a current situation, but which can send them down a memory time hole or a chain of pain. They can be reminiscent of past experiences which have been memory banked or encoded – a bit like an emotional hangover, or a ghost of the past. Some people might be aware of them and be able to make the link, whereas others find them cryptic, subtle, or hard to articulate or remember, although they lead to a response, sensation, reaction, or feeling.

It is important to remember that people might respond in very different ways – there is no checklist or one-size-fits-all response. Some people might be able to name or share them, others might become upset, distressed, and dysregulated; others might retreat, withdraw, feel silenced or immobilized, and so on. Therefore, this is one of the reasons why we need to be curious and mindful, as we don't have emotional and life x-rays and we only see a tiny snapshot of what someone might be experiencing. This doesn't mean as a health professional you should be delving in and asking questions or know what someone is going through (this might be inappropriate and unnecessary), but if you can be more trauma-informed in your actions it is likely to alleviate or reduce some of this distress and, most importantly, will not add harm. Additionally, it will hopefully support people to be more patient, empathetic, and not as quick to jump to conclusions, be minimizing and dismissive, and so on. We explore this further in Chapter 7 where we discuss the rationale for a universal approach in health care, and in Chapter 8 where there are tips and tools around our daily practices.

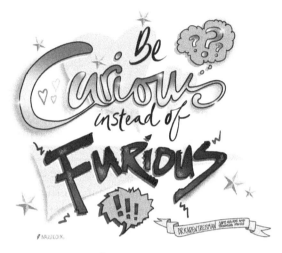

3.6. BE CURIOUS…

It is also acknowledged that 'triggers' and activating experiences can also be associated with positive and feel-good memories (often referred to as a glimmer), for example a perfume might take someone back to a memory of the smell of a loved one or someone who made them feel safe; a song may take someone back to a special time in their life. Moreover, not all activating experiences or hotspots are trauma related; there might be other reasons, for example those within a neurodiversity context, or sensory integration and processing experiences.

Below we explore a series of different types of body-based and sensory 'triggers' or hotspots in a range of health and medical settings and scenarios across the lifespan. Later in this book we go on to think about the environment, facial expressions, tone of voice – small but important ways to tweak interactions, to use this knowledge to inform our way of being.

Please note, these scenarios presented are not intended to blame or shame services – we all have done things that we would do differently with the information we now have, and we are all on a learning journey. These examples are intended to make people stop and think and become more aware of the trauma caused, often unintentionally, by the system.

SOME BODY, MEDICAL & HEALTH CARE TRIGGERS, REMINDERS &/OR HOTSPOTS

SOUNDS & NOISES

- STATEMENTS LIKE 'LIE DOWN', STAY STILL, SPREAD YOUR LEGS & CALM DOWN
- OTHER PEOPLE IN DISTRESS OR PAIN INCLUDING CRYING OR SHOUTING
- ALARMS BEEPING
- SIRENS
- DOORS SLAMMING

VISUAL & SIGHTS

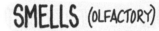

- BLOOD PAIN BRUISES
- TOOLS & EQUIPMENT
- LIGHTING
- FACIAL EXPRESSIONS & FEATURES
- MASKS
- STRANGERS & A STREAM OF NEW FACES
- CLOSED DOORS
- UNIFORMS
- FLASHING BLUE LIGHTS
- THE LANGUAGE ON SIGNS & POSTERS ON THE WALLS

EMOTIONS & FEELINGS

- IGNORED
- MINIMIZED
- PATRONIZED
- OBJECTIFIED
- HELPLESS
- POWERLESS
- OUT OF CONTROL
- SILENCED
- WEAK
- HUMILIATED
- FEELING LIKE A SPECIMEN
- ANESTHETIZED

(THESE ARE JUST A SMALL FLAVOR)

SMELLS (OLFACTORY)

- DISINFECTANT
- ANTISEPTIC
- BLEACH
- RUBBER GLOVES
- BLOOD
- PERFUME/AFTERSHAVE
- 'HOSPITAL SMELL'
- FOOD & COOKING SMELLS
- ALCOHOL ETC

What else would you add?

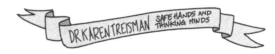

DR KAREN TREISMAN SAFE HANDS AND THINKING MINDS

IMAGISTIC.CO.UK

3.7. SOME BODY, MEDICAL, AND HEALTH CARE 'TRIGGERS', REMINDERS, AND HOTSPOTS – PART 1

SOME BODY, MEDICAL & HEALTH CARE TRIGGERS, REMINDERS &/OR HOTSPOTS

CONTINUED

TASTES OR IN MOUTH

- MOUTH BEING COVERED, MASKED, GAGGED
- OBJECTS OR BODY PARTS INSERTED
- CERTAIN FOODS OR RELATIONSHIP TO FOOD OR CERTAIN TEXTURES
- BODILY FLUIDS LIKE SEMEN
- FEEDING TUBES
- VENTILATORS
- EXPERIENCES WITH THE DENTIST
- BEING HUNGRY STARVED OR MALNOURISHED
- ETC

TOUCH & FEEL

- INTRUSIVE OBJECTS
- BEING TOUCHED
- HUNGRY
- TIRED
- HOT OR COLD
- UNDRESSED OR EXPOSED
- IN PAIN
- CERTAIN BODY POSITIONS
- MEDICATED OR DRUGGED
- TRAPPED OR STUCK IN THINGS LIKE MRI's,
- THROUGH AN EPIDURAL OR IN STIRRUPS

MEDICAL OR HEALTH SETTING ITSELF

- WHERE SOMEONE DIED OR MISCARRIED
- STILL BORN BABIES OR BIRTH TRAUMA
- FEAR OF PAST DIFFICULT EXPERIENCES OF HOSPITAL PROCEDURES, OR WITH HEALTH PROFESSIONALS
- BEING SECTIONED
- BEING DIAGNOSED WITH SAME CONDITION AS FAMILY MEMBER ETC
- WHERE RECEIVED A SCARY &/OR LIFE CHANGING DIAGNOSIS

What else would you add?

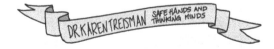

DR KAREN TREISMAN   SAFE HANDS AND THINKING MINDS

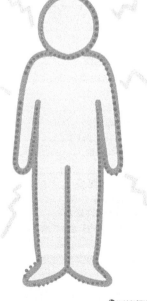

IMAGISTIC.CO.UK

3.8. SOME BODY, MEDICAL, AND HEALTH CARE 'TRIGGERS', REMINDERS, AND HOTSPOTS – PART 2

SOME OTHER EXAMPLES WHEN LOOKING AT A PARTICULAR AREA SUCH AS PREGNANCY.

THESE ARE IN ADDITION TO OTHER IMAGES (OF COURSE EVERYONE IS DIFFERENT & IS NUANCED; & THIS IS NOT AN EXHAUSTIVE OR PRESCRIPTIVE LIST) ARE:

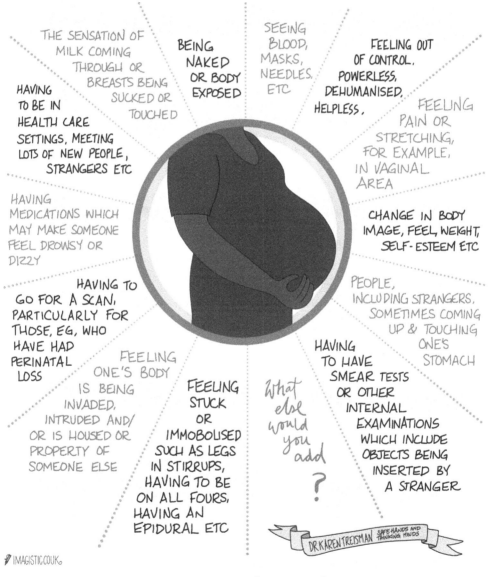

THE SENSATION OF MILK COMING THROUGH OR BREASTS BEING SUCKED OR TOUCHED

BEING NAKED OR BODY EXPOSED

SEEING BLOOD, MASKS, NEEDLES, ETC

FEELING OUT OF CONTROL, POWERLESS, DEHUMANISED, HELPLESS,

HAVING TO BE IN HEALTH CARE SETTINGS, MEETING LOTS OF NEW PEOPLE, STRANGERS ETC

FEELING PAIN OR STRETCHING, FOR EXAMPLE, IN VAGINAL AREA

HAVING MEDICATIONS WHICH MAY MAKE SOMEONE FEEL DROWSY OR DIZZY

CHANGE IN BODY IMAGE, FEEL, WEIGHT, SELF-ESTEEM ETC

HAVING TO GO FOR A SCAN, PARTICULARLY FOR THOSE, EG, WHO HAVE HAD PERINATAL LOSS

PEOPLE, INCLUDING STRANGERS, SOMETIMES COMING UP & TOUCHING ONE'S STOMACH

FEELING ONE'S BODY IS BEING INVADED, INTRUDED AND/ OR IS HOUSED OR PROPERTY OF SOMEONE ELSE

FEELING STUCK OR IMMOBOLISED SUCH AS LEGS IN STIRRUPS, HAVING TO BE ON ALL FOURS, HAVING AN EPIDURAL ETC

What else would you add ?

HAVING TO HAVE SMEAR TESTS OR OTHER INTERNAL EXAMINATIONS WHICH INCLUDE OBJECTS BEING INSERTED BY A STRANGER

DR KAREN TREISMAN SAFE HANDS AND THINKING MINDS

IMAGISTIC.CO.UK

3.9. POSSIBLE ACTIVATING AND 'TRIGGERING' EXPERIENCES
IN A PREGNANCY AND MATERNITY CONTEXT

SOME EXAMPLES WHEN LOOKING AT DENTISTRY
& POSSIBLE TRIGGERS & ACTIVATING EXPERIENCES

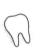

TEETH & THE DENTIST CAN BE VERY SIGNIFICANT IN THE CONTEXT OF TRAUMA. *FOR EXAMPLE:*

35% REPORTED BEING SUBJECTED TO TORTURE INVOLVING THEIR MOUTH OR TEETH (HOVVIK et al 2019). SEXUAL ABUSE & NEGLECT IS ALSO STRONGLY ASSOCIATED WITH DENTAL FEAR. (WILLIUMSEN 2004; LEENERS et al 2007) AND ARE REPORTED TO HAVE HIGHER RATES OF MISSING TEETH, DENTAL CARIES, PERIDONTAL DISEASE, & APICAL PERIDONTITIS (UNELL et al 1999, KUNDEL et al 2014).

THOSE WHO MIGHT HAVE EXPERIENCED TORTURE AROUND THE MOUTH, INCLUDING TEETH BEING PULLED/PUNCHED & KICKED IN THE MOUTH

HAVING FLUID, ITEMS, OR OBJECTS IN ONE'S MOUTH INCLUDING ORAL SEX

EXPERIENCES OF BEING TEASED OR BULLIED AROUND ONE'S TEETH & APPEARANCE OF SMILE

FEELING OUT OF CONTROL / IN PAIN / GASSED / ANESTHETIZED ETC.

NOT BEING ABLE TO BREATHE PROPERLY

BEING GAGGED, HAVING ONE'S MOUTH COVERED, &/OR HAVING SOMEONE WEARING A MASK

NEGLECT AROUND TEETH & MOUTH HYGIENE

ASSOCIATIONS WITH BREATH & CERTAIN DENTIST SMELLS, BRIGHT LIGHTS, MIRRORS, &/OR SOUNDS OF EQUIPMENT & TOOLS

RELATIONSHIP WITH FOOD/ EATING/ VOMITING

HAVING TO LIE DOWN OR BE IN CERTAIN POSITIONS INCLUDING WITH A STRANGER

USE OF SHARP INSTRUMENTS &/OR NEEDLES

BEING KISSED

NOT BEING ABLE TO SAY STOP, OR TALK IF THINGS IN ONE'S MOUTH

?? WHAT ELSE WOULD YOU ADD ??

MIGHT ALSO BE MOUTH RELATED PAST HEALTH OR MEDICAL EXPERIENCES SUCH AS IN THE CONTEXT OF CLEFT LIP & PALATE, TUBE FEEDING, BEING ON A VENTILATOR, DYSPHAGIA, BROKEN JAWS, & MANY OTHER ASPECTS.

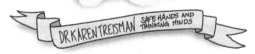

DR KAREN TREISMAN SAFE HANDS AND THINKING MINDS

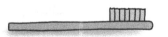

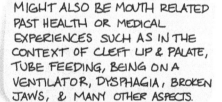

IMAGISTIC.CO.UK

3.10. POSSIBLE ACTIVATING AND 'TRIGGERING' EXPERIENCES IN A DENTISTRY CONTEXT

★ What strikes you from reflecting on possible body-based and sensory 'triggers' and hotspots, including those in pregnancy and maternity and within a dentistry context?

★ Which are you aware of, surprised by, moved by?

★ What might you add to these?

★ How might these show themselves and be activated?

★ Which might you add or apply to your specific context?

★ How might you hold these in mind in terms of service and practice improvements?

These might be layered within a neurodiversity context; for example for someone who is autistic, the noises of the dentist tools and equipment or the texture or taste of the dental paste and drinks might all be 'triggering'.

> As a child, Stephanie had been sexually abused by her uncle. Subsequently, at 16 years old, she had been raped as part of a 'gang initiation' and became pregnant. During the pregnancy and during labour and in prenatal check-ups, her past body memories and sensations from the abuse from her uncle and from the rape were 're-triggered'. She felt that her body was once again being taken over, invaded, and controlled, and she was powerless. The pain in her vagina, seeing blood, feeling breathless, seeing masks, and much more was reminiscent of her past.

Maya froze on the spot each time she heard the ambulance, as this took her back to a time where her child had stopped breathing, and she had had to call the ambulance and unfortunately her child had died before arriving at hospital. Each time she saw flashing blue lights or an ambulance, even toy ambulances, it activated this painful memory.

Ulga found having an endoscopy, where she was constantly gagging, activating and fear inducing. It took her to other times in her life where she had gagged and felt suffocated. When she talked about her experiences with her friends and family, many of them shared how scary this experience was when they had an endoscopy, with issues around gagging and not being able to breathe, and feeling panicked, asthmatic, smothered, and trapped.

Olivia's two-year-old son, Duncan, had begun pulling and tugging at her hair as a way to gain her attention. One day, Olivia was taken by surprise and unintentionally hit Duncan across the face. She was stunned by her actions, but later when debriefing made the connection that as a child her neighbour, when sexually abusing her, would pull her down and restrict her by her hair. This unprocessed memory had been 'triggered' through the physical sensation of having her hair pulled by her son, and she had responded as if she was that child trying to defend herself.

Dan got stuck in the lift and had a panic attack. He later described that the feeling of being trapped and having to bang on the lift doors had taken him back in a scary time machine to memories where he had been physically abused and locked for hours in a tiny laundry cupboard. As he was re-telling this story, he curled up in a ball, making himself small, hidden, and protected – as he must have done all those years ago. He had a similar experience if he felt trapped among crowds of people, for example on the tube.

At age 98, Elsa had a fall in the shower of the nursing home where she lived. She broke several bones and consequently after several major operations and intensive physiotherapy and rehabilitation had to spend most of the time in a wheelchair. She became increasingly distressed and started having nightmares, shouting, screaming, pushing the staff, and fearing that the care staff would harm her. She was previously close to and had trusted the staff for many years. Through an assessment, it was discovered that Elsa had been sexually assaulted as a teenager; she had not told anyone and had tried to forget and push the memory away. However, the recent fall and being in a wheelchair had once again made Elsa feel powerless, trapped, out of control, and disconnected from her body. These unprocessed feelings and intense body sensations had taken her down a time hole to this earlier unprocessed pain and stress of the trauma. She was reliving some of the experiences from her past.

When Simeon heard doors slamming and bells ringing it activated him as it was reminiscent of the noises and sounds during his time as a soldier in Afghanistan. He also found raised voices difficult as it was a reminder of his childhood experience where there was a lot of shouting. This was also worsened when he was in hospital, hearing beeping and constant noises and sounds, as well as people's calls for help and cries of pain.

When Ranni entered a hospital for a routine appointment, she smelled bleach and disinfectant, and it took her right back to a place where she had been repeatedly attacked by her husband and had to clean her face and her house with antiseptic and cleaning products. She also had a similar catapulting experience, when she smelled fresh flowers which reminded her of all the times she had been given flowers as an apology for being hurt. She was very aware of smells, and this had also happened with a doctor whose aftershave was the same as her husband's.

Georgie found it very difficult to be at the back of the food queue at school and to navigate the smells, sounds, and unpredictability of the canteen. As she entered the canteen, she felt overwhelmed, alone, and hungry. This feeling of overwhelm, unpredictability, having to rely on others, and of hunger took her down a memory time hole to a place where she had been starved and deprived of food and left to fend for herself, and where she wouldn't know where her next meal would come from.

Cara was in treatment for a diagnosis of anorexia. Eating was very 'triggering' and difficult for her – it elicited a huge sense of fear. Food had been shoved down her, she was force fed and told to stop being a baby, and that it was just food. She understood that she was very underweight and in a bad place, but how no one ever asked her about her trauma history while on the eating disorder unit all those times. Eventually when a trauma therapist helped her, they were able to connect to the meaning behind this and how each time she ate it catapulted her down to a memory of being forced to give her uncle oral sex.

When Grace was in Rwanda, she was raped several times by Hutu men. When she came to England after a few months she was put into a psychiatric hospital. They hired an interpreter for her who was Hutu, despite her telling them of her rape experiences. She was very distressed and shouted and screamed. It was as if the rape was happening all over again and she was back there – even more so as she felt trapped in the ward and cornered by him. The ward staff said she was 'overreacting and being dramatic'. They told her to 'calm down' and to be 'grateful' they had found an interpreter. For Grace, after that, there was no trust, no care, no belief in them to keep her safe or help.

Sarah received unhelpful and hurtful responses after self-harming due to abuse and pain she had experienced. This included things like: 'You are so beautiful, why would you do this? You don't want to be ugly with those scars', 'Cheer up, it can't be that bad. What have you got to be so sad about? It's much worse for other people, you should be grateful for what you have', 'It is just so attention-seeking, you are wasting our time and taking it away from people who haven't self-inflicted this on themselves.' She was stitched up without pain medicine or anaesthesia and felt as if she was treated as a burden on staff's time and responses. Even many years later, if she went to have her blood pressure taken, she still felt people judge, make assumptions, and look concerned.

Kayla found hospitals very hard. Her mum had died in one when she was young. Her dad had died in one a few years later, and her oldest sister had died too. She felt that hospitals were scary and eerie and each time she stepped into one it terrified her and took her mind to the worst place.

Cece found that so many things echoed and mirrored her early abuse – for example not stopping when they should, not explaining the procedures so she felt like an object, not believing her when she reported symptoms, viewing her negatively, making her feel like an over-exaggerator and not worthy.

When the doctors told Jonny that he needed medication and he politely explained that he didn't want it and felt really worried about taking medication, they were rude and dismissive towards him. If they had been curious, or just a bit kinder, they may have discovered why or what he had been through. As a teenager, he was raped and forced to take drugs and have alcohol thrown into his mouth during the rapes. Also, his mum had been addicted to drugs and so he was worried he would go down that road and be like her.

When Sol's boss at work would roll his eyes or look disinterested, it would remind him of his dad and how he used to make him feel as a child – boring, invisible, a burden. He sometimes had this feeling of going through a time portal or a feeling of unease if someone sounded like his dad or had the same name as him.

Natasha had been sexually abused. She felt that because of what had been done to her she had struggled with life, and was punished by living with the horrors of the abuse, hearing voices of the abuser, and self-harming. Because of this she had been sectioned and admitted to a psychiatric hospital. She was told she was disordered, and once again she felt powerless and entrapped. The staff were worried about her self-harming or hanging herself, so they put her on one-to-one observations. She requested to have a woman, but they ignored this, and she felt 're-triggered' and violated by being constantly watched, judged, and feeling invaded by male members of staff. They would walk into her room without knocking and peer through the glass window on her door. They would stand outside the toilet while she was pooing. This was horrific and traumatizing for her.

Laila had an MRI scan and was impressed with the care and consideration before she went into the tunnel. Sadly, she was deeply 'triggered' as she had previously had an experience where she was unable to breathe and was totally trapped. She had worked hard to stay there and not to press the help button, but when she came out there was no one there to talk to or reassure her, so she left feeling wobbly and in a state of shock. She had a lot of knowledge and skills around trauma and how to regulate herself; however, she wondered how much harder it could have been for others who didn't have this knowledge or skills.

> Lizzie had felt claustrophobic and immobilized having a scan and being constricted within a machine. She felt that the music was intrusive, she felt alone as no one spoke or communicated with her, and she was briskly told to not move and seemed to cause irritation and impatience when saying that she felt panicked or needed to cough.

★ How do you feel physically, emotionally, and from a sensory level when reading these? How might you feel if this was you or a loved one?

★ What others would you add to these examples?

★ How do you view these through a position of power, privilege, fear, safety, trust, communication, injustice, oppression, humility, relationships, collaboration?

★ How might these impact people's relationships to health care, trust, or practitioners, and inform future interactions, following treatment, advice, and so on?

★ What can be done in your own practice, team, and in the wider organization to become more aware of the issues illustrated here, including our own 'blind' spots, and to reduce and try to avoid them?

This chapter highlighted some examples of physical, body-based, and sensory 'triggers' and hotspots. There are of course many other important types of 'triggers' or hotspots which can be overlapping, including *emotional/feeling, social, and relational 'triggers'* and also *autobiographical 'triggers'* (e.g. times of the year and events during the year, topics in school, at work, in the newspaper, or on the TV).

CHAPTER 4

Lived Experiences

4.1. What will be covered in this chapter

- Some feelings and words to capture people's experience within health

- Some examples, stories, and quotes of health experiences

- A spotlight on ill health and the impact on family, relationships, and social support

4.2. Some feelings and words to capture people's experience within health

To bring some of the previously discussed information alive and how these traumas can impact subsequent experiences, this chapter will feature some short examples of stressful, upsetting, and often 'triggering' medical and health scenarios. These have been anonymized, shared with consent, and many are composite and combined examples. Some feature medical, disability, and health trauma, while others explore other cultural, relational, and intergenerational forms of trauma (see also Chapter 1). They also have some relevance to the sensory and body-based 'triggers' and hotspots shared in Chapter 3.

It can be easy to read academic papers or clinical guidelines and lose the person among the text or the statistics, so it is crucial that we hear the voice of the people we serve. People are the experts of their own experiences and they need to be put back into policies; we need to prioritize people over processes, and to humanize services. This also fits within trauma-informed values around collaboration, feedback, and co-production.

It is important to mention that the people in these case studies were asked in equal measure about their positive, healing, and helpful experiences, as much as their difficult and upsetting experiences; however, often more emotive, negative, and difficult memories stay with us and can be easier to recall. Some of the ideas for improvements, positive stories, and examples of best practice are also peppered throughout this book. The words and stories were gathered from a range of contexts, including inpatient, outpatient, and community settings in the UK (the majority), America, Australia, New Zealand, Egypt, Kenya, South Africa, Israel, Sweden, and Canada. The majority of the feedback is from direct experience; however, some is from the perspective of a carer, spouse, parent, and so on. People could freely share but also were given the opportunity to describe their experiences (positive, negative, and all the shades in between) using just a few words or using a metaphor or analogy (see image 4.1). Please take your time to read, as they are more than just words on a page.

★ How did you feel at a cognitive sensory and body level when reading these words and experiences? Which, if any, struck a chord, resonated, were surprising?

★ How do you want people to feel? How would you want to be treated or your loved one to be treated? How do you want people to describe their experiences to themselves and to others?

★ What might the impact of these feelings and thoughts have on their overall experience, on the intervention itself, on future encounters with health care providers? How might these translate into recommendations?

★ How do these feelings align with your own, and with the values of your profession and your organization?

★ How might these experiences reinforce, resurface, and 're-trigger' people's past experiences, for example of feeling powerless? How might these unintentionally add distress or harm? (See Chapters 3 and 7.)

★ Can you think of a positive relational experience with a professional? What did this look like or feel like? What about it made it positive, helpful, beneficial, and important? (You might be able to think of multiple experiences.)

★ What qualities do you think are important in a relationship with a professional (e.g. a GP, a dentist, a surgeon, a psychologist)? What do you feel are some of the key ingredients that support a positive relational experience?

★ What difference do you think it makes when there aren't these qualities or when the experience is not positive?

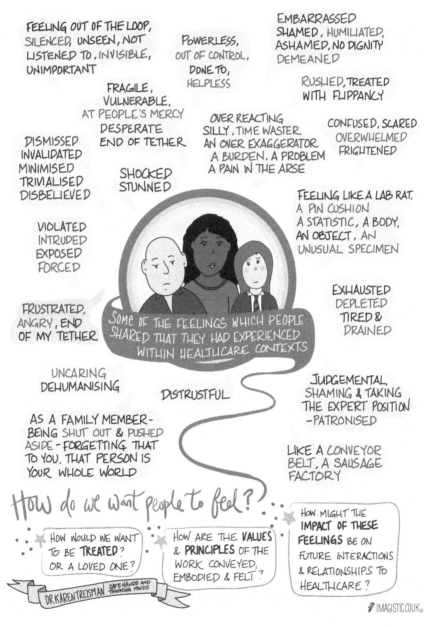

4.1. SOME FEELINGS SHARED BY PEOPLE ABOUT THEIR DIFFICULT HEALTH EXPERIENCES

4.3. Some examples, stories, and quotes of health experiences

To elaborate further on the feeling words shared in image 4.1, some stories are given below. Some of these illustrate the distress around a health and medical situation, including the possible impact a diagnosis or condition might have on a person's life. Others are about the stress and distress caused by the system, treatment, and intervention; and others show the links between the experience and past experiences.

> After I had just delivered a stillborn baby, the hospital placed me on a busy ward of women and their new, healthy babies – it was as if my heart was being stabbed in a million places. Then when I got pregnant again, I was in a constant state of fear but the staff kept telling me to not be silly, and that everything would be fine, and that worrying wouldn't help. I felt so unseen, patronized, and minimized.

> I had tried for four years to get pregnant and finally it happened. I was beyond excited. At my first scan the person looked at me and said they were sorry but the foetus was not viable. I was stunned and beside myself and couldn't believe the robotic and uncaring way it was said. I didn't really understand what that meant. I hadn't even processed the information or had a chance to ask a question and he had walked out of the room. Those words echo to me to this day. I was fortunate to get pregnant again a year later but my whole pregnancy was characterized by fear that I would lose the baby. I was told several times by staff that I was too anxious and should just relax and enjoy it. I felt so alone and hurt.

> I hate needles. I am petrified of them for lots of reasons, but the main one I can think of is that I had a blood transfusion as a kid and they couldn't get it in my arm and then they did but forgot to close the cap and so blood squirted everywhere, like a horror scene. Also, my ex-husband had an addiction to heroin, so needles have a

horrible association for me. I know there are loads of people who are scared of needles – one of my friends because of diabetes, another because of IVF.

When I was pregnant, I found out that my little girl had a cleft lip and palate. I was distraught. I felt guilty and responsible. I know times have changed and surgeries are amazing now, but I didn't want my child to suffer as I had. I had been bullied and mocked. I had and still have difficulties with some of my speech. When I was a kid, food used to come out of my nose, and eating in front of others was terrible. I was called all sorts of names. My mum said she couldn't breastfeed me and I struggled with feeding. It has definitely impacted my confidence, self-esteem, and body image. I had so many operations and still fear doctors and dentists. I missed chunks of school when I had the orthognathic surgery, which was life changing, but involved a really serious recovery too. The thought of my kid going through this made pregnancy so hard. I know I have a long journey ahead but also hope it will be different for her.

It might have scarred her skin, but it's scarred and etched on my brain. (A parent having watched the pain their child endured and the wound aftercare following a burn.)

Every time I see hot water, mugs, or pasta boiling in a pot it takes me back to the fear around hot water that burned me. I feel the panic rising and I am so on edge when other people are drinking hot drinks. I often wake up in the middle of the night still feeling that the gigantic blisters are there, and I have to feel my leg to reassure myself they aren't. Sometimes, I am just sitting watching TV or daydreaming and then I have flashes and can still feel the pain of the wound aftercare and the burning sensation. And sometimes I just get catapulted to the treatment of having the manuka honey put on and the indescribable pain, and it makes my whole body seize up. I also dread going on holiday or swimming for fear of being stared at, and I want to cover my scars.

I had a heart attack out of nowhere. I was fit and healthy, ate well, and had no related health conditions. One minute I was fine, the next I had a major heart attack. I feel unrecognizable. Every time I feel a flutter, or an arm ache, my mind catapults back to 'Oh my goodness, I am going to die, I am going to have another heart attack.' I can't relax and I feel constantly on edge. My world felt turned upside down and inside out. Some people talk about getting a new lease of life and a renewed sense of living, but for me it has made my world smaller. I feel as if I am a ticking time bomb on borrowed time, and I am scared to do anything. I don't feel like myself.

I was 18 when I was in a car accident, and I am now paralysed from the neck down. I've often been told I'm lucky to have survived. I know some people feel thankful and grateful and I sometimes feel guilty that I don't, and I can't be this inspiration, but in the moment, everything changed. My career goals. My love of playing football. My independence and things like my ability to drive. My freedom. My sex life and my attractiveness to women. My relationship with my parents. My ability to do things like go to the toilet or just pop to the shops, or book a weekend away. And so much more. Not to mention the ongoing pain, aches, and sores. Add to that the stares and pity from people, the insensitive questions, the rubbish accessibility in most places. I can't even go to my favourite café or get to the toilet on the plane as it is not suitable for a wheelchair. I still have nightmares of the accident but actually more about some of the aftercare, procedures, and rehabilitation I've gone through. Sometimes, I feel as if I'm right back there even though it is ten years ago. Other times, I wake up and forget and then go to move and it hits me like a ton of bricks: 'Ah, it wasn't a dream.'

My world turned upside down when I was told I had cancer. I froze. I felt as if I was the walking dead. I just couldn't believe it was happening to me. All I could think of was my babies being without their mum. I saw my mum go through it and it was the worst time of my life, and to think I now need to go through it, but even more so my kids, is unthinkable.

When I was diagnosed with HIV I honestly wanted to die, I wanted to jump in front of a train. The doctors told me it was like diabetes, it was chronic. However, all I could think was that it was a death sentence. Where I am from in Africa, the stigma, the discrimination, the shame are indescribable. I was in disbelief. I couldn't comprehend what was happening and then my head was spinning. Where did I get it from, how will I tell my kids, will they be okay, can I still have sex, how will I be able to work, will I get fired from my job?

The anaesthetic didn't work during my operation. It was like a horror show. I can't even talk about it as it haunts me. There are no words. I'm now petrified of doctors, hospitals, needles, even of going to sleep.

Two things come to mind. When I was 18 and at university, I had been going to the GP repeatedly for a year. I was fainting daily, feeling dizzy, and exhausted. I was losing weight as well. I felt that I was not taken seriously, I was positioned as a flaky partying university student, which I really wasn't, and even if I was, it was dismissive and judgemental and beside the point. I was fobbed off so many times, told I was probably just a bit anxious, or a bit image conscious, or partying too much. I also was tanned and naturally have quite dark skin and was told I looked healthy and couldn't have been that bad as I was doing well at university and managing to have a part-time job as well. The symptoms rapidly escalated and a few months later my eyesight went, I could hardly function, and I ended up being hospitalized for a prolonged period. They found that I had refractory coeliac disease, an extremely overactive thyroid, and was so anaemic that I required multiple iron transfusions. A similar pattern occurred about ten years later. I was having numerous symptoms which were impacting me. I am a calm, rational person who just gets on with things, yet possibly because of that I wasn't taken seriously. I was told to stop googling things and that I looked fine. At times, I felt positioned as an annoying, over-exaggerating female. Through persisting and persisting, I discovered that I had gone into early menopause, which not only has lifelong consequences and a devastating impact but could have been caught three years earlier when I was seeking support and sharing the symptoms.

I'm fed up with people being judgemental, shaming, and taking the expert position. For example, 'You will get diabetes because of your weight, your lifestyle choices are killing you.' Or when I share my very thought-out decision about not having kids, 'I'm sure you will want children, you will change your mind eventually. It is the most beautiful blessing in life.'

A doctor called to ask if I would take part in a study around coeliac disease, which involved some invasive testing, and when I politely declined, he said this is why I would probably get bowel cancer because people like me stop research being done and better treatments being created. He said it was selfish.

I was badly burned. I entered the building where there was a strange graphic with fear-inducing images of burns on the wall and a red abstract painting that looked like blood and burns combined; and I had nothing to drink, despite being overheated and dehydrated because of the burn. Then I was stripped naked and left standing in a room while the nurses left to get some cream; they left the door open for anyone on the busy ward to see my naked body. Several people walked by and stared in – it felt incredibly exposing and inhumane.

I weed in the bed due to my bladder issues and was so embarrassed and waited almost an hour to buzz the nurse as I didn't want to be a pain to her and felt like a child. She scolded me and tutted, and changed me in the most rushed, irritated way. It was beyond humiliating.

I was really anxious about having an injection. I realize they are super busy, and most people just do it, but I wasn't trying to be difficult like they labelled me. I'm honestly petrified of needles. My ancestors were medically experimented on, fact. My neighbour's child changed overnight after an injection. And when I was younger a nerve got pinched and I've never felt the same. I get that it's a pin prick to some, but to me it is huge. Being told to man up and stop being silly wasn't the answer.

I could hear the nurses talking in the corridor about me, saying they had seen track marks on my legs and calling me a druggie and a junkie. The looks of disgust and disapproval. When one of the nurses took my blood, she smiled and said you won't mind this, you are used to needles. I last used drugs 22 years ago.

I can't tell you how many times I have felt contagious and othered when people find out my HIV status. I have also had receptionists say it out loud in GP surgeries and heard nurses and doctors whispering about it in the hallways.

Taking my dad to the hospital was so horrific. He had dementia and I felt he was treated with such disrespect. I was so worried for him to be left there. When I arrived, he was often wet and hungry. When he got agitated, they would shout at him as if he was either a child or criminal, which led to his dementia worsening. When I tried to intervene and help, I was told to let them do their job.

After hours waiting in a rammed and freezing A&E, with no food, I finally got to be seen and needed a cannula put in. The nurse had five unsuccessful attempts before she got it in. After the fifth very painful attempt, and feeling very unwell and tired, I fainted. Not only did the nurse not apologize or communicate but she acted as if I was not there and just proceeded as if I wasn't human, poking and proceeding with no eye contact, in silence, and with no sign of empathy or connection. Eventually with no communication or apology (I am not blaming or shaming her as I am sure she was going through a lot) she got someone else who did it the first attempt. This lack of apology and explanation was horrible and made me feel dehumanized and angry. It also added to me feeling sick as I was tensing, feeling uncared for, dizzy, and so on. I used to be scared of needles and had completely got over this fear, but now this has made me very worried about needles and cannulas again. Moreover, while I was sitting in pain trying to tolerate this unpleasant experience with her disconnected lack of care, directly across the room within my eye view was a poster saying 'Welcome to World Class Care'. As you can imagine, that poster did not align with my experience and added to my irritation and disappointment.

I have four live children aged 25-34 for whom I am so grateful, but in the middle of them I lost my twin boys at 30 weeks during the pregnancy. They died of twin-to-twin transfusion syndrome, and I was in labour for two days. When labour really started, I started to shake and cry, and the midwife told me to pull myself together and just to be strong for the births. I was in no fit state to explain neurobiology, but it was terrifying.

★ What is it like to read these? How do they make you feel?

★ How might they contribute to what ghosts and angels of the past people bring into appointments?

★ How might they impact, shape, and influence people's feelings about their health, their body, health professionals, and health settings?

★ How might they impact future interactions?

★ How might these be used to inform practice changes and recommendations? (See also Chapter 8 for more on this.)

4.4. A spotlight on ill health and the impact on family, relationships, and social support

Having shared some of the feelings and experiences of those receiving health care, it feels important to take a closer look at the impact on the family, friendships, relationships, and social support system, including the strain on caregivers. When someone is unwell, it can have a ripple effect and shift the dynamics among the whole family or system. Often the wellbeing and health of carers and family members can be sidelined or not fully acknowledged, yet there are huge financial, psychological, and social implications of not hearing and supporting carers and people who are part of someone's social network.

Of course, each person's situation is unique, and each person functions within a unique context and family culture, and this will also vary depending on the severity, impact, and type of illness, and the family relationships and dynamics before and during. However, it is important to acknowledge some of the possible wider systemic impact that having a disability and/or an illness can have on roles, relationships, and on the whole family. This is by no means an exhaustive list of some of the possible changes and considerations but is intended to give a flavour:

- A requirement for family/friends/social support network to adjust and recalibrate to the illness/disability. There might be numerous changes, transitions, losses, new challenges, and dilemmas to navigate.

- Having to prepare or make sense of the future of a loved one being unwell and/or dying, and/or of their personality or one's relationship changing, which might include anticipatory loss, mourning, and grieving.

◎ Having to live in a place of uncertainty and change. And in some situations, such as in progressive or episodic and relapsing conditions like multiple sclerosis, having to readjust and transition depending on new symptoms, episodes, changes, and so on. There can also be multiple losses at different stages, such as the loss of the ability to drive or be independent, or the loss of someone's bladder control or someone's ability to swallow. There can also be unpredictability around someone's response to chemotherapy or radiotherapy during cancer treatment, or following a stroke or an injury, where you don't know what the future will bring or what someone's new normal might look like or be.

◎ Fear or dread of what is coming next; being hypervigilant for any changes or the presence of warning signs.

◎ Family conflict, disagreement, and discord around how to support or care for the person. This can extend into decision-making, for example when care arrangements are needed such as carers, going into a nursing home/hospice, undergoing certain treatments, doing clinical trials, what the person is able to do or not able to do.

◎ A change in roles and responsibilities such as caregiving, financial contribution, household tasks. There can also be change to daily routine, whether that is around having to attend appointments, cancel plans due to ill health, do tasks which one didn't do before, and so on.

◎ Personality changes, and changes in the relationship dynamics. This can also include change in appearance, confidence, sex life, and much more.

◎ Adjustment to life plans, for example what retirement was hoped to be, or around having children or travelling.

◎ Guilt around being healthy, or being snappy and irritated with the person. There can also be confusion as to how to feel or how to respond. And for some, there can be a sense of needing to be strong or needing to hold it together, or of being forgotten or sidelined as often the focus is on the person going through the illness.

◎ Additional pressure and stress around the role of caregiving, with financial strain and numerous other aspects. There can also be feelings in the person supporting or the person living with the illness of guilt, frustration, fatigue, resentment, hopelessness, helplessness, powerlessness, unfairness, overwhelm, low mood, and fear, among others.

◎ The emotional distress of watching someone you love deteriorate, change, be in pain. There may also be distressing memories of the person being rushed to hospital, or feeling very unwell, shouting in distress, or falling over, and so on.

- An increased level of personal care needed, for going to the toilet, feeding, showering, and so on. This can have an impact on intimacy, physical strength, the power dynamic, and much more. This is particularly the case if the caregiver struggles with being in the carer position or being around someone who is more dependent on them.

- Being faced with their own mortality, fragility, vulnerability.

- Pressure and additional frustration of sometimes having to navigate health care systems and other paperwork, benefits, insurance, medication, and so on. This can be particularly stressful when systems are not in line with one's needs, such as inaccessible buildings.

- Feelings of depression, hopelessness, or suicidal ideation in the person, which can inevitably have a ripple effect on the caregiver.

- Fears of what will happen to the person if something happens to the carer or family member supporting, for example if they die, experience an injury, or lose their job and cannot provide financial support.

- The dynamic of the relationship changing in numerous ways; for example, in the context of dementia, people might want to protect the person and not share as much with them for fear of adding stress or them feeling guilty or going to someone else for support.

Are there any other points you would add?

CHAPTER 5

Organizational Culture and Staff Wellbeing

5.1. Introduction

Having explored in Chapters 1, 2, and 3 some of the different types of trauma, including health and medical trauma, and how they can impact the body, one's sensory world, and a range of other areas such as behaviours, relationships, and sense of self, it seems important to consider organizational, secondary, and vicarious trauma, and within this, the wellbeing of staff.

Organizational trauma is an area within the wider trauma umbrella that is often not acknowledged or discussed enough. A central part of becoming more adversity, culturally, and trauma-informed, infused, and responsive at an organizational level is about understanding organizational trauma and stress, and how an organization itself can become stressed, overwhelmed, unhealthy, traumatized, trauma-inducing, dysregulated, and trauma-soaked. An organization and system can add trauma, harm, and stress to the people who both work in and use the service, through organizational adverse experiences, secondary trauma (Kadambi & Truscot, 2003; Perez *et al.*, 2010; Stamm, 1999), vicarious trauma (McCann & Pearlman, 1990), compassion fatigue (Figley, 1995), emotional saturation, burnout, and work-related stress/strain. Moreover, understanding system, secondary, community, and organizational trauma and dynamics is often not prioritized in people's core and professional development training, team meetings, supervision, and thinking spaces. The focus tends to be on other people's trauma and distress, rather than one's own, and on the impact at an individual level, rather than from an organizational or community lens (community, organizational, and collective care).

Without this knowledge and awareness, a significant piece of the trauma-informed journey is missed. An organization cannot meaningfully become more trauma, adversity, and culturally informed, infused, and responsive without shining a spotlight on organizational trauma, processes, and dynamics, and that is what this chapter intends to do. Not understanding, acknowledging, or responding to organizational trauma and organizational culture are often the things that block or impede progress and development of trauma-informed values, but when these areas are seen and discussed it can really enable trauma-informed ideas to be more meaningfully embedded. This chapter is central to implementing adversity, culturally, and trauma-informed, infused, and responsive practice. However, this is part of a larger puzzle. To learn about the other parts, such as recruitment, policies, and assessments, please see my other books on trauma-informed organizations (Treisman, 2021, 2022).

Please note that although the terms secondary and vicarious trauma, burnout, compassion fatigue, emotional saturation, and workplace strain and stress are often used interchangeably, it is acknowledged that each of these terms has different definitions and slightly different but often overlapping aspects. However, for the purpose of this book I won't go into the definitional maze.

5.2. What will be covered in this chapter

- Organizational adverse experiences, organizational trauma and stressors, and work-related stress and strain

- Why might the work within health care be stress- and trauma-inducing, more difficult, and emotionally exhausting?

- A spotlight on levels and prevalence of burnout for health care professionals

- Some consequences of the high prevalence of burnout and emotional saturation for workers, the organization, and overall care

- Wellbeing is often not prioritized and can be positioned as a luxury or a tick-box exercise

- An organization, like a person, is alive with thoughts, feelings, values, and much more

- What might we see when an organization is in a place of trauma, stress, dissociation, and dysregulation?

- Organizational memory and amnesia

- Mirroring and parallel processes, and mirroring family dynamics and role positioning

- Re-traumatizing, trauma-inducing, and 'triggering' experiences within the system

- Wider system considerations which can make a difference to the trauma-informed organizational culture and overall running of the organization

- Some micro strategies and introductory ideas for improving your own wellbeing and regulation

5.3. Organizational adverse experiences, organizational trauma and stressors, and work-related stress and strain

Staff may also have experienced trauma, harm, toxic stress, and adversity from the work itself, or from the work context, climate, and culture. Remen (1996, p.52) writes: 'The expectation that we can be immersed in suffering and loss daily and not be touched by it is as unrealistic as expecting to be able to walk through water without getting wet.' There can be the cost of caring and of being involved, contributing to, feeling powerless within, and bearing witness to other people's pain and hurt. In addition to the nature of the work itself, there can be an array of other organizational aspects which can create and add to stress, moral injury, decision fatigue, and trauma. If these aspects are ongoing, and if people have a steady diet of fear and stress at work, it can have a cumulative effect, with a person's arousal and fear systems being regularly activated. These effects are also more likely to be felt if the organization is in a place of stress, fragility, dysregulation, and trauma; and, conversely, are more likely to be buffered should there be more organizational protective factors in place.

These will also be impacted and influenced by wider contextual factors, for example things like Covid, Brexit, government and policy changes, insurance factors, Black Lives Matter and racial trauma, redundancies, funding cuts, the privatization of the National Health Service (NHS) in the UK, staff shortages, and much more.

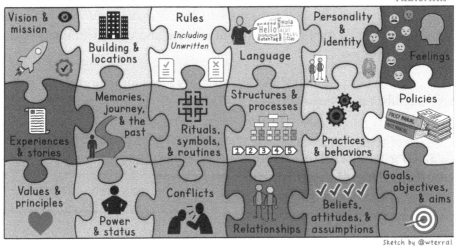

5.1. THE ORGANIZATIONAL CULTURE

Alexander den Heijer has said, 'If a flower doesn't bloom, you fix the environment in which it grows, not the flower.' This doesn't mean that we don't need support for the flower or some additional focus on the flower but rather that what we also need is environmental, cultural, and system change. I would extend this quote further by advocating that we shouldn't label, humiliate, shame, single out, or blame the flower (locate the difficulty or deficit within an individual), nor should we add more stressors to the flower, like flooding it with water, blocking out the sun, or leaving it in icy and hostile conditions (re-traumatizing and oppressive environments and systems). We should instead try to find out what will support the flower to flourish and bloom, and then subsequently we should work towards having a healthier environment that will foster and support the growth and development of all flowers and include everyone who comes into contact with, supports, uses, and works in the garden. This means we are creating healthier conditions for future flowers, fruits, and vegetables as well (Treisman, 2017a). And as educator and author Peter Drucker famously said, 'Culture eats strategy for breakfast, lunch, and dinner' – organizational culture impacts people's behaviours, attitudes, and ways of being, and sets the tone for 'the way we do things around here'.

5.4. Why might the work within health care be stress- and trauma-inducing, more difficult, and emotionally exhausting?

As you read the points below, think about others you might add, which aspects you or people you know have experienced, what they might lead to if they are present, what feelings are evoked, and so on. They could be used for discussion in supervision, team meetings, and reflective spaces.

- Some medical and health settings are marinated in high levels of abuse, pain, pressure, trauma, violence, assault, loss, and death. People in these settings may be immersed in high levels of emotional distress and emotional contagion, often having to operate on an ongoing basis in fast-paced, highly pressurized, emotionally charged, and crisis-led situations. This includes accident and emergency (A&E)/emergency rooms, psychiatric hospitals/teams, forensic units, neonatal intensive care units, and other areas where high levels of violence, self-harm, and mortality rates are prevalent. For example, in a national survey of nurses in Canada, 93% reported being exposed to physical assault, and 77% to a sudden violent death, from direct exposure or by witnessing or learning about the event (Stelnicki *et al.*, 2020). Many staff must deal with situations such as mortality, grief, and death, often delivering difficult, life-changing, and distressing news, and making hard human-cost decisions.

- Staff are often insulted, verbally attacked, criticized, and assaulted. This can be targeted and discriminatory, around race, age, religion, sexuality, and so on. It also might include working with people who do not trust or feel safe with staff, as well as those who might decline care/treatment, or understandably have differing opinions about it.

- Staff, particularly those working with people in distress, must often cope with a high level of unpredictability and uncertainty at work, both on a daily basis and longer term. This might include uncertainty as to what will happen each day, or what they will be faced with, such as legal changes, system changes, and work in emotionally charged contexts. Sometimes, this extends to not knowing where they will have to work or live, such as those on rotation or placement. This uncertainty can also lead to some people feeling uprooted and lacking a secure base. Some might find this exciting and interesting, while for others it can be exhausting and confusing and lead to things like initiative and decision fatigue.

- People have to manage huge pressures, large workloads, and high levels of responsibility, often with complex decisions to be made with a human cost, and within time pressures and restricted environments. This can be even more stressful if there are not sufficient or available services around to signpost to, or if these are available but people don't feel ready or able to access these services. High volumes of patients and high patient turnover can create concerns about compromising their own and others' safety, and there may be limited time to meet basic needs, such as staff being able to eat, go to the toilet, and have time to think and reflect. Other basic needs include access to essentials or things that are seemingly small but make a big difference, such as a working pen, coffee, a mug, cups for water, a chair, equipment that functions properly, and good internet connectivity.

- Staff are often navigating these environments and decisions while contending with high levels of staff turnover, agency staff, staff sickness, unfilled posts due to recruitment issues, including recruitment freezes, funding cuts, short-term contracts, redundancies, and people and teams being 'at risk' for their jobs. This all contributes to role overload and can worryingly lead to compromising the safety of those providing and receiving care, as well as creating further moral injury. Staff may be pulled into roles to bridge gaps or cover other areas which they are often not experienced in or familiar with. And all of this is, of course, influenced and impacted by ever-changing legal, government, and political agendas and changes.

- Staff may have to make decisions which conflict with their own values, ethics, gut instinct, and wishes, and therefore they may be in a double bind. This is often referred to as moral injury, wounding, or decision fatigue. Examples of this include not having enough staff or resources to give proper care in physical health settings; having to deliver therapy in six sessions, even though one's training and instinct say this should be much longer; or having to choose who goes on a ventilator or who is a recipient of an organ, or which treatment is available based on cost or available equipment (sometimes referred to as distributive justice – who should be prioritized for treatment). Moreover, some staff must also navigate the tension between therapeutic activity and management, and safety and risk (Kurtz & Turner, 2007).

- Some of the situations encountered might also cross over with personal difficulties for the practitioner; for example, supporting someone with a diagnosis of cancer while having a family member with cancer or who has died of cancer, or having had cancer themselves; being a midwife supporting others or carrying out an abortion, when struggling to get pregnant or going through IVF; or supporting someone who is a carer for a parent who has a diagnosis of dementia while also being a carer to a parent with dementia.

- Staff may have their own experiences of trauma and adversity, which can be compounded by the work which they are doing or be mirrored or 'triggered' by it; for example, seeing someone who has been raped or experienced domestic abuse, being shouted out, being told they are rubbish or not good enough, or seeing someone in pain or die.

- Difficulties can also occur for staff when trying to support others while feeling depleted and exhausted themselves, or having to juggle home situations and stressors while being present, thoughtful, and empathetic to others. It can be hard for some to know where their work-self starts and finishes, and when and how to switch off – even more so when feeling overstretched so that neither the people at home nor at work get the best version of that person.

- Most people who go into caring/helping professions have a desire to help others and to improve things. Therefore, people can feel frustrated, powerless, and helpless when they cannot help, are restricted in what they can offer, or what they know, and when people don't recover, get worse, or die. For some, this can mean not feeling good enough, feeling deskilled, or experiencing imposter syndrome. In some settings, this can be exacerbated if the staff member is positioned as the person's cause of distress or their 'persecutor'; for example, being responsible for someone's pain through a painful procedure, or when someone has been sectioned against their will.

- Organizations are increasingly driven by performance indicators, financial implications, paperwork, and policies, which can obscure the complex nature of the work and mean that the underlying motivation for being in the caring profession can be lost. Staff often feel that the processes can take over the people, and that the paperwork distracts from the actual work needing to be done. This can be even trickier when there are tasks, expectations, or deadlines which are unrealistic or impossible. Dealing with copious paperwork, tick-box exercises, and the need for duplication can be a poor use of time, compounded by clunky, confusing IT and data systems that are not fit for purpose.

- Some workplaces are toxic, oppressive, chaotic, unsafe, hostile, and silencing. For example, there can be bullying, conflict, sexism, racism (and other forms of discrimination), and harassment in the workplace, between colleagues, from leadership, and in the wider organization. This can include indirect or direct abuse, assault, or aggression, and create a lack of emotional, cultural, and psychological safety in the workplace. Edmondson (1999) discussed some of the questions to consider around establishing psychological safety:

1. If you make a mistake within the team, is it held against you?

2. Are members of the team able to bring up problems and tough issues?

3. Do people on the team reject others for being different?

4. Is it safe to take a 'risk' on this team?

5. Is it difficult to ask other members of the team for help/support?

6. Would people on the team deliberately act to undermine your efforts?

7. Are people's unique skills and assets seen, noticed, valued, and utilized?

This can include being able to call out poor unsafe practice and to whistle-blow, and for this to be responded to effectively and sensitively. Building on the importance of psychological safety and trust in the workplace, Helliwell and Wang (2009) indicated that one unit of trust (on a ten-point scale) was associated with improved wellbeing that is comparable to a 30% salary increase. They stated that this meant that by offering people the equivalent of an extra 20% of their salary or the opportunity to work in a trusting environment, they would likely pick the latter.

- Staff can receive criticism, blame, and negative discourses from external agencies, social media, the media, and the wider public, including allegations, threats, serious complaints, and being sued. They are also likely to be impacted by historical or current events that happen within their profession that can exacerbate blame, shame, fear, shock, doubt, mistrust, and more. Some examples might include things like the cases of Lucy Letby and Harold Shipman, the MMR vaccine fears, the effect of thalidomide on babies, and the fear of contaminated blood samples and infusions.

- Annual leave may not be honoured and protected. In addition, breaks during the day may not be supported, protected, or encouraged.

- Some workplaces have trauma- and stress-inducing team meetings and communications/emails. There may be trauma-inducing debriefing, investigative, and/or disciplinary processes, creating a culture of fear and blame around decision-making and medical errors, and a fear of litigation.

- Some systems, managers, and leaders do not notice, anticipate, or acknowledge the complexities, stressors, and potential impact of the work, including secondary and vicarious trauma, compassion fatigue and emotional saturation, burnout, and emotional stress. The impact of organizational adverse experiences, organizational stress, and organizational culture on staff's work and wellbeing is not acknowledged. There may also be no understanding that staff might have other influencing experiences from their childhood, current, or past lives that are impacting their lives and work.

  Systems, organizational culture, leaders, and colleagues position people explicitly or implicitly as 'weak', 'vulnerable', or 'not tough, strong, resilient, or thick-skinned enough'. An emphasis on 'resilience' programmes can unintentionally feed into these messages and position the difficulties within the individual. In some organizations, there is a belief or narrative that workers are infallible to the same problems which they help others to manage, or that if someone is impacted or struggling in some way, there is a fear, shame, stigma, or an assumption that they will be seen as 'incompetent, unsafe, weak', and that this will impact on them being trusted or promoted. Moreover, there can be a lack of high-quality and regular supervision (*supervision*, not snoopervision). This is supported by studies which show that staff perceptions of organizational support following a traumatic event or for those experiencing trauma symptoms are also associated with PTSD among nurses (Schuster & Dwyer, 2020), and many papers share how perceived lack of organizational support can hinder recovery.

- Following an incident, a death, or distressing experiences there may be a lack of emotional support and meaningful debriefing. For example, medical students report 'extremely inadequate support' after emotionally powerful deaths (Rhodes-Kropf *et al.*, 2005). Many studies have shown that practitioners don't feel prepared or supported to respond to their own or their colleagues' feelings in these scenarios. Often after a serious incident, people quickly come in to offer support and there is a one-off session booked, and then staff are expected to move on and get on with it. But we know that different people process things at different times and sometimes it's when the dust settles or when someone connects with the information, or is in a place to talk about it, that support is needed. For some people, one session is enough, but others may need longer to process an incident and need to be told that this is okay. Some people find groups helpful, others might want a one-to-one space, and others might need a gradual approach.

If there is a culture of people spilling, oversharing, or talking without warning to others, it can unintentionally add to those on the receiving end feeling flooded, overwhelmed, or uncontained. They also might not know how to respond or what to do with the information. And it might be close to the bone or land in a particular way depending on what else they are holding on to or have been going through. So, while it is important that people have spaces to unload, share, release, and be heard, it is a tricky tightrope. Organizations need to create awareness of the forums and spaces which are there for sharing, debriefing, and support. It is also important that if someone is going to share their issues in an informal way, in a corridor or in passing, they are sensitive and mindful as to how it might feel for the receiver, they check if it is okay to share, and don't give unnecessary or potentially activating details.

- Staff may feel ill-prepared and deskilled, particularly if they are students or newly qualified, where their ideals, expectations, and hopes can be mismatched with the reality of the work and contexts in which they are operating. This isn't about doom and gloom and bursting people's bubbles but about having real and realistic conversations and supporting people to feel more prepared and equipped.

- The physical environment may seem unsafe, oppressive, and 'triggering'. For some people, there may be a high level of sensory overload, such as beeping, flashing lights, screaming, a lack of natural light, shouting, machine noises, and so on (see Chapter 9).

- Staff can feel 'done to', ignored, minimized, and silenced, with poor or ineffective communication. There may be a culture or setting which leaves people feeling unable to raise concerns or to whistleblow; or, due to hierarchy and other dynamics, someone not being heard or listened to (sometimes in serious case reviews, someone in a more junior position is not listened to or taken seriously). Staff might feel their concerns are not taken seriously, not believed, are excused, or are glossed over. This feels very relevant in a range of examples, including the more recent case of Lucy Letby. It can also occur during restructuring or regular changes, particularly if these are poorly communicated and done without meaningful consultation or support.

- An organization may have a lack of or blurred vision, mission, meaning, or purpose so that staff do not feel connected or part of something bigger and there are ambiguous expectations around their roles and tasks.

- There may be a culture of unfairness, injustice, or favouritism. This can also fit with organizational justice (Barsky & Kaplan, 2007) which can be distributive (distribution of resources), procedural (contracts, rules, and formal procedures), and/or interpersonal (feeling unfairly untreated by others).

- Some organizations display friction, conflicting messages, and incoherence among the leadership and management team. This might also include dynamics like sibling rivalry, competitiveness, 'favourites', and warring patterns.

- The organizational culture may mean that staff lack appreciation and acknowledgement, and do not feel seen, noticed, heard, and valued. Often people are the organization's greatest treasures, tools, and drivers of change and hope, so it is important to have a culture which also celebrates and magnifies the strengths and positive elements of the work. This should include sharing best practice examples, celebrating progress and proud moments, and learning about and discussing concepts such as adversarial growth, adversity activated development, post-traumatic growth, vicarious resilience, and compassion satisfaction.

- Where there is a lack of understanding and appreciation of each other's roles and skills, this can lead to poor communication, inappropriate referrals, and less effective utilizing of people's skillsets and specialities, as well as less effective multidisciplinary and collaborative working. Shadowing and observing each other's roles, having joint and multidisciplinary learning and forums, and presentations on people's different jobs can all support this process.

- It can be hard to care for others when feeling uncared for by poor quality and unsupportive leadership and systems, or when leaders are talking the talk but not walking the walk or modelling the model. For example, leaders may always talk about the importance of time management and being on time and then themselves turn up late or facilitate a meeting that overruns by 30 minutes. As writer Paulo Coelho states, 'The world is not changed by your opinion, it is changed by your example.'

- Some inspecting bodies and inspecting processes can feel stress-inducing, mismatched to the realities of the work.

- Teams may be unsupportive, fragmented, or not cohesive. Numerous studies have demonstrated that organizational culture and structures directly and indirectly influence team 'outcomes' and that teams flourish when they work in an environment that supports and promotes teamwork, team cohesion, and peer support (Bedwell *et al.*, 2012; Bell *et al.*, 2018; Lemieux-Charles & McGuire, 2006; Rosen *et al.*, 2018).

◎ Access to professional development opportunities and high-quality levels of training may not exist, or these are not meaningful or relevant, and do not help participants to apply the knowledge in the real world and in daily practice.

◎ An organization's culture may be rigid, stuck, and inflexible – the 'we have always done it this way' attitude – and does not encourage learning and development. While of course there must be accountability and responsibility, we also need learning cultures that understand that mistakes happen and use them not to shame or blame but as an opportunity for staff to learn and improve. What is needed is a culture that can adapt, evolve, and grow, is open to change, and has humility around its own limits and areas for improvement; a culture that can think and reflect; a culture that can accept and take ownership and, where appropriate, say sorry and put into place actions for different practice moving forward.

All these stressors of course will vary depending on the context and should be adapted to your specific area of practice. We know that an organization can, for example, have fantastic plans in place, but that this will lack meaning and drive if people don't feel this and have it embodied and modelled; often it will instead feel contradictory, a misrepresentation, and ingenuine. People's words need to be mirrored in their actions and their actions mirrored in the words. As the saying goes, 'Be the change you want to see.' Maya Angelou says, 'People will forget what you say and do but will remember how you make them feel.'

Here are some examples of organizational culture practices which do not model the model, and which illustrate talking the talk but not walking the walk.

> An organization says that it cares about staff wellbeing, but then has a culture which, for example, does not support annual/maternity leave, puts people in unnecessarily unsafe positions, doesn't acknowledge and respond to the impact of the work around secondary and vicarious trauma and burnout, doesn't provide basic needs like a pen, and so on. How can it say that its practices align with the value of wellbeing; and how can it encourage this with the people who use the services if this isn't modelled and encouraged internally? It is hard to provide care when feeling uncared for, or to talk about being a caring organization.

An organization says it puts relationships at the very heart of what it does, but then leaders and managers don't show that they care about staff, don't show appreciation, don't say thank you, and often pass staff in the corridor without smiling or saying hello. How does this model the model and embody the culture and values the organization wants to instil?

An organization talks about being a learning culture which respects and values staff and prioritizes safety and emotional wellbeing, yet there is a blame, fear, and shame culture which doesn't allow for 'mistakes', openness, or humanness.

The points shared above about stress due to organizational culture are not an exhaustive or prescriptive list. However, there are a lot of them, and some important information is included. It is easy to read them as a checklist or to scan them, but please take your time to review and revisit them. You might go through them with your team.

★ What else would you add? How might you expand on them?

★ Which resonate with you and which can you relate to personally, or have seen? Which jar with you?

★ What might be the consequences and ripple effect of these for you/ the work/the people who use the service/organization?

★ How did reading them make you feel?

★ How are these named, acknowledged, and validated in your workplace?

★ Are there things in place to support, acknowledge, and mitigate them?

★ What can you and the wider organization do to boost the organizational immune system and to reduce the fragility factors? To improve things?

★ Which of them do you feel you/your organization are already acknowledging and responsive to?

5.5. A spotlight on levels and prevalence of burnout for health care professionals

Some of the above points and examples given here are likely to have increased
and been exacerbated due to the Covid-19 pandemic. For example, oncology
practitioners have experienced increased levels of distress. This has been due
to several reasons, including numerous practice changes, intensified burnout,
heightened moral distress, and personal circumstances such as family stressors
caused or contributed to by the pandemic (Barello *et al.*, 2020; Hlubocky *et al.*,
2020; Segelov *et al.*, 2020). Oncologists also had to cease in-person visits, delay
critical surgeries, delay or abbreviate chemotherapy administrations, substitute
potentially 'inferior' oral chemotherapy regimens for intravenous therapies,
suspend clinical trial enrolment, and initiate telehealth appointments to deliver
serious news (Desai *et al.*, 2020; Jiang *et al.*, 2020; Kuderer *et al.*, 2020; Schrag
et al., 2020; Ueda *et al.*, 2020).

Given the prevalence of burnout, secondary and vicarious trauma, compassion fatigue, and emotional saturation, there is a clear rationale for trauma-informed practice and for prioritizing and recentring staff wellbeing. We need to
acknowledge the likely ripple effects on patient care and overall outcomes. Of
course, this will vary depending on country, context, organizational culture, and
numerous other factors. Although there are increasing rates of burnout among
clinicians and growing health care demands, implementation of prevention
interventions is lacking among health care organizations. Based on one survey
of 350 clinicians, 66% of respondents felt that they did not have the tools or
resources to handle burnout, and 54% said administrators and leaders were
not actively taking steps to prevent burnout (Studer Group, 2015). An organizational climate that validates and normalizes workers' reactions mitigates the
risk, while one that is perceived as unsupportive increases it (Brockhouse *et al.*,
2011; Dombo & Blome, 2016).

Care and support for all staff is crucial, particularly as we know that there is
a prevalence of trauma and adversity in our communities and societies, which
means that many staff themselves may have experienced trauma and adversity in
their own lives, including adverse childhood, adult, organizational, community,
and cultural experiences. It is not an us and them scenario, and we know from
the literature that experiences of trauma and adversity can be greater for those

who choose to go into the helping/caring professions (Bride, 2007; Dykes, 2011; Thomas, 2016).

There have been high levels of compassion fatigue and vicarious trauma among doctors, surgeons, paramedics, nurses, and many other health care professionals (Drury *et al.*, 2014; Hunsaker *et al.*, 2015; Kelly *et al.*, 2015; Shanafelt *et al.*, 2015; Van Mol *et al.*, 2015). And adding weight to these numbers, literature on physician burnout pre-pandemic revealed an incidence of 51%, with frontline practitioners (e.g. emergency departments, family medicine, internal medicine, obstetrics/gynaecology) at the highest risk (Reith, 2018).

Considering some studies around prevalence and occurrence, research by McFadden *et al.* (2022) used cross-sectional surveys to assess pre-pandemic mental health and quality of work life for 1195 social and health care professionals in the UK and found that 75% of respondents stated mental and physical exhaustion as major factors impeding performance, and 60% shared according to the measures used that they were barely able to cope with daily responsibilities, which included difficulties with focus, attention, completion of patient follow-up, and documentation (McFadden *et al.*, 2022). Furthermore, one study of surgical residents found that 22% screened positive for PTSD and another 35% screened in the at-risk range (Jackson *et al.*, 2017).

Prasad *et al.* (2021) conducted surveys of 20,497 health care workers across 42 health care organizations during three Covid-19 waves in 2020 and 2021. They found that elevated levels of stress and burnout were identified for clinical and non-clinical staff (Prasad *et al.*, 2021). More than 30% of people employed on inpatient units of hospitals had 'high or very high' daily stress scores, 61% noting 'high fears of virus exposure', and 40% of respondents admitted to escalating anxiety or depression. And within this study, almost half of all physicians (49%) self-reported feelings of burnout (Prasad *et al.*, 2021). Similarly, Sharifi *et al.* (2020) found a high incidence and prevalence of chronic occupational stress for health and behavioural health workers (HBWs), leading to the development of more pervasive 'mental health' difficulties, such as acute stress and PTSD.

Additionally, the American Nurses Foundation (2021) assessed using online surveys the mental health of the nursing workforce in the US during December 2020 (N = 12,881). The findings showed that many nurses were experiencing symptoms associated with PTSD and other trauma-related stress and anxiety difficulties, including irritability (57%), profound sadness and depression (47% and 38%, respectively), isolation (37%), feeling life had little to no meaning (35%), disassociation (25%), and increased alcohol use (19%).

Additionally, a study looking at doctors and nurses working in either a newborn or paediatric intensive care unit found that one in six met the criteria for

PTSD and 66% had lower but worrying scores on PTSD scales (Dalia *et al.*, 2013). This was echoed by other studies which found that over half of physicians in the US experienced symptoms of burnout – nearly double the prevalence among the general working population (Studer Group, 2015; Williams *et al.*, 2020). Similarly, Smith (2017) and others have looked at obstetricians and gynaecologists and found that between 40% and 70% experienced symptoms and signs of burnout.

5.6. Some consequences of the high prevalence of burnout and emotional saturation for workers, the organization, and overall care

Amanullah and Ramesh Shankar's (2020) systematic review noted research on physician burnout and found that exhaustion, distractibility, and poor perceived efficacy were among some of the presenting difficulties.

Provider burnout has been identified to double the rates of adverse patient safety events; the greater the levels of burnout, the poorer quality of health care overall (Panagioti *et al.*, 2018; Salyers *et al.*, 2017; Willard-Grace *et al.*, 2019). For example, health professionals may experience impaired attention, memory, and executive function that can decrease recall and attention to details, including medication management, provider orders, patient directions, and timeliness of care. Moreover, Epel *et al.* (2018) described how there can also be preoccupation, rumination, and insomnia. The ripple effect of cognitive consequences can impede the quality of an individual's thinking, creating brain fog, forgetfulness, and distractibility. And we know that stress can impact judgement and the ability to effectively perform tasks, which fits with how brains in pain can sometimes struggle to think.

More than 250,000 medical errors and 100,000 deaths annually are attributed to workforce frustration, yielding poor team member communication and thus fragmented care, order entry mistakes, plus medication and treatment missteps (Garcia *et al.*, 2019; Ozeke *et al.*, 2019; Restauri & Sheridan, 2020).

Research by Norful *et al.* (2021) reviewed the physical and psychological impacts on health and behavioural workers employed in high-stress clinical environments during the pandemic and found reports of severe insomnia, exhaustion, anxiety, and depression. In tandem, ongoing exposure to stress and trauma is associated with practitioner 'dissociation, negative mood, insomnia, emotional exhaustion, and increased medical errors' (Restauri & Sheridan, 2020, p.923).

Bourne *et al.* (2019) carried out a survey study that was sent to all obstetricians and gynaecologists in the UK. Over 3000 clinicians (response rate of 55%) completed the Maslach Burnout inventory. It was found that 43% of trainees and 31% of consultants met the criteria for burnout. Clinicians with burnout were approximately four times more likely to practise 'defensively'. Doctors with burnout were three to four times more likely to report depression, anxiety, and anger/irritability. One in 16 doctors with burnout reported suicidal ideation. This and other studies suggest that avoiding complex 'cases' and procedures, over-prescribing medications, carrying out more investigations than necessary for fear of making a mistake, or missing a diagnosis were common missteps.

Of course, there are various different factors and reasons but there have been high levels of suicide rates among health care workers, and this increased during the pandemic. Approximately 300–400 practising providers die from suicide each year, which is twice the rate of suicide among the general population (Blacker, 2019; Dutheil, 2019; Leung et al., 2021; Schernhammer, 2005).

Both organizational commitment and burnout have repeatedly been tied to a variety of indicators of organizational effectiveness, and burnout has been positively associated with health problems, turnover intention, actual turnover, and absenteeism (Maslach, 2003; Meyer et al., 2002; Schaufeli & Bakker, 2004).

When people feel uncared for by systems and leaders, it can be harder to care for others. This is why we need to care for the carer. As Safe Harbor said, 'In order to be a place of safety you have to become a place of safety.' The effects are far reaching but may include a loss of interest, weakened, crushed, shut-down empathy, avoidance of asking important questions and of being open and curious, more agitation, feeling cynical, emotionally depleted, exhausted, and anxious, and exhibiting low mood, withdrawal, anger, avoidance, hypervigilance, mistrust, frustration, hopelessness, and detachment.

Moreover, if we are in a place of feeling dysregulated, our baseline for being 'triggered' and activated is likely to be higher, and our window of tolerance (Siegel, 2012) is likely to be much narrower, which may mean that we snap more, or find it harder to regulate, or smaller things irritate and push our buttons, or we feel more overwhelmed, or we become more rigid and inflexible. It is also very difficult to regulate others if someone is dysregulated themselves. Additionally, this might also make our attentional bias more towards the negative things and situations; and might make our ability to notice the positives and sparkle moments less. This emotional contagion, mood, energy, or fog can also spread throughout teams and systems. Staff might also experience shifts in the way they perceive themselves, others, and the world (e.g. their narratives, discourses, schemas, and core beliefs); for example, feeling that the world is dangerous and unjust.

For others, connecting with vulnerability and helplessness in the people they are working with can lead to an erosion of self-esteem and a decreased sense of professional efficacy and accomplishment (Dane, 2000). People can feel deskilled, self-doubting, and not good enough. Moreover, people can also develop an overwhelming sense of responsibility and accountability, which can send their rescue valency (their desire to help or make things better) into overdrive. This can lead to a tricky balance between empathic care and empathetic distress and between self-care and self-sacrifice.

Staff may experience symptoms similar to those of the people they are working with, such as intrusive thoughts, nightmares, difficulties with regulating emotions, or feeling helpless, hopeless, powerless, and vulnerable. They might also experience physical symptoms such as headaches, stomach aches, rashes, a compromised immune system, or difficulties with sleeping and eating (McElvaney & Tatlow-Golden, 2016; Motta, 2012; Pistorius, 2006). This can also impact energy levels and personal relationships, and increase certain coping strategies such as drinking alcohol.

5.7. Wellbeing is often not prioritized and can be positioned as a luxury or a tick-box exercise

The irony is that we know the importance of taking care of our own wellbeing, but we ignore or avoid it, and don't act on it. This is about collective care, responsibility, wellbeing, and support. Interestingly, the words wellbeing and wellness both start with the word 'we'. Too often, wellness is bolted on to programmes or interventions. It is often seen as a luxury, or is overlooked or underrepresented in the work, training, and curricula, or it can be there, but is not properly communicated, supported, or encouraged. It can be spoken about but not modelled and so lacks meaning or purpose. It also can be seen as a tick-box exercise, and tokenistic, rather than positioned as a core component and integrated into all interactions. There can also be a lack of practical thinking about existing support programmes, with issues around making the time to attend, and whether it is fit for purpose and available for all staff in all roles.

Wellbeing advice can be conflicting, contradictory, and unrealistic; for example, suggesting that staff attend a mandatory reflective practice group after a 12-hour shift; or advocating an hour of mindfulness when people hardly have access to a pen; or offering 'resilience' programmes which can unintentionally feed into fears and messages of not being 'tough' enough. However, these can be helpful for some, and it is important to have a flexible approach as there can be space for both personal and organizational efforts and accountability.

There can also be a lot of societal, family, media, and organizational discourses around this, which can feed into people viewing self-care as selfish and indulgent, as well as masking, avoiding, or glossing over their needs, and feeling scared, intimidated, and unsupported in sharing these things. People can be worried about being teased, missing out on promotions, or seen as vulnerable, inadequate, or incompetent. People can be positioned (or fear being positioned) as not coping, not trustworthy, not tough or thick-skinned enough. They may feel they should 'soldier on' and 'toughen up'.

Some management and leadership discourses can unfortunately contribute and promote a negative view of wellbeing, with statements such as: 'I don't have time to invest in people', 'It is not my job to pander to people; they are adults', 'I am not a fluffy person', 'I am not a therapist; they need therapy', 'Being too nice will make me a walk over', 'I don't have time to babysit or deal with a Negative Nancy or a Debbie Downer.'

These can also be reminiscent of childhood and adult discourses in which people might have been told: 'Don't air your dirty laundry in public', 'What goes on behind closed doors stays behind closed doors', 'Keep your head down', 'No one will believe you', 'You asked for it', 'You made me do it', 'It is our little secret', 'Others have it much worse', 'It was a lifetime ago, don't hold on to it, move on', 'You are overreacting, or making a mountain out of a molehill', 'It was your choice to drink, you should have known better.'

Such unhelpful belief systems can promote an 'us and them' culture, and lead to deepening feelings of shame and stigma. Early interventions may then be harder to put in place, and difficulties can escalate or be exaggerated, and the consequences can be greater (e.g. work sickness, emotional wellbeing difficulties, impact on sleep/eating/relationships, feelings of inadequacy, impact on patient care and decision-making, possible suicide). This goes against the trauma-informed position of acknowledging the impact of trauma, adversity, and stress, including adverse organizational experiences and emotional saturation.

Paying attention to wellbeing is as essential as brushing one's teeth. It should also be acknowledged that the more we prioritize wellbeing, the more long-term emotional, social, and financial benefits there are likely to be.

Having explored the possible consequences of burnout and emotional saturation, we can now look at how organizations and systems themselves can become trauma-soaked and unhealthy, and how this impacts on people, the work itself, and on the organizational culture.

5.8. An organization, like a person, is alive with thoughts, feelings, values, and much more

Organizations can be emotional and relational places. They are made up of people who come from their own families and a variety of systems, including other organizational families (e.g. other jobs, workplaces, and educational climates). Systems and organizations, just like people, are not machines or blank slates. It can be helpful to see organizations as being alive, and having a collective brain (Bloom & Farragher, 2010). Just like people, organizations develop, grow, evolve, and adapt. They are ever changing and reinventing themselves; they are not still or fixed entities.

An organization, like a person, can become consumed, flooded, and overwhelmed by trauma, adversity, and stress. It can be dominated by survival and protective needs. Dr Sandy Bloom, a trailblazer and leader in this field, defines the term trauma-organized: 'When an individual, family, organization, system, or culture becomes fundamentally and unconsciously organized around the impact of chronic and toxic stress, even when this undermines its adaptive ability' (Bloom & Farragher, 2010, p.29).

Trauma, loss, dissociation, dysregulation, and toxic stress can spread like a wildfire throughout an organization. This can interrupt the organization's flow, the ripple effects can be felt throughout the system's multiple layers, and, if it isn't attended to, it can continue to spread and intensify. We know that the word trauma comes from the Greek word 'traumata', which means to pierce. This is entirely apt when thinking of trauma within organizations, because it can wound, pierce, and permeate individual, family, organizational, and societal layers. Erik De Soir (2012) talks about how the organization's protective emotional membrane can be pierced by trauma. Trauma can also be absorbed, while at the same time leaking and spilling out. Shohet and Shohet (2019) describe how, without reflection, processing, and so on, trauma can be experienced by the organization as ingesting food which is swallowed food, but may have to be vomited out later.

Although these concepts can be applied to any organization, they are especially important to consider in workplaces where staff have to deal with a lot of trauma and stress. We have also seen these processes intensify in the context of the pandemic and other global changes.

Organizations, systems, and individuals are bi-directional – they are dynamic, they interact, influence, and flow with, to, through, and between each other.

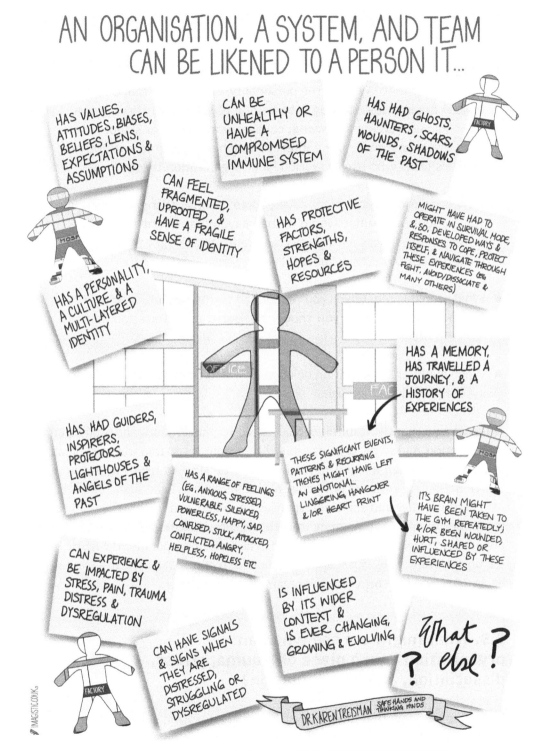

5.2. AN ORGANIZATION, SYSTEM, OR TEAM CAN BE LIKE A PERSON

★ What parallels and comparisons can you see between people and organizations?

★ What images, sensations, and feelings come to mind when you think of your organization? What is the personality, energy, spirit, and feeling of your organization? (It might be helpful to select just three words. You could also create a drawing, collage, word cloud, or sculpture of your responses; this can be interesting when compared with other people's ideas who use or work in your organization/team.)

★ How does the organization leave people feeling? If the building or walls could talk, what would it/they say? What might trauma-informed walls/spaces say if they could talk? What might traumatized walls/spaces say if they could talk?

★ What would it feel like if you responded to the organization as if it was a person? What if you thought about the organization as the 'client/patient'?

★ When might an organization be unwell, have a compromised immune system, or have an injury?

Often when faced with painful feelings, anxieties, uncertainty, threat, danger, dysregulation, and so on, organizations, like people, try to find ways to defend against these. When in survival mode or in toxic stress, organizations often function using survival and protective responses such as fight, flight, or freeze.

These anxieties and survival responses often flow and travel. They can get passed down through the system, from the leaders. If the trauma and stress are not acknowledged and processed, they can be pushed deeper into the fabric of the organization. They can shape and influence feelings, values, attitudes, and behaviours, and the entire way the organization operates.

5.9. What might we see when an organization is in a place of trauma, stress, dissociation, and dysregulation?

Now that we know that a team, system, or organization can itself become trauma-soaked and operate in survival and protective modes, we now need to consider what this might look like.

Organisational Defences

Some responses and coping strategies which we commonly see in traumatised, unhealthy, and at times trauma-induced organisations and systems (Survival mode/ Parallel Processes)

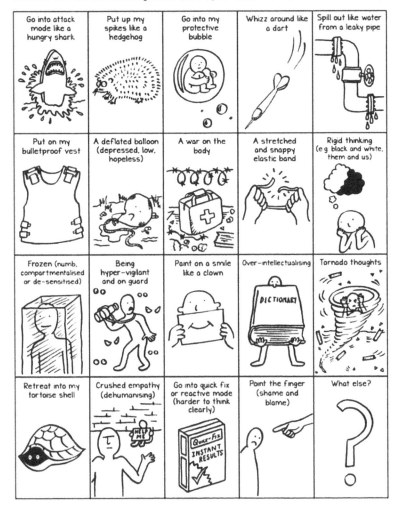

Copyright © Dr Karen Treisman and Emma Metcalfe

5.3. ORGANIZATIONAL RESPONSES

Take a moment to think about the common presentations and signals of trauma and toxic stress at an individual level (e.g. a child or adult who has experienced domestic violence). This might include hypervigilance, dissociation, dysregulation, changes in eating and sleeping patterns, and avoidance. How many of these can also show themselves at an organizational level – in individuals, teams, in the wider organizational culture, and/or between different organizations?

There are many similarities and mirroring processes between individuals and organizations.

Here are some responses to trauma and stress that the people within organizations, or the organizational culture/team, might exhibit:

- Becoming physically and emotionally unwell. People, teams, and the organization can become unwell physically, with more sickness and a compromised immune system, as well as increased levels of stress, emotional dysregulation, and distress. This can manifest in difficulties with sleep, eating, and alcohol consumption, as well as in staff sickness, staff turnover, and staff dissatisfaction.

- Becoming more reactive and crisis driven, including being in quick-fix mode, doing things, and acting without thinking. Being in survival mode, it can be harder to think and reflect, and use more abstract cognitive and executive functions, such as attention, concentration, and problem-solving. Bloom and Farragher (2010) refer to this as organizational learning disabilities. It can be harder to make simple decisions when feeling full up and overwhelmed. People can have their 'minds full' rather than being 'mindful'.

- Going into fight/attack/defend mode. People can respond in more bullying, authoritarian, and aggressive ways. People, teams, or organizations can go into attack, defend, or fight modes. In shark-infested waters, some systems and people can learn to act like sharks themselves, following the notion that it is better to attack rather than be attacked, to be feared rather than fearful, to be powerful instead of powerless. This can also lead to conflict and tension.

- Becoming hyper-aroused, on edge, hyper-alert, and hypervigilant. This can show itself as heightened and reactive responses to something minor, for example when the milk runs out in the kitchen.

- Giving more limbic, emotionally driven responses, or the opposite, as an attempt to avoid emotions. This includes avoidance, withdrawal, numbing, retreating, shutting down, detaching, and dissociating. For example, an organization may become detached from its mission and its purpose, or an organization or person may become detached from feeling, thinking, and reflecting. This might present as someone or the organization burying their head in the sand and not talking about the important stuff like racism, trauma, and political and financial drivers. It can also include people or teams withdrawing emotionally or physically, with people leaving, or people just keeping their heads down. An element of compartmentalization and protective dissociation is often needed, but sometimes this can shift into avoidance, and denial, which can have a range of consequences for the person, the team, and the work itself. This can include displaying flattened, shut down, and/or crushed empathy and compassion; for example, responding to a student who is understandably upset after hearing about a domestic violence experience by saying 'Just you wait, that's nothing to half of my cases I have dealt with' or 'It's just part of the job, you need to toughen up'.

- Being too busy to think or feel, where people or systems operate as if busyness and keeping on the move is the anaesthetic to pain, hurt, vulnerability, and so on; for example, where thinking and feeling are timetabled out or when organizations implement overwhelming changes in a short space of time.

- Feeling confused, lost, alone, and disoriented. The team or organization may feel it has a fragile sense of identity (e.g. who are we, why are we here, what are we doing, where are we headed?), and is not grounded or anchored to a purpose or mission.

- Feeling a sense of splitting or othering – a 'them and us' culture can lead to crushed empathy and compassion, othering, and distancing, idealized or denigrated processes, and so on. This might be between people, such as 'warring' colleagues, or between concepts or approaches (e.g. only one approach, such as cognitive behavioural therapy, can work), or between systems (e.g. child and adult services against social services). These 'them and us' divides not only dehumanize and depersonalize people, but can also widen the power imbalance. Moreover, this might show itself through splitting of aspects, such as our mind from our bodies, or our thoughts from our feelings (e.g. where people are unable to perspective take, show compassion, or empathize), or it can polarize opinions and lack nuance, for example around someone's decision-making, fears about receiving treatment, and views on vaccinations.

- Being rigid and inflexible (including striving for perfectionism). This can include very closed binary thinking, with little room for curiosity and being open to other possibilities. Ideas and beliefs can be clung to and new ideas discounted, disbelieved, or attacked. This rigidity stems from trying to search for stability and certainty but can show itself as a lack of humility and reflection, with responses such as 'We have done trauma', 'We know this all', and 'We are trauma-informed'. It also extends to holding on to processes or ideas even when feedback and new evidence suggest otherwise, for example the links between emotional wellbeing and adversity, oppression, and social exclusion.

- Feeling mistrust and suspicion – not feeling psychologically safe or protected. Often there is a sense of fear, stigma, and shame.

- Becoming more authoritarian, rigid, bureaucratic, and hierarchical.

- Exhibiting crushed or impacted innovation and creativity. The more unsafe and anxious people feel, or the context is, the harder it can be to breathe, create, think outside the box, and innovate.

- Feeling a sense of spilling and leaking out, including operating in chaos, and things feeling very uncontained and unprocessed. Energy and time may be totally consumed by specific issues and tasks, and this can spill out into non-related topics or home life.

- Feeling stuck, frustrated, immobilized, or frozen. It can feel as if the organization is on a hamster wheel or that every day is a Groundhog Day, and staff are unable to act or move forward. One example of this is serious case reviews, where the same recommendations appear over and over again, but are not acted on. There is procrastination and inaction and a sense of nothing moving or progressing.

- Feeling helpless, depressed, deflated, demoralized, and hopeless on an individual, team, or organizational level. This can include grief, mourning, and learned helplessness, such as when teams and organizations want the answers from elsewhere, want to be told what to do, and appear to need to be 'pushed'.

- Becoming disconnected, disintegrated, incoherent, and fragmented. This includes poor communication, where often bottom-up communication decreases and top-down communication increases. Within trauma, disconnection can occur, whether this is the left from the right brain, the mind from the body, the internal from the external experience, or the past from the present and the future. Similarly, an organization can mirror this and become disintegrated and disconnected, with people working in silos.

This is by no means an exhaustive or prescriptive list and should be considered along with the earlier section on the consequences of burnout.

★ As you were reading, which responses resonated? What reflections did you have?

★ What else would you add, or have you observed/felt/learned about?

★ How does your team or organization show its survival and coping responses? What does this look like? Can you think of examples of these responses?

★ When might an organization be unwell, have a compromised immune system, or have an injury?

★ How well can you or others perform, think, and flourish under unsafe, unsupportive, or unthinking situations?

★ In what environments do you best thrive, develop, think, create, and grow?

★ What do you internalize, absorb, breathe in, and feel each day in your work environment (positive, negative, and all the shades in between)?

These consequences and survival responses are naturally likely to have a ripple effect on things such as staff wellness, commitment, morale, spirit, energy, productivity, turnover, and retention, as well as on the decisions made, the feelings shared, the culture felt, and the outcomes achieved.

5.10. Organizational memory and amnesia

Like people, organizations also have their own influencing events, journeys, embedded stories, roots, and histories. They can also have their own historical trauma, as well as their own ghosts (Fraiberg *et al.*, 1975), haunters, scars, wounds, and shadows of the past. They have their own angels (Lieberman *et al.*, 2005), guiders, lighthouses, inspirers, and protectors.

Organizational history and memory can be shaped by so many different things but might include aspects such as medical experimentation, team closures, serious incidents, tragedies, influencing and impactful leaders, organizational changes and restructures, funding cuts, medical errors, formal investigations and court cases, media exposés, responses to key events or times in history like during Covid or terrorist attacks, staff suicides or deaths, organizational and institutional abuse, and so much more. We need to find a way to reflect on this history, as this not only helps us to understand the cultural and wider context of the organization, but also to learn from the past, inform the future, and honour the distance already travelled. This is especially important where there is a high turnover of staff, because this crucial tacit knowledge can be easily lost.

A lack of learning and reflecting on the past can feed into what many people refer to as 'organizational amnesia'. We can see history repeating itself, the same difficulties returning in a cyclical nature, and the same dilemmas and responses repeatedly reoccurring. For example, we see the same issues coming up in serious case reviews over and over again, and we go through stages of closing residential homes and psychiatric hospitals and then later opening them again. Organizations can re-enact the past and get stuck in a loop, leading to staff feeling frustrated and hopeless.

Organizational amnesia can also lead organizations to forget why they are there in the first place. Their mission and vision become blurred and diluted. Just as a person can feel fragmented, uprooted, and have a fragile sense of identity, so too can an organization. This resonates with many of the organizations I support. For example, a GP in a place of distress stated, 'I came into this to make a difference, but somehow we have lost our way. We are in a sea of firefighting and paperwork, and the love, passion, and vision I had seems to have dissipated, or is hanging on by a thin thread.'

An organization's memory and history will inevitably shape and guide its workers and its culture, both positively and negatively. This will be more impact-ful if issues are not addressed, acknowledged, and processed; if the experience is felt, but things are left unspoken. This mirrors what happens in trauma, which is often silenced, unspoken, invalidated, ignored, and avoided. It seeps out in other ways, for example in someone feeling strong feelings but not knowing why, or becoming dysregulated, or learning to minimize or shut down their own feelings. Someone may know something has happened because they sense and feel it, but as they haven't had it confirmed, their imagination may run wild, and they may catastrophize or internalize it. Organizations are similar: these memories and influencing factors, often ignored, can be consciously and unconsciously present and imprinted into the fabric of the organization; their ripples felt bubbling under the surface. This fragmented and unresolved memory and experience can come out in other ways.

It is interesting to think about amnesia in wider society and what comes and goes, is forgotten, or pushed underground, for example HIV, Covid-19, incest, famous people who have abused others, child sexual abuse, the abuse of people with disabilities, famines, and war. Dr Judith Herman (1992), a leader in the trauma field, writes:

> The knowledge of horrible events periodically intrudes into public awareness but is rarely retained for long. Denial, repression, and dissociation operate on

a social as well as an individual level. The study of psychological trauma has an 'underground' history. Like traumatized people, we have been cut-off from the knowledge of our past. Like traumatized people, we need to understand the past in order to reclaim the present and the future. Therefore, an understanding of psychological trauma begins with rediscovering history. (p.2)

5.11. Mirroring and parallel processes, and mirroring family dynamics and role positioning

Due to its piercing and wounding nature, trauma can be passed from an individual, to a family, to an organization, and to a society, in multiple directions. This means that we can sometimes see parallel, echoing, and mirroring processes occur between the work itself, families, and the organization. Britton (1994, pp.79–80) uses a theatre metaphor to reflect this: 'The cast changes, but the plot remains the same.' This is especially true when teams mirror the groups with whom they work.

Additionally, we all come from a primary group, our family. Sometimes our family dynamics and roles can be (usually unintentionally) re-enacted, mirrored, or echoed at work. These processes are crucial to understand, as they can reinforce family trauma and stress. For example, within social services, a traumatized system supporting a traumatized family further compounds the trauma, by creating a triple deprivation (Emanuel, 2002). This can be trauma-inducing and re-traumatizing, which is the opposite of what healing and reparative systems should be doing. Some examples of mirroring and parallel processes, as well as some survival responses, follow:

- Mission mirroring is where an organization can replicate the difficulties it is trying to change or solve. For instance, an organization designed to advocate for social injustice and unfairness instead somehow mirrors the very thing it was designed to oppose, resulting in high levels of injustice and boundary violations which leave employees feeling treated in an unfair and unjust way.

- When a team feels on edge and scared due to fear-based leadership, this anxiety and fear can be passed on to clients. The team, as a defence to the anxiety, might respond in lots of ways, such as becoming more fearful, less containing, and more dysregulated, or more controlling or authoritarian towards the people supporting and using services.

- 'Victim, persecutor, rescuer, and bystander' roles can be played out throughout the system. For example, if the service positions itself as the rescuer, then families are often in the position of victim. If families, such as in social services, are positioned as the persecutor, the person supporting, or the organization, might take the position of victim. This can be even more powerful if it is recreating other dynamics which people have felt at other times and in their own relational experiences.

Additionally, feelings, themes, experiences, and processes can permeate through multiple layers of a system: neglect can get neglected, or dissociation can make people/systems dissociate; we can see a person, their practitioner, and a system feel stuck, helpless, and hopeless.

- The warring and splitting in a family, through domestic violence or interpersonal conflict, or other reasons, can get mirrored by the system. Such warring or splitting can be within or between teams; for example, child and adult mental health services versus school or social services, a team manager versus their deputy, or psychologists versus psychiatrists.

- Teams who work with specific groups may mirror some of the behaviours or ways of being demonstrated by those they support. For example, in teams who work with adolescents, such as residential homes or youth offending teams, staff might show common adolescent behaviours, or those working in inpatient or residential settings may mirror some institutionalized behaviours. One team that was supporting children who had been exploited and trafficked reported that they felt silenced, not listened to, devalued, and ignored, which mirrored the feelings the young people were feeling or had felt.

- As well as being 'live' systems, organizations and team dynamics can be sometimes likened to a family group. As with families, there are unique systems and coalitions within them, and each member can take and be positioned within different roles. For example, effective leadership is crucial for effective teamwork, which parallels the pivotal role parenting plays within a family. So, sometimes the relationship to a manager/supervisor/leader may be likened to some of the dynamics felt in other relationships, including the primary attachment. Also, a person can feel controlled, dismissed, silenced, unseen, criticized, attacked, and so on, which can mirror and echo other feelings and send someone down a memory time hole or resurface or 'trigger' other relational feelings.

Similarly, when a valued manager leaves a team, this can 'trigger' feelings of abandonment and loss within its members, especially if a team member themselves has a history of abandonment. Building on this, leaders, like parents, are commonly polarized; for example, they can be seen as all-knowing or impotent, idealized, or denigrated. Furthermore, these roles can become entangled; a leader might be looked to by an employee to meet a need which was not met in their life, or to re-enact a relationship they previously had with someone in authority, like a parent, for example. Colleagues, managers, and their employees may re-enact rivalrous sibling relationships, or create interesting sibling dynamics such as the favourite child. Because of the powerful and permeating nature of stress and trauma within health and social care, and the personal nature the work often involves, this mirroring and positioning can be profound.

★ What mirroring or parallel processes have you seen, felt, and/or experienced?

★ Why do you think it is important to identify and reflect on these? What might be the hazards of not considering them, on you, the team, and on the work?

★ What was your experience and role within your primary group (family of origin)? How and why did/do you play these roles? How has this impacted your role in teams and groups in the past and currently? Have these roles changed over time?

★ What roles do you currently hold within your team (e.g. mediator, nurturer, peace maker)?

★ What other roles within your team do you align with or find trickier? Do certain team members represent roles in other areas of your life and relational experiences?

5.12. Re-traumatizing, trauma-inducing, and 'triggering' experiences within the system

A central tenet of adversity, culturally, and trauma-informed, infused, and responsive systems is that we acknowledge that the environments and systems we operate in, including the system itself, can add harm and distress and can be (usually unintentionally) re-traumatizing, trauma-inducing, 're-triggering', and dysregulating. They can mirror, parallel, be reminiscent of, and reinforce experiences of trauma, and the related feelings and associations of the trauma. This is more likely to occur in places where the stress is high, and if staff feel depleted, exhausted, and uncared for, and so there is a domino or ripple effect. We need to try to find ways to actively reduce this, and increase feelings of safety and trust, being stress and trauma-reducing instead of stress and trauma-inducing. This is about moving from knowing (that is, having the information) to doing and being – actively responding to the information and doing things differently.

There are numerous powerful and real-world examples of stress-inducing and re-traumatizing health and medical experiences shared in Chapters 3 and 4. Please remind yourselves of these as they are very important to this chapter and the concepts presented, and the scenarios shared are more likely to occur in systems that are struggling.

Having explored some of the key themes around trauma-soaked organizations, and additional traumas and stressors which can occur during the work, you should hopefully now see the rationale for prioritizing staff wellbeing and trauma-informed organizational cultures and have some idea of which organizational aspects are important. While the organizational elements are crucial and organizational accountability is key, it is also important for individuals to have some personal wellbeing plans and awareness in place.

Box 5.1 will explore some reflective exercises which may be useful in considering our own wellbeing.

Box 5.1.

Practical activity and reflection exercise: Wellbeing, empathy, compassion, 'triggers', and hotspots

It may be helpful to break some of the reflection points down, take some time to reflect and explore them, and come back and review them. You may also like to make a drawing, collage, sculpture, or visually depict them in some other way. Some people might find it helpful to do this within a trusting and supportive relationship.

The importance of your own wellbeing

★ If you keep filling other people's glasses up with water, or their bowl up with fruit, how is yours going to get replenished? What can you offer to others, if your glass or fruit bowl is depleted or empty?

★ What do they say on an aeroplane about putting your own oxygen mask on before putting on other people's masks?

★ How can you be there for others, without leaving yourself behind?

★ How can you light and fuel others if you are burnt out?

★ What do wellness, your own emotional regulation, and well-being mean and look like to you?

★ Why is this so important and beneficial (physically, emotionally, financially, socially/relationally, organizationally)?

★ What do you look like, feel like, act like when you are at your 'best and happiest' self? How do others know when this is the case? What do you and others do, feel, say, show, notice, and so on? What personal and professional factors contribute to this?

★ What are some of the physical, emotional, spiritual, and relational hazards of cumulative stacked-up stress? What do you know about the role of stress on someone's health/wellbeing/ cognitive abilities? What do you look like, feel like, act like when you are stressed or depleted at work and at home? How do others know when this is the case? What do you and others do, feel, say, show, notice? What personal and professional factors contribute to this?

★ If the feeling/behaviour/sensation could talk, what might it say? How does your body communicate, show, or share with you when it is… (e.g. full up, overwhelmed, exhausted, stressed, calm)?

★ What advice would you give to your loved ones/those you advise at work around wellbeing?

Blocks and barriers: Questions to reflect on your own and others' relationship to wellbeing

★ How did/does it feel to care for yourself? Do you experience any guilt over taking time to care for yourself? What does 'the guilt' say to you?

★ What are some of the stories and beliefs around wellbeing and taking care of yourself or being taken care of that you have been marinated in? (This includes family, friends, society, media, university, school, work, etc.) For example:

   ★ Wellbeing is 'indulgent', 'a luxury', 'rainbows and fairies', 'selfish', 'time wasting'.

   ★ Toxic positivity: 'Be happy', 'Smile, it can't be that bad', 'Always look on the bright side'.

★ What is your history with, experience of, and relationship to wellbeing, looking after yourself, being looked after, and looking after others (e.g. as a child, at school, in your training, in your relationship, at work)?

★ Where on a scale of 0–10 – with 0 being very poor and almost non-existent, to 10 being excellent all the time – would you place yourself on how well you take care of yourself? Inevitably this will change and evolve and be dependent on a range of factors. What are these factors? What makes this easier and facilitates this time and space (including the context and feelings)? If, for example, you answered 3: Think about what 3 means or looks like; describe 3, and if 3 could talk, what would it say? What is keeping you from being a 0, 1, or 2? (That is, what protective and buffering factors?) What might support or help you to move to a 3.5 or a 4? What might make a difference? How might this be similar or different on a different day, or others close to you were to answer? (Of course, there are many other expanding questions which could be asked.)

★ What blocks and barriers are there to you taking this time? If you were to describe these blocks and barriers, what would they look like/feel like? Where do they come from? If the blocks and barriers were an item/type of weather/something in nature/creature, what would they be? How does it feel when the blocks and barriers are there, compared to when they are less visible? What do the blocks and barriers stop you from doing/achieving/feeling?

★ Can you think of a specific time when you overcame these blocks and prioritized your own wellbeing? What supported this? What did you learn, notice, feel?

★ What could you do today that your future self would thank you for?

★ What messages do you want the people you love and support and/or those you work with or manage/supervise/train to pick up from how you model wellbeing? (Remember that, as writer Paul Coelho says, the world isn't changed by your opinion, it is changed by your example.)

★ How would you want people to describe you/remember you if you weren't there? What could they have learned from you?

Hotspots, activating experiences, prickly parts, and 'triggers'

When working with people who have experienced traumas and losses, our own 'triggers', hotspots, and prickly parts can understandably be exposed (we are all human, so we all have some). This is even more likely as many people come into this type of work with their own ghosts of the past, and human nature means that there is more likelihood of there being crossovers and associations with their own life and experiences. Hawkins and Shohet (2012) share a powerful question for people to reflect on:

★ Why am I a helper?

Many people go into caring/helping professions because they have a desire to help others, to improve things, and to make things better. Therefore, people can feel frustrated, powerless, and helpless when they cannot help, are restricted in what they can offer, or what they know, and when people don't recover, or get worse, or die. For some, this can mean not feeling good enough, feeling deskilled, feeling stuck, or experiencing imposter syndrome. In some settings, this can be exacerbated if the staff member is positioned as the person's cause of distress or their 'persecutor', for example being responsible for someone's pain through a painful procedure, or when someone has been sectioned against their will.

Within this, people in these professions are often the containers for others' complex, painful, and intolerable feelings, and their coping resources, buffers, and protective factors can be weakened, making their own ability to think and respond effectively and mindfully more challenging.

These powerful and complex feelings, responses, and relational interactions, at times, can 'trigger' surrounding people's survival modes, hotspots, and prickly parts. This is particularly the case when these experiences, feelings, and memories remain raw, unresolved, and unprocessed (e.g. themes of abandonment, rejection, inadequacy, secrecy, being silenced and oppressed, abuse, powerlessness, fear, injustice, unfairness, vulnerability, shame, worthlessness, and helplessness). Past experiences and relational patterns are inevitably, to some degree, brought into current relationships, and subsequently can colour and shape people's perceptions, attributions, and responses.

For example, when we are reminded of our own experiences and history, we too can become dysregulated, activated, 're-triggered', preoccupied, or absorbed in our own trauma and loss. In these moments, when lost in a sea of emotions, or when we may have fallen through a time hole (Hobday, 2001), we can then understandably struggle to read, connect, and respond to others' emotional states and needs in a regulated way. This can pose a block to being able to practise mindfully.

★ How can you respond mindfully and reflectively, or make effective decisions, when you feel full up, burnt out, underappreciated, and are in survival mode?

Here are some examples of professionals' own hotspots (many more are shared in Chapter 3):

Justine had been working with a teenager who had died by suicide. This experience had largely remained unprocessed and unresolved, yet had left a lasting impact on her. Years later, when she was working with another young person who was speaking about suicide, she found herself back down a time hole. Her levels of panic became pervasive and overwhelming, and she understandably struggled to not entangle the two experiences.

Karine heard a racist comment being said between two people, and it catapulted her back to all the times she had been on the receiving end of racism; the words hit her like a bolt and cut through her. She understandably responded to the people from that survival and protective place.

Lionel was struggling with a manager at work. He felt this manager picked on him and bullied him. This understandably felt very difficult. On later exploration, he realized that this relationship experience felt even more wounding and impactful as his manager reminded him of his father, who also made him feel not good enough, silenced, and dismissed.

Simon found it very frustrating to be on the receiving end of a patient who declined medical treatment or who was not listening and acting on his advice. Many people would understandably find this difficult and frustrating, but for Simon it felt like emotional dynamite and really got under his skin. It not only took him back to a place where a family member had not listened to medical advice and died from something preventative, but it also fed into his feelings of inadequacy and not being respected or listened to. These were feelings he had experienced both in his relationship and when at school.

Rukmini was brought up with a 'soldier on' attitude, and she found it hard to connect with her own vulnerability and to be on the receiving end of what she saw as 'needy, wimpy' behaviours. This made it difficult for her sometimes to empathize, show compassion, or be curious about what was going on for her patients who might respond very differently to how she would have done.

When Vanessa was supporting someone during labour it could be both beautiful and painful due to her own experience of having a baby who died during labour and her subsequent struggles with getting pregnant.

Kaia found the dad of one of her patients incredibly hard to work with. He had the same name as her dad, some of the same characteristics, and some of the same qualities.

★ Is there a particular behaviour/difficulty/theme/person currently that is worrying/distressing you/getting under your skin?

★ What is your relationship to, connection to, experience of, and history to that theme/issue/experience/difficulty/behaviour? What is the significance or meaning of that behaviour/difficulty/theme/person to you?

★ What, if any, experiences or themes does it stir up in you? Does it take you down a time hole or feel similar to another time/theme/person/feeling/sensation in your life?

★ What ideas/values/themes/beliefs/hotspots do you have that are being evoked/'triggered'/challenged by the theme/issue/experience/difficulty?

★ How can you reduce/notice/respond/understand these? How
can you also try to find ways in the moment to recognize, and
stay regulated and grounded, when a hotspot is activated?

It can also be useful to think about some of the different types of
'triggers', hotspots, and things that can get under our skin (Chapters
3 and 4 provide some more examples). Some can be much harder to
identify than others or seem to have less meaning or fewer explanations. Some can be helpfully explored in therapy or through other
reflective forums that are trusting and supportive.

The more we understand why we react as we do, the more it
makes sense, and subsequently the less personal and more resolvable
it can become. Moreover, once these 'triggers' have been identified
(an ongoing work in progress, and dynamic process), coping strategies and multi-model tools can be sought, which aim to identify ways
to stay regulated and empathetic, to manage high levels of affect,
and to regain emotional equilibrium, rather than getting hooked on,
or engaging in, mutually escalating arousal patterns.

5.13. Wider system considerations which can make a difference to the trauma-informed organizational culture and overall running of the organization

These ideas are not exhaustive and prescriptive and are not presented in a
particular order. Each context is unique, so no one size fits all, and many of
these are impacted or prevented by changes and barriers. Please take the time
as you read these to adapt and apply them. Many of them are expanded further
throughout this book, and some of the daily and more tangible interactions
which can be done are shared in Chapter 8.

- A focus on increasing psychological, cultural, and relational safety and
  trust within teams. This includes leaders that model the model and walk
  the walk instead of just talking the talk. It includes a culture that can say
  sorry, learn from 'mistakes', and be human, avoiding blaming, attacking,
  and shaming responses. And this can be aligned with a growth mindset
  and a learning culture that encourages, where appropriate, out-of-the-box
  thinking, creativity, experimentation, and innovation.

  This means that there needs to be support and places for leaders to
  be vulnerable and connect with their own fallibility, to be able to share

and release, think, and reflect. This includes modelling and promoting curiosity, compassion, and empathy, and creating a sense of identity, connection, and belonging within the team and to the organization. Having meaningful feedback, consultations, and communication loops is also important, as is creating clear expectations, boundaries, and ways of being which are aligned with values, and making sure that breaches are responded to.

- Access to the essentials such as a chair, a working computer, refreshments, a pen, and so on.

- Encouraged, supported, and protected breaks and lunch breaks, as well as annual leave. Where possible, some flexibility in working patterns is helpful.

- A culture of thanks, appreciation, acknowledgement, and validation.

- Best practice forums and spaces that celebrate great practice and enrich it.

- IT systems that are user-friendly, that work, and that connect with each other and avoid duplication or added stress.

- Emphasis on staff wellness and wellbeing, to increase staff morale, cohesion, satisfaction, health, retention, and continuity of care, and to reduce staff mistrust, staff sickness, and staff leaving. This includes validation, normalizing, naming, and acknowledgement of the complexity of the work and the contextual factors that contribute to this, particularly around secondary and vicarious trauma, emotional saturation, compassion fatigue, and burnout, and meaningful action to alleviate, reduce, and where possible prevent and respond to these.

- Meaningful access to relevant high-quality training which applies to the real world and infuses into applicable change and action. The concepts and ideas must be embedded throughout, and the information not just tokenistic or a one-off. This training from a trauma-informed position should ideally include a spotlight on different understandings of trauma, trauma-informed values, organizational trauma, secondary and vicarious trauma, staff wellbeing tools and theory, cultural humility, and organizational culture. Additional training might be specific, such as around self-harm, emotional regulation skills, and trauma within a maternity setting, and for this training should be infused into core medical, nursing, midwifery, dentistry training, and so on.

- Access to a menu (as there is no one size fits all) of high-quality, well-matched support, which could include things like supervision, reflective and thinking spaces, meaningful debriefs and check-ins (see Chapter 7), peer support groups, and policy reviews of whistleblowing and staff support.

- An optimizing, supporting, and acknowledging of wider roles, such as volunteers, hospitality staff, nursing assistants, janitors, security staff, and domestic staff.

- Careful thinking about the physical environment (see Chapter 9).

- Thinking about the daily interactions, including things like the language that is used and the feelings that are conveyed (see Chapter 8).

- Processes, policies, and practices reviewed through a trauma-informed universal lens (see Chapters 7, 8, and 9), which includes improving recruitment and induction procedures to get the right people in post and keep them there. It also involves looking at change, restructuring, investigation, and disciplinary processes from a trauma-informed lens.

- Opportunities to meaningfully reflect and improve on the patient's journey, from entry to exit and from a trauma lens.

- Active and creative listening to complaints, feedback, and suggestions, and involving multiple voices and perspectives in the designing, running, and improving of services.

- Reflection on and consideration of some of the biases, disparities, and inequalities within services and actively putting into place strategies to reduce and combat these (Chapter 6).

- Reduction of silos and fragmented working. This includes a deepening understanding of each other's roles through shadowing, observations, joint working, multidisciplinary working, being co-located, and having shared forums and trainings. This also includes thinking about local services and the relationships and understanding between them, the referral processes, the shared language, and so on.

- A trauma-informed view of communication and media for staff and people using the service. This might include podcasts, blogs, emails, newsletters, and conversations that highlight key messages and keep the momentum up but also humanize services and reduce some of the 'them and us' divide that can occur.

- Advocating for trauma-informed ideas and values and knowledge to be integrated into core training, such as medical or nursing university courses, as well as into work inductions and refresher training.

- Trauma working groups and implementation committees to drive, monitor, and shape the ongoing implementation.

- Things put in place that support continuity of care and relationship-based care, particularly in areas such as maternity and general practice – and thinking about ways of avoiding retelling and repeating information, or information getting lost.

- Careful thinking about the presence of students and meaningful consent (see Chapter 8), particularly centred around safety, dignity, and integrity.

- Where possible, access to psychologists and emotional wellbeing staff; however, this doesn't mean, for example, that a psychologist is needed every time difficult news is delivered or when someone cries or is a bit upset.

- Clear information about services to refer on to or liaise with. If services are not available, how there must be a plan for how this information is escalated and advocated for.

What else would you add? Which would you add or change or highlight in your service?

5.14. Some micro strategies and introductory ideas for improving your own wellbeing and regulation

5.14.1. What to be mindful of

Having discussed some of the overarching team and organizational areas, we will now look at some more specific individual strategies for supporting one's own emotional wellbeing, regulation, and wellness. The strategies and ideas shared below are to support professionals to look after and care for themselves. These are in the context of wider organizational changes and are by no means a replacement. We know collective and community and organizational care is essential but sometimes this needs to go hand-in-hand with some individual strategies too.

The ideas shared here are by no means an extensive or rigid list, and are just intended as ideas. What works for one person will not work for another person, and so they need to be tailored to the unique individual. We all have different needs, likes, interests, sensory profiles, outlets, and so on. For example, one person might find physical exercise and going to the gym helpful and enjoyable, whereas another person might find this stressful, exhausting, activating, impossible, or dysregulating; or one person might find mindfulness or breathing exercises incredibly useful, whereas another might find them 'triggering', frustrating, and evoking of their asthma or feelings of panic. Therefore, there is not a recipe book or one-size-fits-all approach.

It is also important to be realistic within this. For example, someone might find going to the spa very useful, and so it is great to integrate this into their routine, but it is unlikely that this can be done on a daily basis or in the moment when they are feeling overwhelmed, or in between appointments, meetings, or sessions. So, it is about having a range of tools and go-to options that can be applied depending on the context and on the person. It is also about finding things that can be integrated into someone's daily practice and regular rituals. It is helpful to get it into their muscle memory. Finding a breathing exercise that works for a person is fantastic, but it is unlikely to be remembered and effective unless it is practised regularly so that it is in their muscle memory. It needs to be integrated, like brushing one's teeth. Early intervention, before things reach crisis point, is also crucial. It is a bit like blowing up a balloon and releasing some air, and then blowing and releasing, rather than keeping on blowing up the balloon and waiting for it to pop.

We also need to remember that we will need different things to up- and down-regulate, depending on our arousal and regulation levels and the task. For example, if I am running a training session and need to keep the energy up for my audience, I often need to use regulation strategies to fuel me up, to pump me up, to energize myself, and to get me into the zone; whereas after the session, I often need to find things to help me unwind, release the energy, and calm down. It's the same when I have been with a young person who is presenting as sad, dissociated, and depressed. When I leave the room and before I see my next person, I need to find a way to shift into being more present and to release some of the heaviness and tiredness I might feel. Whereas after I have been with a young person who is, for example, shouting and throwing items and in a place of high emotional expression, I need to find a way to bring some calm and peace in. Otherwise, this emotional contagion will spread and likely spill out into other interactions.

What follows are just a few strategies that you might like to try.

5.14.2. De-roling and releasing – integrating brain break and mindful moments

It can be helpful and important to separate oneself from work and to mark the beginning and end of each day and the transition between home and work, and work and home. Many people like to cognitively de-role and debrief after the visit/day, and to have some micro strategies and brain breaks to do before and after the day, and even during it. We need to find strategies that stop any negative effects from work permeating our feelings and the mood we take home or into our next appointment, meeting, or interaction, and spilling out too intensely.

★ What do you do at the end of the day or at the beginning of the day to de-stress and to de-role?

Everyone has different rituals which they do – there is no right or wrong way – and these will probably change depending on the day and need. It is about exploring options and finding what works for you, and then ensuring that you make a commitment to integrate them into your routine. I like to do two or three, which only take a few minutes, but can make a huge difference. Here are some that might be helpful:

◉ Physically shake it off, often to music, shaking legs and arms. There are numerous studies about the benefits of shaking and moving one's body.

◉ Clapping/tapping different rhythms. Things that are rhythmic, regulating, and repetitive can be helpful in shifting one's arousal state. This can also use the left and right sides of our brain, which can be helpful for bilateral stimulation. Other ways of left- and right-brain stimulation include a butterfly hug (tapping left and right sides of the body) from eye movement desensitization reprocessing (EMDR) therapy, left and right breathing exercises, bilateral drawing, using fidget items like a stress ball, or moving it from one's left hand and then switching to the right hand, back and forth, walking, pacing, or moving around, sitting on a rocking chair, tracing with a finger or moving around a maze or labyrinth, dancing, and brain gym exercises.

◉ Going to a 'safe/calm' place, moment, or memory and then using creative reminders of this 'calming' place. For details on this exercise please see my *Presley the Pug Relaxation Activity Book* (Treisman, 2019), my grounding and soothing cards, or my treasure box for creating trauma-informed organization resources (Treisman, 2021, 2022). I also teach and show these in some of my trainings found through www.safehandsthinking-minds.co.uk.

- Using items from your sensory/grounding/soothing box/bag/jar. This will vary for each person but ideally will be things which utilize the different senses. So, for example, you might have things which bring a feeling of calm, via things you can smell, things you can do, feel, or touch, things you can hear or listen to, and so on. It is not just about having these items but thinking about which items you need at that time to up- or down-regulate and how you might enhance or enrich their effectiveness, such as incorporating a different sense while using the item. So, for example, there might be something tactile like a stress ball, but you could bring in another sense by moving it between the left and the right hands, or choosing a particular coloured ball, or writing or drawing a calming word or image on it, or putting hand cream or a scent on the ball.

- Listening to a particular song.

- Changing out of work clothes or taking off your ID badge.

- Doing some muscle tensing and 'calming/relaxing' exercises. Two of my favourites are hand breathing and rainbow breathing, but each person will have different preferences. Importantly, a lot of breathing exercises are not about the exercise itself but the way you do it. Small tweaks can make a big difference, such as the pressure on your hand being ticklish or deep pressure, having eyes open, lowered, or closed, the way you position your body, the pace of your breathing. It is important to find one that suits you and then adapt it according to your own needs.

- Applying a particularly regulating, grounding smell to the wrists, as hand cream, or to an item like a squishy stress ball.

- Leaving the work mobile phone at work.

- Putting a personal limit on the amount of time you speak about work outside work.

- Talking to, emailing, texting, or leaving a voice note for a trusted colleague.

- Taking a brain break – moving around, having a change of scenery, going for a walk, listening to a podcast, flicking through a magazine, watching something that makes you laugh or puts a smile on your face.

- Reminding yourself that tomorrow is a new day, and of all of the things that put you in home mode rather than work mode – in essence where work stops, and you start.

- Writing a list of things which are worrying you or the tasks for the next day and putting it away until the next day. One colleague told me how they pass a tree on the way home from work and they pretend they are hanging up the worries and the tasks of the day on the tree, and then in the morning they pick them back up. Some people find it helpful to also remind themselves of the things they did do and did achieve, including the minute detail, in line with 'every interaction is an intervention' (Treisman, 2017a).

- Having mantras or affirmations which you might say; some people might say a prayer or a well-known saying.

- Where appropriate, identifying and writing down some of these thoughts or worries and imagining getting rid of them. This might be by putting them in a bottle or a balloon and watching them float away, putting them in a rubbish bag, or writing them on a piece of paper that is then burned, ripped-up, or buried. Others may want to write down the words on a tissue and watch them fade away when placed in water or flushed down the toilet.

- Releasing feelings through journalling, diary keeping, or expressing them through art, music, and so on, or channelling them into social action.

- Incorporating some feel-good and regulating factors and items into our everyday routine. These will be unique for everyone, but we know that small things can often make a big difference. For example, having a small, pleasing item such as a specific mug, key ring, door sign, screensaver, mouse mat, diary, pencil case, phone cover, image, or messages on the back of your lanyard.

- Using some cognitive behavioural, compassionate mind, acceptance and commitment, or narrative therapy questions to support your thoughts, especially when these thoughts, feelings, and sensations might be tangled and fused, or blocked or spilling and leaking out. I use some of these if I have a particular worry or upsetting thought, am falling into a thinking trap or mind loop, or to externalize things like self-doubt or hope or stress, as well as to connect to things like guiding values. Different questions, perspectives, and approaches will resonate or jar with different people, and everyone has different ways of supporting their wellbeing. So, for example, after a tricky day or situation, and having had space to debrief, it can be helpful for some people to try to reflect on some of the following questions:

★ What other difficult situations and times have you been through that were or felt worse and how have they improved? What other things personally or professionally have you navigated or overcome? How did you get through those times? What skills, strengths, resources, resiliencies, and positive qualities did you use? How can you build and reconnect with these skills and resources?

★ If the hope/compassion/empathy (the positive quality) could talk, what might it say to you? What advice might it give? What does it look or feel like? What has been your history or relationship with, for example, hope? What might make it bigger/more present? (Types of therapy such as Narrative Therapy, Compassionate Mind, Internal Family Systems, and others have a series of exercises and questions to explore these emotions further.)

★ How can you borrow hope, courage, strength, or wisdom from other people, from your motivators, supporters, role models, inspirers, or life cheerleaders? (See section about support systems below.)

★ What advice would you give to a friend/colleague/family member/ person you are working with in a similar situation? And what might a trusted colleague/supervisor/mentor advise or say to you? How are you modelling and showing compassion to yourself, as you would hope to do for a loved one?

★ What does it look like when you step back or look at the situation from a different perspective? (See a situation differently and you can see a different situation.) From a cognitive behavioural perspective, it can be helpful to reflect on some of the thinking traps, for example are you over-generalizing? Catastrophizing? Using all-or-nothing thinking? Filtering? Mind-reading?

★ Will this still seem important and be worrying you in a week, month, or a year? Are there things you can remember from the past that consumed your thinking and took up a lot of time and worry, but now seem like a distant memory or less relevant or important? What aspects of it do you have control over and what aspects don't you have control over?

★ Are there ways you can break it down into smaller steps? Which tasks can be achieved? (Think SMART goals – are your expectations realistic and manageable?)

★ Are there things which you have already done within this, things that are moving in the right direction, even if only slightly?

Some of these strategies are described in more detail in *A Therapeutic Treasure Deck of Cards: Grounding, Soothing, Coping, and Regulating* (Treisman, 2017b), and I deliver specific training on this around emotional regulation.

5.14.3. Motivation and satisfaction

Sometimes, amid the noise and the stressors of the work and the wider context, the reason we came into the role can get lost or diluted. This can be difficult, particularly if you have spent years investing in your work, when it is a large part of your identity and you have taken a lot of time, effort, and sometimes sacrifice to get there. Therefore, it can be helpful to remember why you do what you do, and what keeps you in it. This is about your journey, your motivation, your drivers, and your values. This is your roots, your anchor, and your compass.

Remind yourself why you do what you do, and what fills your emotional, social, spiritual, and physical buckets and pushes your reward buttons. It can also be helpful to actively take your brain to the gym by noticing and paying attention to the bits which you have achieved, enjoyed, and felt satisfaction in. It can be helpful to keep a diary recording of all the changes and achievements that have been made on a daily or regular basis. These can be seemingly small, or parts of things. You can even have things like a sparkle or proud moment, a feel-good book or diary, a bank of positive memories book, and a treasure box or jar filled with positive post-its. This could be extended to a team wall of pride or an art gallery of celebrations and successes. We can recall and reflect on the good bits and the things we want to remember, but it can also be there as a reminder when having a difficult day or need a boost.

Another activity which can be very powerful in connecting us to our motivations is the professional tree of life from Narrative Therapy, which was originally created by Ncazelo Ncube but has been adapted to numerous professional contexts. This should be ideally facilitated by someone trained in the methodology but can be a wonderful activity, especially when done as a team, where together a community of trees and forest of trees to weather the storm are created.

Similarly, you could write a letter or make a video or message for yourself about why you came into the work, what fuels you, what keeps you in it, what you have navigated through, what advice you would give your younger self, your future self, or others in the profession, and what those who have learned from you, been supported by you, and been impacted by you might say. This can be done in all sorts of ways, from a letter, to a tree, to a path, and whichever other ways resonate. For example, image 5.4 shows a photo of a patchwork I created to support myself. The top left corner represents some of the aspects of the job that I love and enjoy. The upper right-hand patch represents some of my biggest sparkle moments and sources of encouragement; the lower left-hand patch represents some of my roots

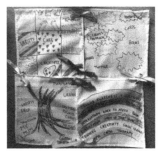

5.4. A PROFESSIONAL
PATCHWORK

and journey and what people, events, and experiences inspired me and led me to becoming a psychologist. And the lower right-hand patch represents some of my hopes and wishes for the future of the work. Now there are eight patches as it is a journey which I add to and review. I regularly look at this to remind myself of my roots and what keeps me in the job.

5.14.4. Personal and professional team of support

Working with complexity, in isolation, or with people where you often feel an overwhelming sense of responsibility can feel at times quite lonely and hard. This is why having a cohesive and supportive team, alongside high-quality supervision, thinking spaces, and leadership support, can be so buffering; however, we know this isn't necessarily the case for everyone. And there are also people who work in more isolated roles, or virtually, from home. Where possible, trying to find ways to increase one's support network whether through special interest groups, peer groups, social media forums, and so on is a good idea. When we do experience this sort of support it is important to show our appreciation and thanks for our colleagues and those who make a difference to us.

Additionally, it can be helpful and powerful to reflect on and draw inspiration, hope, wisdom, encouragement, and strength from our own life inspirers, helpers, cheerleaders, feeders, motivators, and supporters. As the well-known proverbs say, 'It takes a village to raise a child' and 'Sticks in a bundle cannot be broken'.

These inspirers, motivators, supporters, and cheerleaders might be people from our personal or professional lives: people who are alive, dead, real, imagined, creatures, spiritual figures, celebrities, random encounters, teachers, authors; they might even be people whom we want to prove wrong, or who have showed us what not to be. It could also be the whole person or parts of a person, or certain attributes or qualities of theirs. Having this safety net and circle of support can help us to feel more connected, encouraged, and less alone; we can draw on their support, relational gifts, and messages of hope, and see ourselves through their eyes. It can feel as if we are connected by invisible string, and we carry these people with us in our inner voice, in our inner cheerleader, in our hearts, and in our minds.

★ Who are some of your past and present role models, inspirers, help-ers, supporters, motivators, and life cheerleaders? (Remember these can be personal or professional, they can be alive, dead, imaginary, famous, spiritual, from history/books/TV, etc. And they can be whole people or parts, qualities, or attributes of people.)

★ How can you utilize and expand on this support? Are there times that your connection with the person or people feels stronger?

★ How can you draw on or borrow some of their positivity, strength, hope, values, energy, inspiration, and encouragement? What strengths and qualities do they have which you want to keep close to you?

★ How can you drink them in, breathe them in, and internalize them?

★ How can you see yourself through their eyes? What do you think they would say to you about...? What do you think they admire, notice, and appreciate in you?

★ Within the notion that relationships should be reciprocal and activate our social engagement systems, what more can you do to support others in your system or to show your appreciation to them? Who do you think might put you as one of their life cheerleaders and supporters if they were going through the questions here?

Sometimes, it can be helpful to have some visible and tangible reminders (e.g. on a keyring, lanyard, pencil case, picture) of these life supporters, as this helps to bring the ideas alive in a multi-sensory and fun way; it can be particularly helpful when you are in your survival brain and struggling to access some of the positive thoughts or memories. Taking the time to make such an item can also help us to reflect on the questions above, and gives us a tangible item to help us feel anchored and supported.

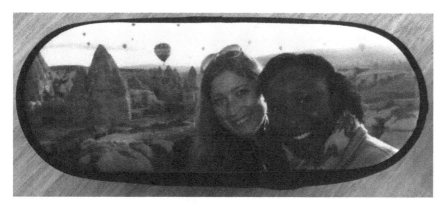

5.5. A PENCIL CASE WITH A MOTIVATING PERSON AND CALMING MOMENT

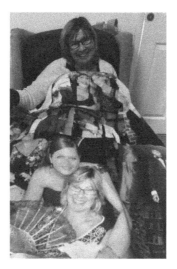

5.6. A BLANKET OF SUPPORTERS AND HELPERS

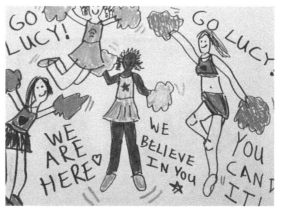

5.7. A CHEERLEADER OF SUPPORT

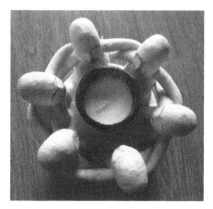

5.8. A CANDLE AND CIRCLE OF FRIENDS (YOU CANNOT LIGHT OTHERS
IF YOU ARE BURNED OUT; WHO LIGHTS YOU UP AND FUELS YOU?)

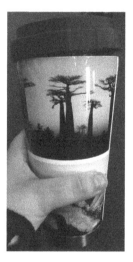

5.9. A TRAVEL MUG WITH IMAGES OF A CALMING PLACE
(IT COULD ALSO BE PEOPLE OR QUOTES)

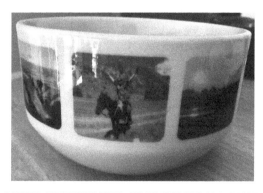

5.10. A BOWL SHOWING FEEL-GOOD IMAGES AND REMINDERS

5.14.5. Wellbeing and wellness planning (and things to be mindful of within this)

Creating a wellbeing plan can be a helpful way to support yourself and for others to take some time to reflect on their and our own wellness and regulation. This is also intended to be a working document, not a one-off or tokenistic task. The whole point is that it is meaningful, useful, and relevant, and that it is personalized and tailored to your unique and evolving needs. If it collects dust on a shelf or is used as a tick box or weaponized against you (e.g. 'Do this because you aren't resilient enough or coping well enough'), then it doesn't model the model and can do the opposite of supporting your wellbeing. This can also be useful, when it is safe and appropriate, during reflection, supervision, and so on. However, it is based on having a trusting relationship and is around choice; it should not be a mandatory or forced activity.

A wellbeing plan can also help when used as a communication tool to support people to think about what they need and how similar or different this might be to others. For example, I can feel dysregulated physically and emotionally when I don't eat or when I am hungry, for a range of reasons, but if my colleagues don't know this, they might take my responses as being distracted and they might be less aware of the impact of things like planning back-to-back meetings over lunch, without lunch, and so on.

Some people like to display their safety and wellbeing plan to keep it present and at the forefront of their mind during the day. For example, they might put an image on their lanyard or ID badge, on a mug, a mouse mat, or in the front of their diary, on a sticker on a note pad, or have it as a recording or audio on their phone.

One example of a wellbeing plan follows; however, this is a springboard, so feel free to adjust the questions or add new ones.

Worksheet 5.1. A wellbeing plan

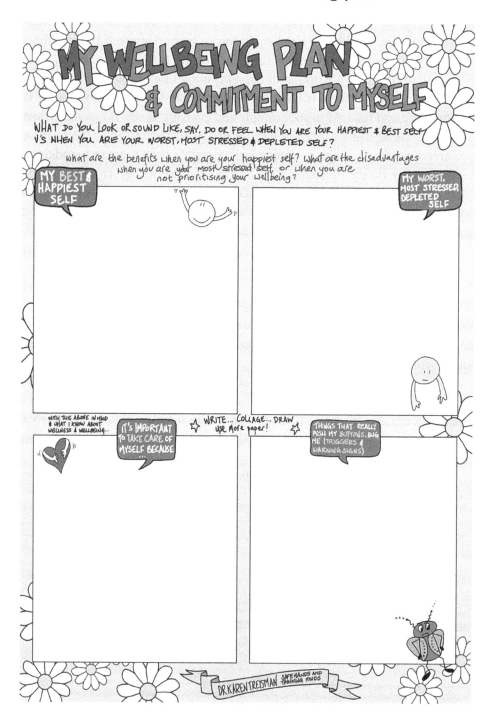

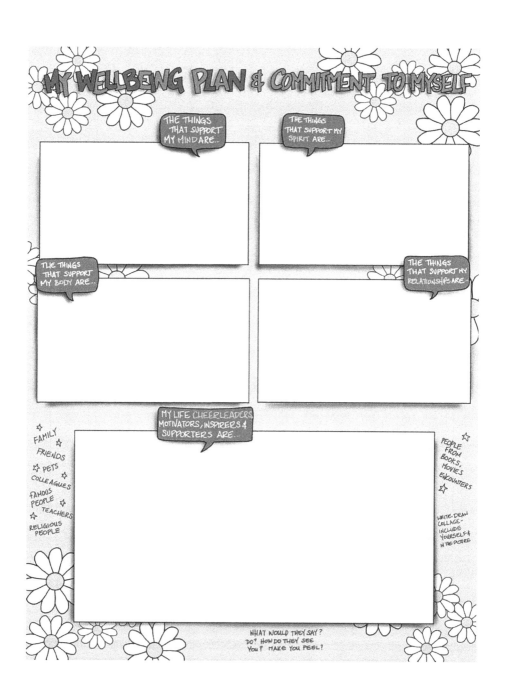

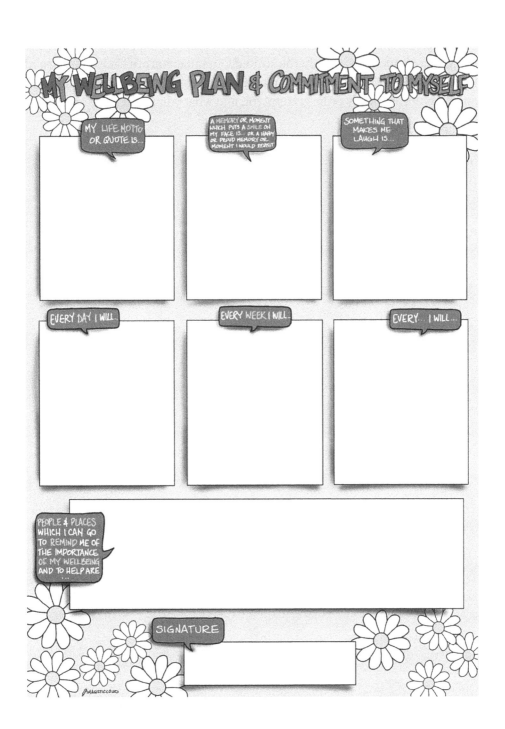

5.14.6. Take what you need tokens

While these do not constitute an exhaustive list, they can act as a reminder that you are important, you are the strategy, and that you are likely holding and navigating a lot. So, take a mindful moment and a brain break to consider what you might have already or be grateful for, and what you might need or want.

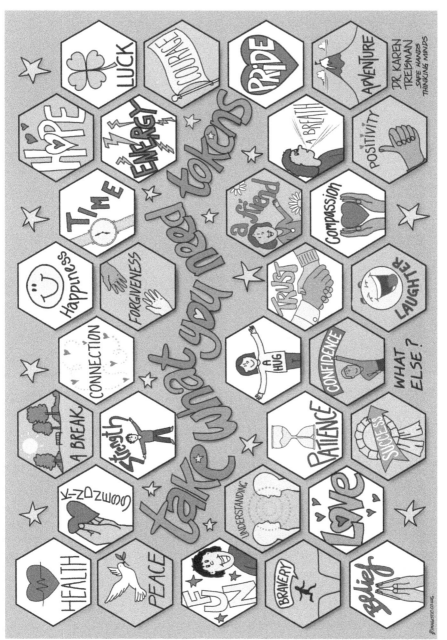

5.11. TAKE WHAT YOU NEED TOKENS

CHAPTER 6

Health Injustice and Cultural Humility

This book has covered different types of traumas, including medical and organizational trauma, and some key parts of the relationship between trauma and health, including sensory and body-activating experiences. It feels important before going on to explore trauma-informed practice in more depth that we have a chapter on cultural humility – partly because culture influences all that we do but also because cultural humility is a core part of trauma-informed practice.

6.1. What will be covered in this chapter

- An introduction to the concept of cultural humility

- How cultural humility fits in with the trauma-informed journey

- Some things to be mindful of when transferring these concepts to your own context

- Intersectionality and multiplicity of identities

- Biases, inequalities, and disparities in service provision and system experiences

- A spotlight on some cultural idioms, scripts, and perceptions of aetiology

Please see Chapter 2 for sections on some of the links between poverty, discrimination, and health.

6.2. An introduction to the concept of cultural humility

Cultural humility is the ability to maintain an interpersonal stance that is other-oriented (or open to the other) in relation to aspects of cultural identity that are most important to the person. It is an active engagement and a lifelong process of self-reflection and self-critique, whereby the individual not only learns about another's culture, but also starts with an examination of their own beliefs, biases, assumptions, values, and cultural identities (Kumagai & Lypson, 2009; Tervalon & Murray-García, 1998). Cultural humility differs from the term cultural competence (often referred to in organizations, such as the NHS in the UK, as the aim), which is about competence.

Cultural humility involves taking an active interest in and making an ongoing commitment to curiosity, self-awareness, critical thinking, reflectiveness, and reflexiveness. It also is about the lens through which we view ourselves, others, and the world, and about being respectful and open. We need to be mindful that culture is ever changing and dynamic, and that no one size will fit all, and it is important to be open to learning from the person we are working with. Being 'culturally responsive' means being proactive and intentional, considering how we move from knowing to being and doing. We translate what we know and feel into action and infuse it into the fabric of the organization. It is also about a feeling, the looks, the facial expressions, the body language, the level of interest felt by someone.

While culture refers to numerous different layers and is much broader than race, it is important that the term 'anti-racist' is highlighted here. This generally refers to actively doing the work to challenge racism, not just responding when faced with it, or simply passing on the message. This concept extends to other aspects of othering, prejudices, oppression, discrimination, and so on. This includes the active process of identifying and eliminating racism by changing systems, organizational structures, policies, practices, and attitudes, so that power is redistributed equitably.

Cultural humility and responsiveness within an organization also are about acknowledging and considering the impact and presence of community, collective, social, cultural, structural, institutional, political, and historical trauma, violence, exclusion, social dislocation and rejection, othering, and oppression. This might involve the following complex and multi-layered areas:

- Racism and racial trauma/slavery/imperialism and colonization.

- Segregation and apartheid/discrimination, oppression, and persecution (including institutional racism, sexism, homophobia, ageism, islamophobia).

- Medical racism, including medical experimentation (e.g. Tuskegee experiment, experiments during the world wars and by the Nazis, forced coercive sterilization and other contraceptives).

- Genocide and war.

- Political regimes of fear, oppression, othering, splitting, and so on.

- Immigration, migration, and displacement.

- Poverty, including famine, housing, unemployment.

- Marginalization, social exclusion, chronic loneliness, and othering, including social stratification. We know that people's position in society can affect health outcomes by impacting on psychosocial factors. Social identities may influence and interact with these, such as ethnicity and gender; different levels of power, prestige, and access to resources between groups in society can in turn affect health and other related outcomes.

★ Which others would you add?

★ Which resonate with you?

★ To what extent are these areas acknowledged, named, and reflected on? Is any training given on these areas?

Thinking about cultural humility and responsiveness at an organizational level means considering the social, political, and cultural context and history of the organization, and of the populations being served, and intentionally shaping, designing, and delivering the service with respect and collaboration. This includes reflecting on institutional racism/sexism/ageism/classism/ableism (and so on) and how power imbalances and inequalities can impact the employees and the communities being served, often on a daily and ongoing basis. This can be within the practices, policies, structures, cultures, and laws of an organization and system. Cultural humility and responsiveness mean taking organizational accountability, which includes being more intentional and proactive. After all, if staff can't do this at an organizational level, how will they be able to do this within the work itself? We need to model the model. As Martin Luther King said, 'Injustice anywhere is a threat to justice everywhere.'

Cultural humility and responsiveness also need to consider and reflect on power differences, positions of power, identity, privilege, and access, status comparisons, and interplaying social norms. This also includes how inclusive and diverse the organization is, across all aspects, and encompasses white, male, and other forms of privilege. However, it is also important within this to see the nuances, and to also try to understand the different layers of identity and of the individual person.

Moreover, cultural humility and responsiveness also include reflecting on how and what our own biases, meaning-making, values, judgements, actions, traditions, beliefs, expectations, attitudes, behaviours, assumptions, and perspectives are based on and influenced by. This really can colour everything we see, think, and do. As Shotter (1993) says, 'Meaning is never freely chosen, it is always made and found.' Culture, like oxygen, is everywhere, even if it can't be seen, and it needs to be thought about, for example in our:

- relationship to support/help/services

- family roles and constellations

- conceptualizations of wellbeing, coping, illness, death, and health

- assumptions and representations around things like parenting, gender, marriage, child development age and stages, and development stages and roles, such as in ageing

- conceptualizations around trauma, adversity, hardships, loss, and abuse

- cultural idioms and representations of illness (see section below)

- terms, understandings, and expressions of emotions, distress, pain, hurt

- language and way of communicating

- connection to spirituality.

The list is endless. And there are many more aspects!

Cultural humility is not about a deficit or problem-saturated model, it is about celebrating, learning from, and respecting diversity, as well as magnifying and honouring individual, family, community, and societal strengths, resiliencies, legacies, survivorship, and resources. However, this does not mean avoiding or overlooking areas of concern and worry (e.g. safeguarding in the context of culture).

6.3. How cultural humility fits with the trauma-informed journey

The area of cultural humility and responsiveness is often overlooked or seen as separate when considering the shift towards becoming more adversity and trauma-informed and responsive. Many organizations discuss trauma but exclude it when actively thinking about culture and wider contextual areas. It is often positioned as separate or as an afterthought, or organizations have a separate team or role around trauma-informed practice and around anti-racism or cultural humility, yet these often are not working in collaboration. However, cultural humility is a central tenet of adversity and trauma-informed, infused, and responsive practice; they go hand-in-hand and are difficult to disentangle from each other. We need to infuse cultural humility and cultural responsiveness into this journey and way of being, ensuring that conversations about trauma and adversity include those around culture, and vice versa. Definitions of terms including culture, ethnicity, and race can be confusing, but rather than go into the minutia of these, this chapter will focus on some broader overlapping themes and areas. Image 6.1 should help provide an idea of the intersection of identities. This book is advocating for the centrality of intersectionality, and for re-contextualizing – in essence, seeing a person within their context.

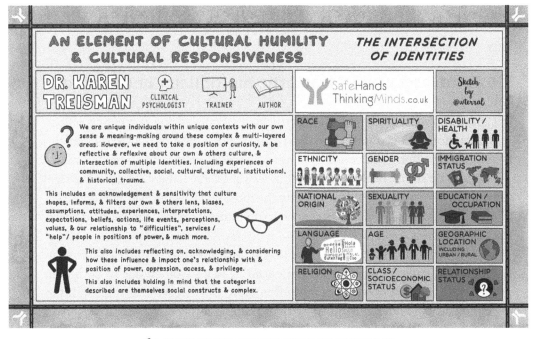

6.1. SOME OF THE INTERSECTION OF IDENTITIES

6.4. Some things to be mindful of when transferring these concepts to your own context

It also feels important to acknowledge that this book is being written by myself whom has, I have worked internationally, including in different parts of Africa, Asia, the Americas, and Australasia, but I am based in London, England. Therefore, I am mindful that different contexts have different words, terms, and specific contextual considerations. We need to be careful to not over-generalize concepts and directly translate ideas or assumptions or programmes from one place to another. In my work across the world, the contextual differences have been huge, whether between countries or on a smaller scale, between one London borough and another.

These differences are multi-layered, varying from the health systems, the education systems, the economies, the politics, the demographic needs and makeup of the sub-population, the histories, the governments and legal structures, the criminal justice systems, the cultural idioms, the access to resources, the competing agendas, the access to public funds, the geographical landscape, the training and different roles of, for example, social worker, surgeon, and psychologist, and the dominant discourses, powers, and narratives the countries are marinated in. Therefore, my hope is that you can absorb and reflect on this chapter and then creatively apply and critically consider it in relation to your own specific setting and context. I am just planting seeds and providing a springboard for further learning and action.

6.5. Intersectionality and the multiplicity of identities

Cultural humility and responsiveness include acknowledging, respecting, reflecting on, honouring, and responding to the intersection of multiple identities (e.g. age, gender, socioeconomic status, religion, spirituality, race, ethnicity, relationship status, health, sexuality), as well as other elements of difference and identity. This means that highlighting the multiplicity of individuals' and communities' lived experiences is central to an intersectional analysis (Hankivsky et al., 2010).

The term intersectionality was originally coined by Kimberlé Crenshaw around the experience of bias experienced by Black women due to both their race and gender; however, it is now often more widely used and applied. Intersectionality includes the multiplicity of these identities and narratives, like a kaleidoscope or a tapestry. This lens sees people as unique individuals, within their wider context, and among the landscape of their experiences, and not as an homogenous group. Marsella (2011) uses the term 'society as a patient', which is about not locating all things within the individual, and understanding that someone's wellbeing or struggles are often about wider contextual issues and the external environment. This also fits with the concept of re-contextualizing.

Seeing people through an intersectional lens also considers layers and the possible spiral of oppression, exclusion, and devalued identities. For example:

- Being a woman, being Black, being unemployed, and being in a wheelchair.

- Being a woman, wearing a hijab, seeking asylum in the UK from persecution for being part of the LGBTQI community.

- Being an elderly man from the Irish travelling community, who is also deaf.

- Being a teenage parent who is also pregnant and is Black, who has speech and language difficulties, and is in the foster care system.

This intersectionality and re-contextualizing also extends to layering of experiences and contexts; for example, my grandparents survived the Holocaust and escaped to South Africa where they then lived in Apartheid; or there were those who fled Syria and then had to live in a refugee camp, and then were moved to a different context such as inner-city London or Northern Ireland. We should also consider the nuances within these threads of identity; for example, someone from Rwanda might be seen by services as Rwandan, or even broader, as African, but in Rwanda, there are numerous different ethnic groups, religions, and languages, and then there are all the other threads that make up a person's unique personal, family, cultural, and societal identity. And to each person, these aspects will mean different things and hold different weighting. So we need to think about the different aspects of identity, and within them which may be visible, voiced, invisible, and unvoiced, and the different weight and meaning different people give to the different parts of their identity, at different times, and when communicating to different people. Another example is the views, assumptions, and expectations around sex, sexual expressions, and sexuality (everyone will be different and attribute different meanings and levels of importance and influence) and how these might change for someone with a learning disability, or for a woman, or someone who identifies as transgender, or for someone in a wheelchair.

There are also other aspects which are often neglected in discussions around culture, such as whiteness and how the nuances within this are often overshadowed, different religions (e.g. Catholic, Jewish), country of origin (e.g. Bosnia, Russia, Northern Ireland), being from a travelling community, and so on. This intersectionality and disparities in health care and systems will be expanded on throughout this chapter. What also is crucial is to think about our own biases, hotspots, interest areas, personal experiences, and so on. While writing this book and throughout my work, I have constantly reflected on my own privilege, blind spots, attentional bias, and so on, and I invite the reader to do the same, in a safe and compassionate way.

★ Pause for a moment, to think about some of the intersectionality and nuances within these different aspects of identity. What assumptions, biases, expectations, and so on do we have within these? Hold in mind the different meaning and weighting people and others place on these aspects; and the ones which are visible, invisible, voice, or unvoiced. Consider these things further as you move through this chapter and in the encounters that you have.

6.6. Biases, inequalities, and disparities in service provision and system experiences

Remember that it is acknowledged that these are far more nuanced than presented here and will differ depending on the context, the individual, the setting, and many more factors.

When a person or team or organization is working towards cultural humility and responsiveness it is important to consider social inequalities, differences, biases, disparities in the intervention, engagement, and approach towards different people. This also includes the blocks and obstacles people might have in accessing and utilizing the services. Often, it is not the people but the services that are 'hard to reach', particularly as there can be huge cultural invisibility and overrepresentation within these areas. This is often not given sufficient attention in the trauma-informed world, but it is important when undertaking a baseline assessment of one's organization/team to support the direction of travel and the needs analysis.

6.6.1. Learning/intellectual disabilities

There are many reports and studies of disparities in service provision for those with a learning/intellectual disability. For example, when studies have looked at those with a learning/intellectual disability accessing mainstream services for their physical health, a range of barriers have been highlighted, including communication difficulties, resulting from individuals with intellectual disability being excluded from consultations (Ward *et al.*, 2010; Wullink *et al.*, 2009), GPs not conducting certain blood tests and investigations, a lack of health promotion and screening (Broughton & Thomson, 2000), and a lack of transport and accessible buildings (Gibson, 2010). Studies have also shown an inadequate knowledge of doctors about the health needs of people with an intellectual disability (Fisher *et al.*, 2005; Minnes & Steiner, 2009), which has contributed to diagnostic overshadowing. Diagnostic overshadowing occurs where signs and symptoms arising from physical or emotional health difficulties are misattributed to the individual's intellectual disability. Studies have also found that some health professionals exhibited more negative attitudes and behaviour towards individuals with an intellectual disability (Dinsmore, 2012; Webber *et al.*, 2010). Also, in line with this, Thiara and colleagues (2011) shared that unless women who were disabled made explicit disclosures of abuse, social workers and other professionals were unlikely to recognize signs of partner abuse because they tended to focus on the disability and minimize or discount other possible factors and experiences.

6.6.2. Gender-specific and race differences

There are also numerous studies of how intervention and treatment decision-making can be impacted by factors including race, disability, gender, weight, and many more biases. One disparity worth mentioning is gender-specific differences; for example, women in pain being positioned as 'emotional' or 'psychological', whereas men in pain were positioned as 'stoic, brave, strong'. There are also numerous reports showing how women are more likely to be viewed or described as 'hormonal', 'menopausal', 'sensitive', 'exaggerating', 'highly strung', or 'hysterical'. Other studies show that women are more likely to be disbelieved and have their symptoms invalidated or minimized. There are also several papers about the androcentric (focused or centred on men) bias within health care, with differences and omissions in research where women have been included, and about women-specific conditions, with a lack of inclusion of aspects such as hormones, periods, and menopause. We also know that there are lots of reports of how women going through menopause have their symptoms missed, minimized, or attributed to depression, and are often treated by anti-depressants. Moreover, 'borderline personality disorder' can be seen as a highly feminized diagnosis, with more than 75% of those diagnosed being women (Ussher, 2013).

To illustrate a gender-specific disparity, an example is offered in myocardial infarction presentation and survival; however, this could also be considered in a range of other areas where there has been little funding or examination as to how different conditions might present differently in women. While members of both genders present with chest pain, women often present with what is known as 'atypical' symptoms such as nausea, vomiting, and palpitations (Kawamoto *et al.*, 2016; Mehta *et al.*, 2016). The mention of 'atypical' in the literature is misleading given that women make up half of an average population. However, some large cohort studies have found increased in-hospital mortality of 15–20% for female patients compared with male patients. Interviews with 2985 patients under the age of 55 who had suffered myocardial infarctions revealed that women were 7.4% more likely to seek medical attention and were 16.7% less likely to be told their symptoms were cardiac in origin. This indicates a need for education of public and health care professionals alike about the symptoms of a myocardial infarction in women (Hannan *et al.*, 2020; Hao & Liu, 2019; Her *et al.*, 2018; Wei *et al.*, 2017). For a fascinating and important spotlight on women and health with a focus on the historical context, I recommend Elinor Cleghorn's (2021) book, *Unwell Women: A Journey through Medicine and Myth in a Man-Made World*.

This, alongside other economic and race disparities, was echoed in a study by Schulman in 1999 who asked thousands of doctors to test their clinical acumen by reviewing a medical history given by an actor who acted out the symptoms of potential cardiac syndrome. There were eight elderly patients. Four were men, four were women, two identified themselves as white, and two identified as Black. Doctors were asked to recommend a cardiac workup. They were also told if the patient was insured or not insured (or course, there are system differences depending on whether the country requires insurance or offers free health care). Based on the gender, race, and insurance of the patient, doctors recommended different medical workups. Men of both races were more likely to be referred than women for angiograms, but those who were Black were less likely to be referred for further tests. Those who were insured were more likely to be referred, which demonstrates some possible disparities.

6.6.3. Black maternal health, some diagnoses, and Covid-19

Other examples of disparities are around medical racism, discrimination, and biases which are likely to influence health care at a range of levels, including unequal treatment/access and differences in decision-making; and around which populations, medications, symptoms, and treatments are studied, included, or excluded in clinical trials, and researched. For example, research done in the US (echoed in many other countries) indicated that across virtually every type of diagnostic and treatment intervention people who are Black and from other minoritized backgrounds receive fewer procedures and poorer quality medical care than people who are white do (Smedley *et al.*, 2003; van Ryn & Burke, 2000). It has also been suggested that providers' implicit bias is also associated with poorer quality of patient-provider communication, including the provider's non-verbal behaviour (Cooper *et al.*, 2012). It has also been shown in some studies that those who are Black are less likely to be prescribed pain medication in emergency and A&E departments (Tamayo-Sarver *et al.*, 2003).

Similarly, in 2018, the MBRRACE-UK report revealed that maternal and perinatal mortality in pregnancy was five times higher in Black women compared with white women, and these findings have been replicated in US data, with a similar order of magnitude of three to four times. There have been numerous reports, TV programmes, and books written around some of the inequalities and medical racism within maternity care, including lower levels of quality care, poorer experiences of maternity care, and possible adverse perinatal outcomes (Henderson, 2013; Knight *et al.*, 2018; Lewis & Drife, 2004; Patrick & Bryan, 2005; Pollock, 2004; Puthussery, 2016; Straus, 2009).

In line with this, the Covid-19 pandemic emphasized existing health inequalities among numerous areas for marginalized and underrepresented communities (Niedzwiedz *et al.*, 2021; Raharja *et al.*, 2021; Sze *et al.*, 2020). Additionally, Brooke and Jackson (2020) found that some public discourse during Covid devalued older people through media reportage, where some of the deaths of older people in nursing homes were not reported. This created the impression that some lives were not as significant as others or that deaths were expected and inevitable.

Moreover, some of these differences and disparities can also be seen around diagnosis. For example, diagnoses of schizophrenia have consistently been found to be elevated in African and Caribbean groups within the UK when compared with their white counterparts (Bhui *et al.*, 2018).

6.6.4. Those without a home or often referred to as 'homeless' and from a lower socioeconomic position

Those who might be living without a home or who are living on the streets are likely to be experiencing additional social and structural inequalities, including social exclusion, rejection, and dislocation and possible chronic loneliness. We know that those who experience homelessness often have poorer health outcomes, including higher incidence of ill health, head and body injuries, and chronic pain, as well as often not having access to a consistent primary health care provider and being less likely to be able to access preventative interventions such as cervical screenings, blood pressure checks, eye examinations, and so on. Discrimination and stigma can be common among those experiencing homelessness. In one study, people described unwelcoming health care encounters, including these feeling rude, rushed, and dehumanizing. People shared about the felt impact of gestures and microaggressions, such as moving away, disgusted facial expressions, sniffing. Some reported feeling dismissed, or having their complaints minimized or trivialized (Rae & Rees, 2015; Upshur *et al.*, 2006, 2010; Wen *et al.*, 2007). These people are also more likely to be exposed to harsher weather conditions and have less access to nutritious food and medication. Additionally, when homeless, people are more likely to experience trauma, such as being a 'victim' or witness of an attack, a sexual assault, harassment, or any other violent event.

These biases and differences can also be extended to stereotypes and negative responses and perceptions of those in a lower socioeconomic status/class. For example, some common descriptors used to describe people living in poverty or of a lower economic status include uneducated, lazy, dirty, stupid, immoral, criminal, and violent (Cozzarelli *et al.*, 2001; Kemeny *et al.*, 2012). Anecdotal reports and studies have also shown that some health care providers also hold these stereotypes. For example, they may perceive people with lower socioeconomic status as having more negative personality characteristics, lower levels of intelligence, and being less likely to be adherent to or to want an active lifestyle (van Ryn & Burke, 2000). While this is a complex and multi-layered area, studies also show that children living in poverty and those identified as having a low economic status are more likely to have contact with social services and to be taken into care (Drake *et al.*, 2003; Fluke *et al.*, 2003; Sinclair *et al.*, 2007).

See Chapter 2 for more on poverty and health.

6.6.5. Racism and disparities across the board, including in hospitals, child welfare, prisons, and schools

We see disparities and inequalities throughout all areas of society and in numerous contexts; for example, in countries such as the US and the UK, the overrepresentation of people from Black and other minoritized communities in child protection and at risk of being removed or known to social services/child welfare, in prison and/or known to the youth justice system, being sectioned and restrained in psychiatric hospitals, being detained, being restrained in residential and children's homes, and being excluded and secluded from school. There have been shown to be differential outcomes within child welfare for children and families, and this includes racial bias being present in decision-making and seen as a key factor in the differential outcome (Dettlaff *et al.*, 2011; Rivaux *et al.*, 2008). Moreover, Black children are less likely to be identified by and provided with access to early intervention services and programmes, such as those for autism spectrum disorder (Boyd *et al.*, 2018). And similarly, McManus *et al.* (2020) found that Black children were less likely than white children to be referred for early intervention, and practitioners were more likely to minimize parental developmental concerns and developmental screening results and attribute them to social factors such as poverty rather than clinical factors.

There have also been numerous studies and reports that people who are Black are more likely to be positioned as 'angry and aggressive' and to be criminalized. Moreover, it has been found that there is more likely to be harsh and punitive treatment of Black children, with Black children more likely to be viewed as older, more culpable, and less empathetic, leading to possible adultification (Cooke & Halberstadt, 2021), as well as the lower expectations and learning opportunities provided to Black children (Gardner-Neblett *et al.*, 2021).

More on the impact of discrimination and racism on health is shared in Chapter 2.

6.6.6. Refugees and asylum-seekers

Another example of health care biases and disparities occurs with refugees and asylum-seekers. Of course, there is huge variation in this area. However, Gee and Ford (2011) showed how immigration policy can influence health disparities both by modulating direct access through the introduction of different levels of coverage and through indirect obstacles stemming from racism, including xenophobia. This messaging around scarce resources, abuse, and fraud of the system and many others can bias practitioners and lead to institutional discrimination, which is likely to impact practice (Haider *et al.*, 2011; Shavers *et al.*, 2012; Stepanikova & Cook, 2008; van Ryn & Burke, 2000). Moreover, people from culturally and linguistically diverse backgrounds (particularly those who do not speak the language of the 'host' country) have often received disparate quality of care, with their access also limited by a range of factors.

Some of these biases and disparities are highlighted in a report by the Equality and Human Rights Commission (2018) called *The lived experiences of access to healthcare for people seeking and refused asylum*. The first category of findings is titled 'We are people too'. This discusses how some people felt they were treated inhumanely, unequally, or with little respect or dignity, and often were not believed. The second category of the report describes some of the barriers that the people in the study experienced in accessing health care that met their needs. This included things like lack of information, difficulty navigating the system, immigration interviews, proceedings and dispersal taking precedence over their health, not having enough money to access services or pay for them, 'living in fear' about how their personal data might be used, and being unable to overcome language barriers.

6.6.7. The LGBTQI community

Members of the LGBTQI community have often reported discrimination, stigma, negative stereotypes, and detrimental biases within service provision and health care. This includes perceived and actual discrimination which impacted seeking support and trusting practitioners.

Within the disparities, many clinicians and practitioners shared that they felt they lacked the skills, training, or confidence to work to their best ability with people from the LGBTQI community (FitzGerald & Hurst, 2017; Grant *et al.*, 2010; Lambda Legal, 2010; Shires & Jaffee, 2015); including understanding aspects such as pronouns and use of language. Of course, this will vary depending on person, context, and time of research, but there have also been more reports of judgements and negative attitudes, as well as people feeling uncomfortable among some health care professionals (Burke *et al.*, 2015; Khan *et al.*, 2008).

Additionally, and holding in the mind the intersectionality, qualitative research has found that those who identify as being lesbian and gay and who are also seeking asylum are subjected to inappropriate questioning by staff from the UK Visas and Immigration Agency (Danisi *et al.*, 2021). Another example of this is barriers found within accessing domestic and sexual violence services, where services are primarily designed with heterosexual, cisgender women in mind (Harvey *et al.*, 2014). Moreover, Stonewall (Aldridge & Somerville, 2014; Guasp, 2010) found that those who identified as LGBTQI and who were also older adults were more worried about the prospect of going into a care home compared to heterosexual people, and were more likely to feel as if they could not be themselves in an older adult residential or nursing setting. In addition, 41% of respondents reported that they would expect to be discriminated against at a residential home; and one-third of respondents stated that they would be uncomfortable being open about their sexual orientation or gender identity with social care staff.

6.6.8. Being in a wheelchair

A survey of over 2300 primary care facility sites in California between 2006 and 2010 found that only 3.6% had a wheelchair-accessible weight scale, and 8.4% a height-adjustable exam table and the basic equipment necessary for people with a range of mobility needs to transfer safely for examinations (Mudrick *et al.*, 2010). Equipment inaccessibility in many outpatient provider offices led to fewer preventive tests, missed diagnoses, and delayed care.

I have personal experience of this form of bias and inequality through my mother, who has multiple sclerosis and is in a wheelchair. She was told she could not have a mammogram as they could not adjust the equipment for someone in a wheelchair, and they only had access to standing scales. They did not offer a solution or recommend how this could be done or signpost to where it could be done, but rather were dismissive. Not only does my mum have a family history of breast cancer and so it is crucial to be screened, but this also left her feeling like a burden, embarrassed and uncared for. This is someone who is articulate, patient, and accommodating. Thankfully, we persisted and were able to get the mammogram; however, some would not have done so and their loved one would have gone unseen or been put off future health encounters. Sadly, my mother had a similar experience where she was told the clinic didn't have the facilities to give her a smear test as they couldn't move her onto a bed to carry out the procedure.

Moreover, she recently broke her leg from a fall from the toilet. She received a range of responses around not needing pain killers, not being able to be lifted into a hospital bed, and not having surgery which other people would have had to support their recovery, as well as experiencing some minimizing, non-creative, and ableist ways of thinking. There are endless other examples, such as hospital transport not arriving or arriving two hours late, resulting in missed appointments and then her being blamed or labelled as 'not wanting treatment', 'not turning up', and so on; or encountering buildings that are not accessible and incredibly difficult to navigate, with narrow corridors, broken lifts, non-automatic doors, unreachable leaflets, high desks, and so on.

6.6.9. Those who are deaf

Many studies report that people who are deaf can encounter communication barriers when accessing health services. They experience fear, mistrust, and frustration, as well as difficulties exchanging information, understanding treatment and advice, and expressing symptoms (Chaveiro *et al.*, 2009; Pereira & Fortes, 2010; Scheier, 2009; Smeijers & Pfau, 2009).

Various reports reveal that people can feel patronized and treated as if they are stupid, or made to feel like a burden or a source of irritation. One report from the UK showed that 44% of those patients who identified as deaf found the last contact with their GP or health centre to be difficult or very difficult, compared with only 17% from a general population patient survey (NHS England, 2015; SignHealth, 2013).

Getting in contact with emergency services has also been a challenge for deaf people for many years. Research about people with disabilities in acute care settings found that the presence of a physical communication problem (deafness and blindness) was significantly associated with an increased risk of experiencing a preventable adverse event (Bartlett *et al.*, 2008). Harris and Bamford (2001) noted that the NHS routinely operates systems which rely on hearing, such as shouting patients' names when the health practitioner is ready to see them or when it is their turn. Moreover, during the writing of this book, some colleagues who are deaf shared with me how confusing, stress-inducing, and difficult it can be when, for example, undergoing a procedure or having to have an emergency caesarean and they couldn't communicate or hear what was happening to them and had to rely on either a stranger or a family member to explain.

There can also be less access to information about health, for example on the radio or TV, as well as fewer education materials provided in sign language (Pollard & Barnett, 2009). For example, knowledge and awareness related to the spread of HIV was found to be lacking among deaf populations in Nigeria, Swaziland, Brazil, and the US (Bisol *et al.*, 2008; Goldstein *et al.*, 2010; Groce *et al.*, 2007). Among a sample of 203 adults who were deaf in the US, over 60% could not list any stroke symptoms, whereas in hearing adults only 30% were not able to list any stroke symptoms; only 49% of the people who were deaf could list chest pain/pressure as a heart attack symptom, whereas 90% in a US population-based survey could do so (Margellos-Anast *et al.*, 2006). There have also been similar concerns raised in other areas, for example cancer, dementia, and pregnancy.

6.6.10. Some additional and concluding thoughts

Sometimes, these biases are much more subtle – a look, a comment, an assumption. At other times, they feed into the set-up and running of a service, such as how someone is supported when form-filling if they can't read or write, or how accessible interpreters are, or how a waiting room or physical environment considers different cultural experiences.

These are just a small selection of how disparities and biases can be seen within our systems. There are many more I have not discussed as they are beyond the scope of this book. These examples are simply shared to give you a flavour, and to increase your awareness, before you reflect on your specific organization.

It is important to consider how these biases might shape or influence relationships, decision-making, and other health-related behaviours. For example, a 2017 review and meta-analysis of studies on discrimination and health service utilization revealed that perceived discrimination was inversely related to positive experiences with regards to health care (e.g. satisfaction with care or perceived quality of care) and reduced adherence to medical regimens and delaying or not seeking health care (Ben *et al.*, 2017). We know this can also lead to difficulties with trust, which inevitably can have multi-layered consequences on someone's health and health care.

★ Having read the above section on disparities and system biases, what reflections have you had? How can you proactively respond to these and take them forward? Which others would you add?

★ Think about what values and characteristics preference someone over another person, and how our own biases and lenses colours these. For example, if the world was coming to an end and there was a room where people could be saved, who would you save and why? Would it be an elderly priest, a pregnant woman, a doctor, a person in a wheelchair, a person who has just got out of prison?

★ Think about some of the labels, words, sensations, biases, stereotypes, images, songs, movies, headlines, and so on that arise when you reflect on a particular group of people. How does your own lens, background, experiences, beliefs, and attitudes influence, shape, and guide this? Which groups are brought to the forefront and given more weight? Which are neglected, avoided, or attended to less?

6.7. A spotlight on some cultural idioms, scripts, and perceptions of aetiology

We know that there can be very different perceptions of the aetiology of ill health, and expressions of distress can vary across cultures, as can roles, rituals, beliefs, scripts, narratives, discourses, and explanations (this refers to socially and culturally resonant means of experiencing and expressing distress in local worlds; Nichter, 2010, p.405). This includes the variability and nuance of meaning attached to aspects such as wellbeing, healing, health, and trauma. These perceptions of the aetiology of ill health can also influence how events, concepts, and experiences are appraised, expressed, and experienced.

One example of this was given in one of my research theses, which explored women from different countries in Africa and their meaning-making around being diagnosed with HIV during their pregnancy at their 12-week check. One of the key qualitative findings was around how influential people's individual, family, and wider representations, discourses, narratives, and scripts were in their subsequent coping, attributions, and assumptions about HIV. For example, there were differences in whether they saw HIV as a chronic illness, like diabetes, or as a death sentence, or as being a punishment from God, or a message from an ancestor, or a condition that was only for certain types of people, like 'prostitutes' or 'gays'. These discourses, assumptions, and narratives also seemed to be influenced by different linguistic labels, adding weight to the power of language and the meaning it conveys. These findings were echoed in research by Koku (2010), who illustrated how HIV was often referred to in various African countries by certain linguistic terms, such as *maiti inayotembea* (a walking corpse), used in Tanzania; *makizi yaku mochari* (the keys to the mortuary), used in Zambia; and *menfese mute* (a ghost), used in Ethiopia.

Some other interesting examples of cultural idioms which could influence and impact what we see in health care settings include those seen in Traditional Chinese Medicine, where some illnesses are ascribed to a lack of balance between pathogenic factors of yin and yang; in Ayurveda, one of the main traditional healing systems in India, 'mental health difficulties' (as seen in the western world) may be perceived to be a product of karma or one's actions (Haque, 2010; Kirmayer, 2004). And among some Native American people, ill health is thought to be caused or contributed to by imbalance, loss of harmony, and being dispirited with oneself due to a loss of vital connectedness.

Other people and cultures may ascribe the onset of 'disease' to possession by spirits, the 'evil eye', black magic, or the breaking of taboos. For example, in Northern Uganda, for some people, ill health is seen through a version of 'cen', which is referred to as 'spiritual possession'. Some young people who were abducted and forced into recruitment (often referred to as child soldiers) have shared that their identity has been taken over by the ghost of the dead person who the child was forced to kill. Some of these behaviours and presentations might be seen as psychosis in other contexts and when viewed through a different lens.

Religion, belief systems, and spirituality can also play a key part in these perceptions (Hechanova & Waelde, 2017). For instance, in the UK health care systems, and many other countries, albinism is generally seen as a skin condition. However (this is shifting and of course is more nuanced and doesn't apply to all people), in Tanzania, albinism can be seen as the result of a curse, or as the omen of a disaster (Bucaro, 2010). In Namibia, people with albinism can be thought of as cannibals and as being contagious (Ntinda, 2009); and in Zimbabwe, as well as other countries in the region, some believe that having sex with someone who is identified as being an albino will bring a cure for those living with HIV/AIDS (Baker *et al.*, 2010), along with many other explanations (Taylor *et al.*, 2019). Similarly, in some countries, epilepsy can be viewed as the person being possessed by evil spirits and is often thought to be highly contagious; whereas, in other countries, it is generally seen as a neurological condition.

Another example of a cultural idiom is where emotions often labelled in the UK as sadness or fear are known in Zimbabwe by some as *Kufungisisa*, which is a Shona-language term that translates as 'thinking too much'. This is regarded as both a cause and a symptom of illness. Some people believe that 'thinking too much' can cause pain and feelings of physical pressure on the heart and they offer responses and interventions according to this belief.

Similarly, another instance of where symptoms are felt or described differently is from Cambodia where some people talk about 'kyal cap' or 'wind attacks', manifesting as dizziness, palpitations, shortness of breath. This is based on the belief that 'kyal', a wind-like substance, rises in the body and causes various problems and that it is 'triggered' by worrying thoughts, specific odours linked to bad memories, being in crowded spaces, and so on. Similarly, many people described kyal and also 'thinking a lot' as their more common trauma reactions and responses following the Cambodian genocide than most of the DSM-5 PTSD symptoms (Hinton *et al.*, 2015), which argues for being mindful of some of these idioms in the assessment of trauma reactions for this group of people.

Building on the above around conceptualizations of trauma, in a study in Nepal, Kohrt and Hruschka (2010) found that some survivors of trauma conceptualized 'negative' events as karma, related to past life sins, which caused certain feelings, including guilt. In Japan, however, social image (e.g. maintaining face) for some people was a prominent theme in the context of trauma, and in other cultures, there was more emphasis on aspects such as honour (Mesquita & Walker, 2003); in others, the trauma was interpreted by some as ancestors withdrawing their favour and protective function from an individual (Eagle & Kaminer, 2013). These beliefs, discourses, conceptualizations, and explanations are likely to shape how someone might feel, think, and respond.

Another area of interest is how the concept of trauma and the diagnostic category of PTSD varies across cultures. As shared in Chapter 1, many people have become increasingly critical of the universal applicability of a narrowly biomedical model, based on western notions of trauma (Papadopoulos, 2007; Quosh & Gergen, 2008; Summerfield, 2004). This is not to deny that trauma can be usefully conceptualized in biological and psychological terms, but that an over-emphasis on symptomology can result in the divorce of the mind from the body, the individual from the community, and the community from the environment. It is essential to consider the cultural, historical, familial, political, and individual meaning of the symptoms and signals, which are shaped by a range of factors, including history and culture. For example, in many countries, nightmares are designated as a symptom of PTSD, yet whether they are reported will depend on whether an individual or a society regards them as problematic. In some cultures, nightmares are viewed as conveying ancestors' messages, and as indicators of the person's spiritual status.

This wider and differing conceptualization of trauma is highlighted by Afana *et al.* (2010), in a study of how Palestinian communities have processed continual exposure to war (ongoing insidious trauma) through particular linguistic constructs of trauma, such as *Sadma* (trauma as a sudden blow with immediate impact), *Faji'ah* (tragedy), and *Musiba* (calamity). *Sadma* is used metaphorically to refer to painful events that happen suddenly, *Faji'ah* is used to describe the reaction to an extraordinary event (mainly the loss of a loved one), and *Musiba* is used when traumatic events are persistent and have long-term consequences. Interestingly, Honwana (1997) explains that the local understanding of post-war trauma in both Mozambique and Angola can be associated with the anger of the spirits of those people killed during the war. Individuals who have been in a war therefore can be believed to be 'polluted' by the social transgressions of the war, therefore they must be 'cleansed' to ensure collective protection against this pollution and to facilitate their social reintegration into society.

In addition to this, and family, cultural, and societal discourses, there can also be the lingering impact of medical racism, institutional racism, and historical racism, such as medical experimentation and eugenic programmes like the Tuskegee experiment, and experiments during the world wars.

Variations are also reflected in the terms or words used, for example people are more likely to use the words 'suffering' and 'hurt' than 'trauma'. It also has been found in many studies that in different cultures people can be more likely to describe somatic and body-based feelings and symptoms; for example, in Salvador, feelings that might be described in the UK as anxiety, fear, and anger were talked about as an intense body heat. Similarly, Weissbecker *et al.* (2018) described how words and terms related to the heart – some of the idioms used were *poil-heart* meaning 'heavy hearted' in Krio in Sierra Leone; or in Somalia, *qalbi-jab* meaning 'broken heart'; or *qalb maaboud* meaning 'squeezed heart' in Arabic (referring to dysphoria and sadness), and *houbout el qalb* meaning 'falling or crumbling of the heart' (referring to the somatic response of sudden fear).

These examples give a small indication of how important it is to be respectful and curious, and mindful of our own biases, and for the person, family, and community to be able to define for themselves the meaning of their culture and cultural experiences.

These differences have implications for people's meaning-making, for the appropriateness, adaptation, and sensitivity of assessment and measuring tools, for engagement with services, and for the interventions offered. This includes consideration of the complexities around language, choice of words, use of acronyms, choice of practitioner, and accessibility of language and materials, as well as aspects such as the applicability, inclusiveness, and appropriateness of the materials and approaches used. These are also likely to shape and influence people's relationship to illness, help, and professionals, and much more, including their feelings and ability to trust.

Having explored a range of different areas of cultural humility and responsiveness, we will now consider a range of reflective questions.

Box 6.1.

Value and principle – cultural humility and responsiveness expanded

Please read the explanations given in this chapter before considering these questions. They also are multi-layered questions, and each one could take a long time to explore, so are intended as starting platforms and as part of a longer reflective process. Some are practice based and some focus on teams/organizations.

Remember that practising cultural humility and responsiveness is not a formulaic process and needs to be tailored to the unique context and culture of the organization, and thought about through collaboration, curiosity, and reflection. These concepts and ideas will also vary depending on your specific population and demographic.

★ How are people's intersectionality of identities acknowledged, reflected on, and responded to in your team/organization/in the practice? Looking at image 6.1, which areas are brought to the forefront? Which are less prioritized? Are these viewed in multi-layered ways or in stereotyped tick-box ways?

★ How are experiences of community, collective, social, cultural, structural, institutional, and historical trauma, violence, poverty, and oppression, and the different areas of power acknowledged, reflected on, understood, and responded to in your team/organization? How is the political, social, historical, cultural, and financial context being considered?

★ How might these influence and impact on a person's health and relationship to health care and health practitioners?

For example, how might someone's legal status, living situation, and language level be impacting on their health/life/experience?

★ What differences, biases, disparities, and inequalities might there be in the treatment, engagement, and approach of different people? (Read the section on service disparities earlier in the chapter.) For example, the different responses to a young girl who has self-harmed versus a young boy who has; or a Black man who seeks support for hearing voices versus a white man who does the same. What factors may influence a decision, for example around treatment? What obstacles and barriers might there be for certain people or 'groups' around engaging with and accessing the services? How inclusive is the service? How is meaningful feedback gathered to be guided and shaped by a multiplicity of views?

★ What implicit and explicit assumptions/beliefs/attitudes/expectations/biases might there be about… (e.g. someone who identifies as transgender, someone who has a diagnosis of Down syndrome, a man experiencing domestic violence, someone who identifies as being Muslim or Jewish, a single mother of five children)? How might your own biases, meaning-making, judgements, actions, traditions, beliefs, expectations, attitudes, behaviours, assumptions, and perspectives be influencing you?

★ How might your lens and identity be informing how you are approaching…and viewing…? What is your own and your team's meaning-making around… (e.g. mental health, religion, natural healing practice, parenting, gender roles, power dynamics)?

★ What is the cultural meaning of an event or experience for someone? How does their culture see them due to this (e.g. traumatic experience)? What are someone's explanations, attributions, beliefs, attitudes about…? How might… (e.g. nightmares/emotional expression/emotional wellbeing/suicide) be seen differently depending on someone's culture?

★ If there is a cultural difference, where appropriate, is this explored and reflected on; and if there is a similarity between the worker and the family, is this also explored and reflected on, including holding in mind the possibility of over-identification?

★ What aspects of delivery and practice might be representative/ significant/'triggering' for someone else? (See the section on hotspots, activating experiences, and 'triggers' in Chapter 3.) For example, having buildings that are not accessible for those with a disability, which might make them feel like a burden; or making someone fill in forms about their sexuality without options which are inclusive or allow them to opt out.

★ How 'safe' do people feel culturally (in their work as employees and for the people being served)?

★ How is safeguarding still prioritized in the context of cultural differences? What are some of the complexities around this given how so many safeguarding practices are based on western and Eurocentric models? How is there thought, reflection, support, and training around this?

★ Are you considering people's cultural idioms of distress, for example in descriptions about the service, in assessments, and in interventions?

★ How are you supporting each person's own way of defining their own experience?

★ Where appropriate, are you considering and asking questions about, for example, someone's experience of oppression, racism, sexuality?

★ What are the individual, family, community, and societal strengths, resiliencies, and resources? How can these be respected, honoured, learned from, and magnified? What beliefs, resources, or practices support the person in the hardship which they have faced?

★ Is there reflection on the role religion and spirituality might play (e.g. a belief in a higher power, strengthening of faith, a protective factor, a coping resource, access to aspects such as prayer, chanting, meditation, but also, at the other end of the spectrum, institutional abuse, religion being the source of the abuse or trauma, being shunned by a community, negative attributions about the person, such as being sinful or going to hell)? How are ideas around spirituality and cultural scripts considered and interwoven into therapy? How are the arts, the body, and nature interwoven into interventions?

★ How might someone's understanding of a role (e.g. a social worker, nurse, dentist, police officer, foster carer), or of intervention options (e.g. traditional healing, voodoo, mind-body techniques, community approaches, spiritual leaders) differ depending on their intersecting identities?

★ How do you/the team adapt your approach to tailor it to the unique individual (e.g. if they are blind, if they are in a wheelchair, if they have executive function difficulties, if they pray several times a day)?

★ Do intake and outcome forms/reports/IT systems allow for how someone would like to be described and identified? Are there provisions for those who need another option, such as those who don't speak English, those who can't read or write, those who are blind? This also includes aspects such as how someone wants to be described, the country they are from, or a subsection within this.

★ Is there interest in how the person would like to be called, including things like prefixes, personal preferences, and pronunciation? This includes those who have changed their names or parts of their identity.

★ What language and choice of words are used in all documents, including consent forms, assessments, and letters, and in phone calls, on posters, and so on? How relevant and accessible are these? This includes considering local knowledge required, jargon, acronyms, and so on. Are these mindful of stereotyping and negative biases and discourses? Are materials available in different languages/braille? What about those who cannot read or write/those who are blind/those with learning disabilities and so on?

★ Is there access to suitable matched interpreters when needed? Are staff trained in how to work effectively using best practice guidelines of working with interpreters?

★ How are people communicated with via the telephone and/or through the automatic phone system?

★ Is it held in mind that some languages don't have a particular word (e.g. in some languages there is no word for depression)?

★ What materials/website/magazines/leaflets/posters/pictures/art/toys/books/food/spaces are available? How do these consider people's culture and intersection of identities? How accessible and inclusive are these? (It can be helpful to do a walk-through in your mind and then an actual walk-through, and think about different scenarios, as well as get other people in those positions with direct experience to do that walk-through – use worksheet 9.1 in Chapter 9 to support this process.)

★ These will differ depending on need and context but, for example, do doors open easily or have buttons to open them automatically? Is there braille on the lift buttons? Are there prayer rooms? Are the snacks and foods available considerate of different needs and diets? Are the buildings wheelchair accessible? Are signs in different languages? Is there thought around the artwork, posters, and brochures?

★ Is there, where possible, a choice or preference of intervention (e.g. gender or race of therapist, timing of appointment, having another person present)?

★ What tools, models, assessment measures, programmes, and therapies are used? (Most therapies and the disciplines and models we draw on are from western, ethnocentric, individualistic ideas and notions.) How do these account for cultural, identity, learning, and linguistic differences? What population have these measures and approaches been normed and validated on and for? What barriers and hazards might there be with these? How suitable and sensitive are these approaches? Who has been included, or more importantly excluded, in data and research around these treatment options and approaches? Is there an interest in and openness to more culturally sensitive healing processes and forums?

★ How are cultural humility and responsiveness present, infused, and prioritized in the following organizational areas – and what could be improved?

* Performance reviews, appraisals, and human resource processes.

* Team meetings, thinking spaces, reflective practice, and supervision.

* Recruitment and induction.

* Feedback processes and meaningful consultation/co-production.

* Panels, committees, and decision boards.

* The physical environment.

* Policies and procedures.

* Training and professional development.

* Staff wellbeing and wellness.

* The materials, signs, brochures, letters, and the website.

* Assessments, tools used, services available, approaches offered.

* Evaluation and monitoring processes.

* Interactions.

* Treatments and options.

* Type and choice of language.

- ★ Leadership and management style.

- ★ Organization's vision and mission.

★ Which identities and voices are given preference, included, silenced, avoided, neglected, and so on? Who in the organization is often misrepresented, silenced, denied, ignored (within the organization and staff team, and the people being served)? What in the organization gives someone status, power, preference, privilege, access?

★ How are people asked about their identity and their different feelings about different parts of their identity and experience? How curious are we about the whole person? How do services account for considering people's intersection of identities, including in supervision and reflective practice? (Hold in mind that different people will attribute different meaning and weight to different parts, and that these may change and evolve.)

★ Who was the service designed for? How were those people at the forefront of the design, shaping, and delivery of the service? Whose voices are missing? (Hold in mind co-production and partnering.)

★ What is people's experience of power imbalances and inequalities (organizationally and at a service level)? How are aspects such as institutional racism, ageism, and sexism acknowledged, reflected on, named, and responded to? How seriously does the organization act on reports or observations of discrimination, oppression, and so on?

★ Are you/staff members/supervisors 'comfortable' and trained in asking questions and having discussions in ways that reflect an openness, respect, curiosity, and interest in learning about what is important to people about their experiences, culture, and identities? Is there meaningful training on aspects such as racism, cultural humility, and ways to effectively use interpreters?

★ Are you/staff supported to have a space to think about your expectations and assumptions around, for example, someone with Down syndrome, or someone from a particular religious background?

★ Are you/staff able to understand the distinction between gender identity, gender expression, sexual orientation, and so on? Are you able to think about your own biases, values, beliefs, and attitudes around these, and respond fairly and respectfully? Are you able to think about the different pronouns, and be open to the person's preference and feedback around this?

★ How inclusive and diverse is the workforce and recruitment? Are there ways to diversify the recruitment and hiring strategies and to make them more inclusive?

★ Are there meaningful questions in recruitment about cultural humility and responsiveness?

★ How reflective is the organization's workforce of the population being served?

★ How seriously does the organization act on reports or observations of discrimination, oppression, workplace bullying, and so on?

★ Does the induction include aspects such as cultural humility?

★ What are the policies and flexibility around things like Ramadan, Yom Kippur, and Christmas, or different practices around death and mourning, or around timing and choice of meetings or appointment times? Are there provisions in place to support rituals, routines, and traditions (e.g. prayer rooms or separate utensils for cooking)?

★ How does your organization learn from, liaise, connect, and collaborate with influencers and key people in the community?

★ What is in place or needs to be put in place to support the organization to become more culturally responsive? How is culture kept at the forefront? Is there a working group around this or space within an existing working group to discuss and explore the above areas?

★ Is there an organization commitment to be culturally responsive? Is this reflected in the mission, vision, and values of the organization?

★ What are the process, feedback, policies, and procedures should someone feel the above is not being achieved? Do people feel 'safe' to voice and raise these concerns?

What else would you add? What reflections and questions have these stimulated?

This is by no means all that is needed, and it needs to be in collaboration with people who use the service and adapted to the context, but it demonstrates how small changes can make a big difference. For example, here are some suggestions from the literature and surveys of things that could really help those who are deaf. It is hoped that each area would be looked at and considered:

- Accessible ways to make appointments.

- Flashing light or number system for when waiting for an appointment or for the name to be called. Often names are shouted or called out.

- Professionals themselves who are deaf or proficient in sign language (of course, not all people who are deaf use sign language, so there is variation within this). Be mindful that some medical terms are less familiar or harder to interpret to sign language.

- Information, including videos, available with subtitles, captions, and/or in sign language.

- Access to sign language interpreters, including possible on-call interpreters.

- Training for staff on effective use of interpreters, including around seating, eye contact, timing, etc.

- Minicams and text phones.

- Access to be able to text or email health professionals.

- Training and awareness-raising about some of the additional barriers people who are deaf might face and some tools to support improved care.

- Rooms ideally being well lit, quiet, so that they are less distracting and don't have a glare which might interfere with vision.

- Where possible, longer appointment times to allow for a greater quality of communication.

- Thinking about things like fire alarms or evacuations.

- Respect, dignity, compassion, and empathy (as should be the case for all people).

- Specific tailored health education days or preventative check-ups. Some people have found these useful.

CHAPTER 7

What Do We Really Mean by Trauma-Informed?

This chapter presents some of the **definitions, key questions, dilemmas, and myths and misconceptions around trauma-informed change**. Remember that the examples given in this chapter are by no means exhaustive or prescriptive, and need to be expanded on in conversation, practice, training, and consultation, but should provide a springboard for further thought.

7.1. What will be covered in this chapter

- Why do we need a universal trauma-informed approach? How do I apply this?

- What is the difference between trauma-specific and trauma-informed?

- What is the difference between trauma-informed at a practice level and trauma-informed at an organizational level?

- I am a doctor, a nurse, a midwife... I am not here to talk about trauma. What has this got to do with me?

- Does being trauma-informed mean excluding or missing other important aspects? Does being trauma-informed mean that everything is about trauma?

- Is being trauma-informed just for frontline practitioners in the organization? Why is this relevant to people in roles such as business support or domestic staff?

- Is being trauma-informed just about being sweet, nice, and kind?

- Is it enough to just train people in trauma-informed ideas and values?

- What are some of the benefits and strengths of trauma-informed practice and organizational cultural change in health and medical settings?

- What are the key elements of adversity, culturally, and trauma-informed, infused, and responsive practice at an organizational and system level?

- The nine R's.

- What are the core values of trauma-informed practice?

- How are these values linked to trauma and why?

- Some of the anchoring and guiding values.

7.2. Why do we need a universal trauma-informed approach? How do I apply this?

We don't need to know that someone has experienced trauma, adversity, or stress to hold trauma as a possibility and to use a trauma-informed lens.

An adversity, culturally, and trauma-informed, infused, and responsive approach generally advocates for a universal, inclusive, and integrated approach. This is important as it acknowledges the widespread occurrence and systemic nature of trauma, stress, and adversity (including poverty, medical and health trauma, cultural and racial trauma, discriminatory experiences, system and organizational stress and trauma) (see also Chapter 1).

We often don't know (nor do we need to know depending on the context) who has experienced trauma, stress, or adversity, because it isn't within our role, and because trauma can be invisible, silenced, camouflaged, denied, or marinated in secrecy and shame, and it can show itself in many different forms. Due to the very nature of trauma and the sometimes ill-equipped individual, system, and societal responses, it can be difficult to name or disclose, and is often understandably not shared. Furthermore, trauma might have occurred during the in-utero experience or when the child was pre-verbal, or the person may not choose to use the term or label it as 'trauma' or may not conceptualize or view it as such. Therefore, there are multi-layered benefits for everyone at every level of an organization of becoming more adversity, culturally, and trauma-informed, infused, and responsive, and of being more preventative, proactive, compassionate, and healing.

This universal approach is also about stopping people from falling off the radar, as well as preventing people being re-traumatized or having new stressful or traumatic experiences. It doesn't rely on someone having to report or revisit something painful. We don't need to know someone's history to be mindful, empathetic, and to tread gently, to not add hurt or harm unnecessarily. It is helpful to liken this universal approach to how hospitals respond to infections. For example, hospitals assume that everyone receiving services may have a blood-borne infection, so, to reduce the harm, staff take various precautions such as wearing gloves, changing syringes, and cleaning or disposing of items, rather than trying to identify the few people at entry to the hospital who may be infected. They employ a strategy that supports all, is inclusive, prioritizes safety, and aims to reduce time wasted, and avoids people being singled-out and stigmatized. Similarly, it is helpful to use a universal adversity and trauma lens with everyone, especially as we don't know who has experienced adversity and trauma, and this approach is unlikely to cause further harm.

Another example is going to the hospital, and being expected to wear a gown when you are going to have an x-ray, a mammogram, or other procedure. The gown is often see-through, white, or a pale colour, with a string or Velcro fastening at the back, so your body is often exposed and not fully covered. Sometimes, people are also required to walk through the corridors of a clinic or a hospital or stand or sit in rooms waiting to be seen. For some people, being naked or poorly covered can be extremely stressful, humiliating, and 'triggering'; it can make them feel vulnerable and undignified. It may be reminiscent of other experiences or 'trigger' certain feelings or sensations from their current or past experiences (see Chapters 3 and 4). For others, it is uncomfortable and unpleasant but tolerable, and there are some people who are indifferent to the experience and feel relaxed and happy, and will go with the flow.

We don't know who is coming to the hospital that day, but we can take a universal approach and make the gown procedure much more comfortable. The people who don't notice and are indifferent won't be bothered or impacted by these changes; for the people who were uncomfortable with it, changes will hopefully increase their comfort; and importantly, for the people who were feeling exposed, distressed, and 'triggered', it will likely make a big difference to their experience and engagement with the service, which will also have a ripple effect on the staff's experience, on the efficiency of the procedure, and on the person being willing to engage in future interactions. This is the essence of a universal approach. You could apply this to so many processes, from assessments, to searches, to transitions.

Now let's look at another example of a universal process, in the context of doing a smear test and how this can be done differently. This also illustrates some of the differences between a trauma-informed approach and a trauma-specific intervention.

A person undertaking a smear test is not expected to deliver a trauma-specific intervention or to process or work on someone's trauma. Nor are they expected to ask probing or inappropriate questions about, for example, the person's history or experiences of trauma. They are not expected to be a therapist or to know the intricacies of how trauma might impact that person. It is not within their skillset, their role, or the time slot in which they have been allotted to do the smear test. However, a trauma-informed approach involves the person doing the smear test using their knowledge of trauma (including how it might impact the body, regulation, 'triggers') and bearing in mind the values of trauma-informed practice, such as safety, trust, communication, transparency, choice, cultural humility, agency, and mastery to improve and support the task.

For most people, a smear test is likely to be unpleasant, but for some having an item inserted into their vagina by a stranger in a clinical environment, with their legs spread apart, can be exposing, painful, activating. When someone comes in for a smear test, we don't know what their past experiences might have been around:

- previous smear tests and other internal examinations

- possible sexual abuse, sexual assault, sexual violence, or rape

- their relationship to touch, sex, or to their body

- their experiences within health, sexual health, and medical settings

- their possible family, friends, or own history of cervical cancer and worrying news after a smear test

- pregnancy, fertility processes, abortion, or other gynaecological issues

- their experiences with periods and/or going through menopause

- possible experience of female genital mutilation.

For some, it might be uncomfortable and unpleasant, but for others – and we don't know who this may be – it might 'trigger' feelings of fear, vulnerability, powerlessness, and helplessness. Moreover, many people are likely to be in a more heightened state, having to undergo an uncomfortable procedure, done by a stranger, and so might feel their stress levels rise and might experience things like tensing their muscles.

The person undergoing the smear test does not have a responsibility to share their past history with a stranger they are seeing for just a few minutes – and in many cases, the person doing the procedure doesn't need to know. So, we can take a universal approach that everyone coming in might find it uncomfortable, unpleasant, and stressful, and some might find it 'triggering' or trauma-inducing. The people who are fine and less worried about smear tests won't be harmed by a more thoughtful approach, but it will make a big difference to those who are worried, not just for that smear test but potentially for future smear tests. They may go home and share their experience with friends and family members to encourage them to have smear tests, and it will benefit their overall relationship and future engagement with health practitioners.

A trauma-informed universal approach (different from trauma-specific) might involve things like thoughtfulness and transparency in the information provided before the smear test (e.g. letters, phone calls, on the website, in infographics, and possibly in videos); the set-up of the room and the physical environment; the positioning of the chair and the person; the way touch and consent are discussed; the use of regulating and grounding items or activities before and during the procedure; the language used (e.g. not saying things like 'spread your legs'); showing the person empathy, validation, and compassion around the procedure; clearly communicating with the person what is happening; the person doing the procedure being regulated and grounded themselves; giving options and choice; and thinking about the person's privacy and who they might like with them. Many of these ideas are expanded on in Chapter 8.

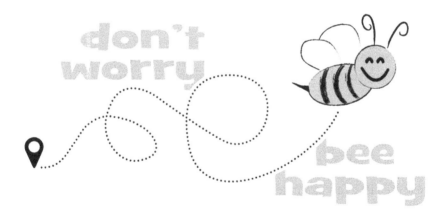

7.1 EXAMPLE OF POSTER

Similarly, a universal lens can be used for posters or signs on the wall (see image 7.1). Imagine walking into a waiting or treatment room and seeing posters on the wall with the messages 'Be happy' and 'Keep calm and carry on'. I am sure the person who put it up on the wall had good intentions and from their lens it is positive and welcoming (I am not criticizing these posters, which many find inspirational, but merely offering them as an example of the need to take a universal approach to avoid inducing stress or trauma). Some people entering the space will probably like the poster or be indifferent and not even notice it; however, here are some examples from a possible a trauma and remember we don't know who will be entering our spaces including ourselves and colleagues as not us and them; we do not have emotional x-rays:

- Someone was raped last night, and now needs to have a medical examination and speak to the police about the trauma about the trauma and they look at the wall and see 'be happy, keep calm and carry on'.

- Someone has just had two family members die of Covid and another is on a ventilator. 'Be happy, keep calm and carry on.'

- Someone has just been diagnosed with terminal cancer. 'Be happy, keep calm and carry on.'

- Someone has just had to catch three buses to get to the hospital, doesn't have electricity in their meter, hasn't eaten for two days, has a broken boiler, and is likely to get hit and hurt by their partner that evening. They are then told they have missed their appointment, or the doctor has called in sick. 'Be happy, keep calm and carry on.'

- Someone has just had a stillborn baby after years of IVF. 'Be happy, keep calm and carry on.'

- Someone has just attempted to jump in front of a train and is talking about suicide. 'Be happy, keep calm and carry on.'

- Someone has been told their whole life to 'grow a pair', to 'man up', and that 'big boys don't cry'; or they have been marinated in messages around the need to smile and say they are fine, but the person working with them says it's okay to be not okay, it's okay to cry. 'Be happy, keep calm and carry on.'

These are just a few examples to illustrate why universal approaches are important. Another example of breastfeeding posters is shared in Chapter 9. This is not to say that there shouldn't be additional support, assessment, and specific trauma interventions for those who might want or need them, but we can take a universal approach as well. This is about connection and integration (a core value of trauma-informed practice).

This is the same when applied organizationally. For example, I might be a manager who has to support a change process or a restructure. I might have some team members who love and welcome change, and they might be excited and champion it. I might have some team members who are ambivalent or on the fence. I might have some team members who are apprehensive, worried, and less keen about it. I might have some who are not on board and who disagree and oppose it. I don't know which of my staff members struggle with change or what change means or represents to them, or how for some change can be activating. But if I take a universal approach as a manager, using trauma-informed values to support and navigate the change process, the ones who are happy may think it is a bit much, but it is likely to do no harm to them; for those who might be struggling, this approach can make a big difference to them and this will likely have ripple effects on the work, the team, the group dynamics, and future changes.

7.3. What is the difference between trauma-specific and trauma-informed?

It is important to understand the distinction between trauma-specific and trauma-informed, as we know people can often be worried about saying the 'wrong' thing, making things worse, and 'opening a can of worms' (Copperman & Knowles, 2006).

Trauma-specific is generally applied to individual, family, group, or community approaches, models, programmes, and therapies which are designed to specifically address, target, and/or directly intervene with the symptoms and signals resulting from trauma. Examples of trauma-specific approaches are things like EMDR, or testimonial psychotherapy, trauma-focused cognitive behavioural therapy (these are not necessarily always done in a trauma-informed way) Or a group that is specifically focusing on the experience of domestic abuse, or a service that supports survivors of rape to process their trauma, etc.

Trauma-informed refers to applying the knowledge and lens of trauma, and the guiding values of trauma-informed practice, to one's role and way of being. Anyone can apply trauma-informed principles – it doesn't have to be a clinician or practitioner. For example, it can be a security guard, a business support member of staff, someone in human resources, a janitor. This means that an organization can be trauma-informed without providing trauma-specific services. Similarly, an organization can provide trauma-specific services without being trauma-informed.

In the previous section, the example of the smear test illustrates the difference between a trauma-informed and a trauma-specific approach.

7.4. What is the difference between trauma-informed at a practice level and trauma-informed at an organizational level?

Trauma, adversity, and culturally informed, infused, and responsive practice on an individual and intervention level (trauma-specific), although very aligned, is different from trauma, adversity, and culturally informed, infused, and responsive practice at a whole-system, wider, organizational level. Being trauma-informed and responsive, in the context of this book, is about the wider system and organizational culture. As Fallot and Harris (2009) said, it is about 'creating cultures of trauma-informed practice'. It is about whole system-wide transformation, cultural change, and viewing and responding to an organization as a whole.

While they can be interlinked, it is important to be mindful that there are differences within trauma-informed at a practice level and trauma-informed at an organizational level. For example, you might be a trauma-informed practitioner working within a non-trauma-informed team or hospital; or a trauma-informed teacher working within a non-trauma-informed school. Trauma-informed at a practice level is often about what is done in the clinic and therapy room, and in interactions with the person (see Chapter 8 for some examples of this type of change). It's about how a nurse undertakes a smear test, or how a cannula is placed in someone's arm, or how difficult news is delivered.

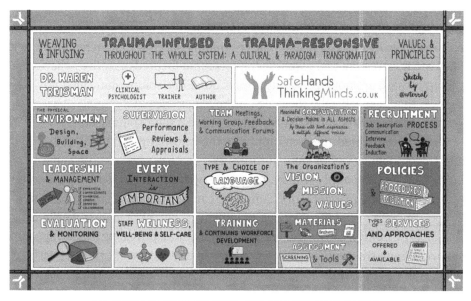

7.2. BEING TRAUMA-INFUSED AND TRAUMA-RESPONSIVE
THROUGHOUT THE WHOLE SYSTEM

At an organizational level it is much more about infusing trauma-informed values into aspects such as the overall work culture, the physical environment, staff wellbeing, access to quality supervision, the HR processes and policies, the language used in meetings/emails/handovers/brochures/website/assessment forms, the organizational mission and vision, performance management and disciplinary processes, training, assessment and referral processes, induction and recruitment processes, and leadership.

Of course, organizations can take both a trauma-specific and trauma-informed approach but it is important for people and organizations to be clear about the difference because strategies, targets, outcomes, choosing and training, and so on, will be different depending on which approach is chosen.

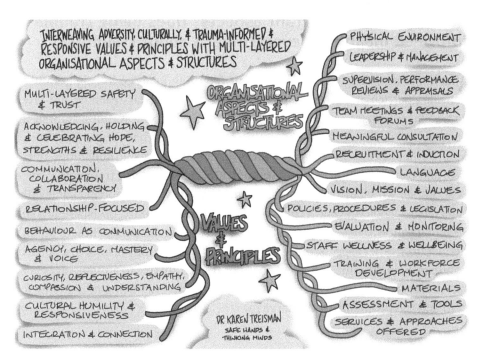

7.3. INFUSING VALUES INTO ORGANIZATIONS

7.5. I am a doctor, a nurse, a midwife... I am not here to talk about trauma. What has this got to do with me?

While not everyone in an organization is expected to be a trauma specialist, we have seen in Chapters 1–3 how stress and trauma can impact on health and wellbeing; therefore, being trauma aware is everyone's business. We also have seen how trauma can impact a person's relationship to health care and health care practitioners, with aspects around trust, safety, communication, disclosure, adherence, and engagement, as well as around early intervention, screening, and prevention strategies and approaches. We know that ignoring or discounting these aspects can contribute to unintentionally harming people and missing or worsening situations and symptoms. And it is important for ourselves and our colleagues as practitioners too, as we might also have had similar adverse experiences. If you are still wondering why trauma and stress are important, go back and re-read Chapters 1–4 to reconnect with some of the consequences of not infusing this information and knowledge.

7.6. Does being trauma-informed mean excluding or missing other important aspects? Does being trauma-informed mean that everything is about trauma?

Absolutely not. Trauma is an important factor and can be hugely helpful to consider, particularly given its prevalence and possible far-reaching and often camouflaged consequences; it can be hazard to discount it. But a trauma-informed lens is certainly not suggesting or advocating that people discount or ignore other key factors, such as neurodiversity, other organic difficulties, nutrition and diet, head injuries, or developmental aspects. Being trauma-informed is about showing curiosity, reflection, and humility. It is applying values like safety, trust, choice, agency, collaboration, cultural humility, transparency, and communication to how we support people and the organization. These shouldn't detract from other aspects, or cause harm; they are generally helpful in a range of contexts. Being trauma-informed does not reduce anyone to any singular event but rather seeks to prevent trauma, stress, and adversity being minimizing for staff and the people using the services.

7.7. Is being trauma-informed just for frontline practitioners in the organization? Why is this relevant to people in roles such as business support or domestic staff?

These are common questions and can often be a barrier to getting people on board. Adversity, culturally, and trauma-informed, infused, and responsive organizational transformation is about creating, facilitating, and sustaining a cultural and paradigm shift throughout the whole fabric of the system. It is about creating a healthier organizational culture, one which is more mindful, humanizing, and reflective. This doesn't just apply to the people using the services, or to 'frontline practitioners', or the leaders, it is for everyone. There should be no 'us and them'. Everyone should be valued, and everyone should contribute to the culture and interact with each other. And we should remember that each person might also have experienced trauma or stressors in their childhood, adulthood, working life.

To create a cultural and paradigm shift in an organization, everyone has a vital role to play. Everyone shapes and contributes to the overall culture, feeling, language, personality, spirit, messages, energy, and fabric of an organization and system. As Dr Bruce Perry has said numerous times, 'It is the people, not programmes, who change people.' Understandably, in order to change the whole, there needs to be a focus on nurturing and strengthening all the parts, and the relationships between those parts. This includes creating a shared framework, language, and direction of travel. Everyone involved has a stronger sense of identity, and they are more likely to contribute to unity and consistency. This approach being held by everyone also means that it is far more likely to be sustained and hardwired into all areas of the organization, rather than just pushed by one person or a small group of people.

This universal approach fits with the notion that 'every interaction is an intervention' (Treisman, 2017a); and that 'people need to be therapists to do therapy; however, people do not need to be therapists to be therapeutic' (Treisman, 2017a). It can be the small things that make the difference and set the tone. These contribute to the overall feeling, personality, culture, energy, and experience of an organization. It is about creating and supporting a sense of community, connection, and belonging, which we know is more likely to support people to develop and flourish. It is about humanizing services.

Take business support staff as an example; they are often the glue of the team. They are the first impression of the service: the person who answers the phone; the person who greets someone; the person who assists if certain things go 'wrong'. Therefore, their responses and way of being can make a huge difference. But also, they might be the person taking minutes in stressful meetings, reading graphic details of stories, transcribing letters, or being the first port of call when the printer isn't working, a room isn't booked, or the IT system is down. They are often the person who is not included in the away day or doesn't have access to reflective practice or clinical supervision. So how this person is treated and supported and how they greet someone or answer the phone or deal with a complaint inevitably will lead to a series of consequences and have a ripple effect.

While there might be different levels and requirements for training or access to supervision for different people in different roles, everyone is human, everyone contributes to the overall culture, everyone can model the values or misrepresent them, and everyone is valuable in the contribution they make. So, it is important, for example, for a security guard to know how valuable their role is and how the trauma-informed values apply to them and their role.

Here is a list showing the ways in which everyone in an organization contributes to the overall culture:

- How someone is greeted and welcomed when entering the building by volunteers, or the security team, or the business support. And how someone is supported to find where they are going or to navigate the building or service (including the personal response and the signage). This is their first impression of the service.

- How someone feels when they phone or arrive to make an appointment for the service or to ask questions, including how accessible it is.

- How language and choice of words are used in meetings, in interactions, on the phone, in letters, on signs, on posters, on the website, on assessments, on referral and screening tools, and so on.

- How a security guard or other staff responds to a potentially escalating situation, as well as their general way of being; or how someone feels welcomed, or judged or criminalized.

- How human resources, leadership, and management support someone when their pay doesn't come through or is incorrect, or supports someone in returning to work or through performance management and disciplinary issues, incidents, complaints, grievances. How restructures, changes, and returning to work processes are handled and communicated.

- How someone is treated and supported in the canteen/kitchen/grounds (particularly as food can be a 'triggering', multi-layered, nuanced area in care and wellbeing).

- How someone is treated when they are moved somewhere, for example moved on a bed or in a wheelchair by the hospital porters.

- How the maintenance and cleaning team respond to, for instance, property damage, mess, bodily fluids, or a fire alarm.

- How the physical building feels, is decorated and maintained. This includes the small but important touches, like supplying toilet paper in the toilets, water to drink, a range of magazines in a waiting room, and up-to-date and organized bulletins on the notice board. (See also Chapter 9.)

- How people interact with each other as colleagues and within teams and between services, as well as with external agencies and partners – the organizational personality, culture, and identity.

- How people have access to technology and IT support and the quality of this support.

- How leaders make their team feel seen, heard, and cared for, and how they model the model.

There are many more. What others would you add?

7.8. Is being trauma-informed just about being sweet, nice, and kind?

While it is hoped that people are kind, empathetic, compassionate, and thoughtful, this is not what being trauma-informed should be summarized or defined as. The following bullet points share some thoughts discussed by me and Dr Mandy Davis in a trauma-informed online thinking space as to why trauma-informed is far more than being 'sweet, nice, and kind'.[1]

- While we ideally want and advocate for people to be compassionate, empathetic, curious, thoughtful, and, where possible, helpful, it becomes potentially problematic when it is suggested that being nice and kind is all trauma-informed is about or requires, or when statements are made such as: 'I don't need to go to training on trauma-informed practice because I am already nice and sweet.'

- Trauma-informed is not just about being sweet and nice. It is about having the trauma knowledge and theoretical background to apply a trauma lens. It includes different forms of trauma, such as intergenerational, medical, cultural, and relational, and is about knowing how these experiences can impact on someone's body, brain, emotions, belief system, behaviours, and relationships. It also uses various values such as safety, cultural humility, collaboration, and choice, among others. Just saying it is about being sweet and nice dilutes the knowledge and skillset required and the value base it is anchored to.

---

1   For a 17-minute free video conversation around this topic see www.youtube.com/watch?v=vFR1MyznXW4. More details can also be found at www.safehandsthinkingminds.co.uk under the online training tab.

◎ In many situations, being trauma-informed is not being sweet and nice. It can involve difficult and painful decisions and discussions. For example, a social worker removing a child from their parents and home is not sweet, nice, and kind; a police officer arresting someone is not sweet, nice, and kind; a doctor sectioning someone into a psychiatric hospital is not sweet, nice, and kind; a manager having to take an employee through a disciplinary process or firing them is not sweet, nice, and kind. However, it is how these things are done and applying trauma-informed values to them that makes them trauma-informed. It is about doing these things in a trauma-informed way and trying to reduce and mitigate harm, not just being sweet and nice. Similarly, in parenting, sometimes you need to make difficult decisions or deliver difficult information or discipline a child. That is not about being sweet and nice but is about being authoritative, demonstrating high levels of love, warmth, and connection with limits and boundaries.

◎ To claim that trauma-informed is just about being sweet and nice reduces the need for certain resources, strategies, and proactive support. For example, being sweet and nice to someone who is hearing voices, or who is self-harming, or who has just been raped may be helpful and supportive but is unlikely to be all that person (and the people around them) need to support their recovery and healing.

◎ It is important to recognize that sometimes our roles or situations will cause, add to, or need to sit with pain, hurt, and harm. Being trauma-informed often is about being with and sitting with the hurt and the pain, having uncomfortable conversations about abuse, difficult news, someone's behaviour, or experiences such as racism, sexism, ageism, and so on. It is not about putting a pretty bow over something, saying that it is okay not to be okay; it is about how this is recognized, honoured, and acknowledged, and doing our best to prevent, support, and where possible restore.

◎ We don't want to feed into toxic positivity, gloss over experiences and feelings, or be inauthentic. This can invalidate or minimize the person's experience but can also be likened to some of the feelings experienced or conveyed during other traumas; for example, messages like I love you, but I hurt you; or you are in pain, but you need to show the outside world all is okay with a smile. It is important that we don't encourage pushing things underground or adding to people feeling minimized, oppressed, or silenced. Moreover, sometimes people's wish to be sweet and nice can add to distress in the long run; for example, a manager may be unable to be transparent about performance concerns with their employee, but when these concerns are brought up in a formal permanence management review or disciplinary process, the person can feel shocked, unprepared, deceived, and confused.

- Being sweet and nice can be helpful but also hazardous. Sometimes we need to be able to say no, or be assertive, or have clear boundaries, or say or share difficult things.

- It is not correct to imply that the only people who can be trauma-informed are sweet and nice people. There are numerous different ways to implement and embody the values beyond a person having to be sweet and nice.

7.9. Is it enough to just train people in trauma-informed ideas and values?

In short, no, and sadly this is often being done, where training is seen as ticking a box or as sufficient in itself. Of course, this will vary depending on the team and organizational aims – there is a difference between wanting an introduction to being more trauma sensitive or to gain a bit of knowledge and awareness and a team or organization saying that it wants to commit to using this knowledge to change practice or the organizational culture.

Training is a key step and often one of the first pillars in the trauma-informed journey for establishing foundational knowledge, conveying the direction of travel, galvanizing interest, creating a shared language, and conveying the organizational message that this is important and necessary thinking and knowledge. However, training is not sufficient for most people to mobilize change and it is easy to get lost among the storm of other information and tasks. People only remember a small chunk of information, so refreshers and repetition are crucial. While training is one step, to make it worthwhile, the concepts need to be meaningfully embedded and applied. It is about moving from knowing to doing to being and to feeling. Training needs to provide real-world examples and tangible ways of how the concepts can be actioned in everyday situations. This will also be hugely influenced by the ability of the practitioner delivering the training, who should have practical experience as well as the knowledge and skill to convey the issues in a trauma-informed way.

Moreover, we know training is not effective as a standalone and needs to be consolidated through supervision, reflective and thinking practice, team meetings, debriefings and informal conversations, consultations, and so on. While a short training may be helpful and encouraging, inevitably training that allows more time for reflection, a deeper set of knowledge, and for practitioners to be marinated in the information is likely to be more effective (Purtle, 2020).

7.10. What are some of the benefits and strengths of trauma-informed practice and organizational cultural change in health and medical settings?

It is difficult to share the benefits of trauma-informed practice and trauma-informed organizational change as there are so many and of course they will vary depending on what weight the person perceiving them places on the context itself, on what is measured or measurable (Albert Einstein famously said, 'Not everything that counts can be counted, and not everything that can be counted counts'), and much more. What one person describes as 'trauma-informed' someone else might not. Within this, many people confuse or use interchangeably trauma-informed on a practice level and trauma-informed on an organizational level, or what might be trauma-informed compared to trauma-aware, trauma-sensitive, and trauma-responsive.

However, some of the possible benefits and strengths seen within the existing literature base, qualitative reports, and my own experience of supporting numerous organizations on this journey are summarized below. This is not an exhaustive list and I hope that you will personalize and contextualize them within your setting and continue to add to, expand, and evidence them.

- Improved wellbeing, team cohesion, and staff morale. This can have a huge ripple effect, increasing the protective and buffering factors for staff, and decreasing staff burnout, compassion fatigue, emotional saturation, secondary and vicarious trauma, moral injury, workplace stress, and the impact of exposure to trauma (see Chapter 5).

- A positive impact on staff satisfaction and staff commitment, as well as on staff turnover (intended and actual), staff retention, staff sickness, absences, and the need for agency or temporary staff. This has huge financial and health implications, as well as an impact on service capacity and effective use of resources. It also retains and enhances the skills which have been invested in, while supporting professional development, and continuity of care/relationships. A positive work culture can also be a more attractive place for people to choose to work and so there can be increased job applications and an enhanced organizational reputation (see

Chapter 5). Both organizational commitment and burnout have repeatedly been tied to a variety of indicators of organizational effectiveness (Meyer *et al.*, 2002; Schaufeli & Bakker, 2004). Additionally, meta-analyses and systematic reviews have repeatedly found that organizational cultures that are based on collaborative decision-making styles and increased staff autonomy are positively associated with organizational innovativeness and organizational effectiveness (Greenhalgh *et al.*, 2004).

- A positive impact on decision-making, on our ability to think and to be more curious, reflective, creative, and innovative, to show more compassion and empathy, and to be more patient. This includes creating a culture of learning and development as opposed to fear, rigidity, blame, and shame. Also, staff are less likely to be as frustrated, agitated, cynical, and depleted, and underappreciated, devalued, and unseen (see also Chapter 5). Moreover, with increased wellbeing and the ability to think and learn and be present, people are less likely to make mistakes and errors, and the likelihood of brain fog, forgetfulness, lack of attention and concentration, and distractibility is reduced (Amanullah & Ramesh Shankar, 2020; Epel *et al.*, 2018; Keesler, 2020 ; McFadden *et al.*, 2022). More than 250,000 medical errors and 100,000 deaths annually are attributed to workforce frustration, yielding poor team member communication and thus fragmented care, order entry mistakes, and medication and treatment errors (Garcia *et al.*, 2019; Ozeke *et al.*, 2019; Restauri & Sheridan, 2020). Moreover, burnout in practitioners has been shown to double the rates of adverse patient safety events and contribute to the poorer quality of health care overall (Panagioti *et al.*, 2018; Salyers *et al.*, 2017; Willard-Grace *et al.*, 2019).

- Reduced conflict, assaults, and complaints internally and externally.

- A decrease in workplace violence and abuse (including the conditions that exacerbate and contribute to it), as well as an increase in the quality of support for those impacted when it does occur. Studies that looked at critical and violent incidents also reported overall decreases following trauma-informed approaches (Baetz *et al.*, 2021; Barnett *et al.*, 2018; Goetz & Taylor-Trujillo, 2012).

- Better outcomes on so many levels, including treatment adherence, appointment attendance, reduced levels of distress during appointments, people seeking help and support earlier. Moreover, services become more accessible, increasing communication and trust, improving the quality of relationships, and contributing to a better relationship to 'help' and 'helping professionals', supporting people to feel seen and heard, reducing the likelihood of medical and health trauma occurring or of mirroring, echoing, or activating past traumas and distress (Chapters 1–5), and much more. Green *et al.* (2016) found that, following a trauma-informed training for primary care physicians, there was significantly improved patient perceptions of shared decision-making.

- Staff feeling more prepared and skilled in understanding trauma, and in ways of supporting and responding, including aspects such as having more effective conversations, delivering difficult news, increasing someone's comfort, and responding when someone is distressed or dysregulated (Hales *et al.*, 2019; Niimura *et al.*, 2019; Palfrey *et al.*, 2019).

- Practical implications for people using services. For example, a trauma-informed approach can help if someone is feeling tense or in a heightened state, making it easier for them to undertake procedures. Likewise, when someone is worried or feels judged, shamed, or hurt, if staff are trauma-informed, they might be more likely to share concerns or symptoms or make disclosures and be more likely to come for preventative procedures like blood tests, mammograms, and cervical screenings.

- Positive effects on the incidence of seclusion and restraint. Numerous studies evaluating trauma-informed organizational interventions within psychiatric settings evaluated effects on incidence of seclusion and restraint. For example, Blair *et al.* (2017) found significant reduction in the incidence of seclusion at a psychiatric hospital two years after implementation of a trauma-informed training intervention. And similarly, in a cluster randomized controlled trial, Borckardt *et al.* (2011), in a study of 340 staff and 446 patients, also observed a significant reduction of 82.3% in the rate of seclusion and restraint.

- Better outcomes in child and adolescent psychiatric settings. Hales *et al.* (2019) found that within a child and adolescent inpatient psychiatric setting a trauma-informed programme provided alternative interventions but, more importantly, brought a heightened level of staff self-awareness when interacting with children. Staff began to see the child in a different way, which allowed them to not take the child's behaviour as personal or as a reflection of poor care. Staff began using trauma-informed language and approaches consistently during crisis incidents, using de-escalation and debriefings, and were able to see that this approach was successful in maintaining the dignity and care of the child. They also found an overall reduction in crisis interventions of holds and seclusions of more than

41%; and staff developed an increased sense of pride knowing they had more effective and less trauma-induced strategies to use. Additionally, research has discovered that implementing trauma-informed approaches has increased client retention in treatment (Amaro *et al.*, 2007; Hales *et al.*, 2019).

◉ Staff are supported to be more curious instead of furious – and can see the person behind the behaviour, label, or diagnosis. They are less frustrated, agitated, and impatient and less likely to take things as a personal assault. For example, Purtle's (2020) review of 14 studies that assessed the effects of a trauma-informed organizational intervention on staff knowledge, attitudes, and behaviours revealed that 12 found a statistically significant improvement in one or more of these outcomes.

★ Why might adversity, culturally, and trauma-informed, infused, and responsive organizational change be relevant and beneficial for you or your context/team/organization/population being served?

★ What difference does having some knowledge of trauma and stress and using the values as anchors and guides make to you and the people you support?

★ What are the emotional, physical, social, moral, and financial costs of not becoming more culturally, adversity, and trauma-informed, infused, and responsive? What might be the hazards?

★ Why do you exist? Why are you here? What do you believe in? What drives you? What is important to you? Where do you want to be and to travel to? What do you want to see/achieve/accomplish/be part of? What is your vision?

To read more about adversity, culturally, and trauma-informed systems, see my book *A Treasure Box for Creating Trauma-Informed Organizations* (Treisman, 2021).

7.11. What are the key elements of adversity, culturally, and trauma-informed, infused, and responsive practice at an organizational and system level?

7.11.1. The four R's and Ken Epstein's notion of trauma-informed systems

We will now move on to explore some of the guiding values, principles, and definitions of being an adversity and trauma-informed, infused, and responsive system at a wider organizational level. Ken Epstein offers an explanation, saying that trauma-informed systems are about: 'Reflecting instead of reacting, self-care instead of self-sacrifice, curiosity instead of numbing, and working as a collective instead of in silos.' This also means having services that are healthy and mindful, using their thinking brains, as opposed to their survival brains, and that seek to increase safety, regulation, and trust.

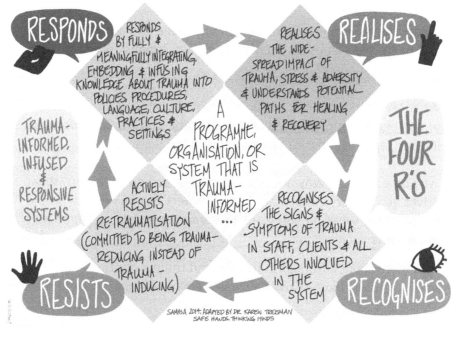

7.4. THE FOUR R'S

Another helpful definition and some guiding aspects of trauma-informed practice have been created by the Substance Abuse and Mental Health Services Administration (SAMHSA). These are referred to as the four R's: *realizing, recognizing, resisting,* and *responding.* I have expanded on these four R's (SAMHSA,

2014) in the image above, as well as in the following sections (the explanations are my take-home messages and way of applying the R's, not the ones directly offered by SAMHSA). They can provide a useful framework to apply to lots of different aspects of an organization.

7.11.2. Realizing

The first R is about *realizing* and accepting the multi-layered and widespread impact and common occurrence of trauma and adversity, and of the pathways of recovery and healing. This involves active engagement with this knowledge through training and reflection. This realizing also includes acknowledging that anyone – people and their families using the service, staff working in the service, and people in agencies the work interfaces with – may have experience of trauma, stress, and adversity which may or may not be known to others. This could be current, ongoing, and historical trauma at an individual, family, team, community, organizational, and society level. These traumas and adversities may be wide-reaching and include intergenerational, cultural, collective, medical, health, disability, relational, and developmental trauma, alongside crucial aspects such as poverty, discrimination, chronic loneliness, and stigma.

It is also about realizing that there might be resurfacing, 'triggering', and stressing experiences; for example, people might also be in pain, feeling scared or vulnerable, feeling powerless, being in a new and unfamiliar environment, seeing a stream of strangers' faces, or being in an environment with lots of possible 'triggers' including sensory ones like hospital smells, bleach, flashing blue lights, being stuck in an MRI or scanning machine, being undressed, and seeing masks, needles, or blood (see Chapters 3 and 4).

This realizing aspect also includes considering and acknowledging the importance of relationships within the organization and how influential they can be, as well as the possible impact of power imbalances and dynamics, and of harmful, re-traumatizing, and stress and trauma-inducing experiences. Within this, realizing is also about how historical practices and experiences can inevitably shape and influence people's present feelings, relationships, and experiences (e.g. past medical experimentation, previous experiences when in hospital or sectioned, harm caused during treatment).

Staff and families may have their own trauma, stress, and adverse experiences, and these might also be compounded by the emotional pulse of the work and the possible impact of organizational adverse experiences and organizational trauma (Chapter 5), such as emotional exhaustion, secondary and vicarious trauma, empathetic strain, moral injury, decision and compassion fatigue, burnout, caregiver stress, and workplace bullying.

If we don't acknowledge or realize these things, we are just ignoring the elephants in the room. As the writer James Baldwin says, 'Not everything that is faced can be changed, but nothing can be changed until it is faced.'

7.11.3. Recognizing

This second R is for *recognizing*. This is about recognizing how trauma, adversity, and stress can influence or impact people, systems, and organizations. We can notice certain signals, signs, flags, or behaviours, such as sleep difficulties, self-harming, headaches, dissociation, crushed empathy, fear, and anger. It is also about being curious and mindful about how the trauma or stress might show itself and communicate, considering what the behaviour or presenting focus might be communicating. If the body, feeling, or behaviour could talk, what might it say? This follows a trauma-informed philosophical shift which moves away from the position of 'What is wrong with you?' to 'What happened or is happening to you/us/our organization'; and similarly away from 'What is the matter with you?' to 'What matters and is important to you?'

We also need to recognize how our own actions, power, 'triggers', beliefs, biases, values, training, experiences, and attitudes can influence and shape things, and potentially influence others (including possibly contributing to harm or added stress).

7.11.4. Resisting

The third R is about actively recognizing and acknowledging that the systems themselves can add, reinforce, perpetuate, and exacerbate stress, pain, and trauma; and this can be re-traumatizing, dysregulating, stress- and trauma-inducing, and 'triggering'. This might be through things like the posters on the walls or how procedures are done (smear test and poster examples were shared earlier in this chapter), the physical environment (see Chapter 9), the language we use, the way someone is or has been treated, the organizational culture which can add harm to its employees and people who use the service, and so on (see Chapter 5). Therefore, the third R is about finding ways to reduce and *resist* re-traumatization, and aim to be trauma-reducing and healing, instead of trauma-inducing and harmful. This is about trying to mitigate or reduce the likelihood of activating new or further stress or trauma.

7.11.5. Responding

The fourth R is around actively *responding* to what we know about adversity and trauma by trying to find ways to embed and integrate this information, understanding, and knowledge into the culture of an organization. If we have the knowledge around trauma and stress, how do we move from knowing and being informed, to feeling and doing? How do we not just talk the talk but walk the walk?

For example, we might know about different learning styles and ways of processing information and how trauma can be a multi-sensory experience which can have a multi-sensory impact on, for example, communication and language. However, if we do not incorporate this multi-sensory knowledge into the interventions we offer, into our interactions, into our facial expressions and body language, into the design and feel of the physical environment, into making our communication more multi-method and accessible (see Chapter 8), into our team meetings, then it is just words and knowledge without action.

Another example of modelling the model and moving from knowing to doing involves the knowledge of the power of language and the impact of the words which we use. How do we take this knowledge and actually infuse and respond to it? How do we speak to each other in team meetings, how do we write our notes and our letters, what do we say in handovers and informal conversations, what language do we use on the website, on the posters which are on the walls, in the brochures and leaflets we give out, in emails, in assessment and screening forms and questionnaires?

How do we respond if we know the prevalence and possible impact, for example, of secondary and vicarious trauma, moral injury, emotional saturation, burnout, and compassion fatigue on ourselves and on staff? How do we acknowledge and respond to this impact by prioritizing wellbeing, putting into place systems that support and aim to reduce this?

Responding is also about sustainability and hardwiring the ideas and values into the fabric of the organization. It is about moving from 'This is what we do' to 'This is who we are'. If you have an amazing leader or a phenomenal trauma-informed champion and then they leave the team or organization, it will likely leave with them, be diluted, or lost unless the trauma-informed ideas and values have been woven into the fabric of the organization and have become the culture so that they will live on, and be more sustained.

7.12. The nine R's (expanding on the four R's)

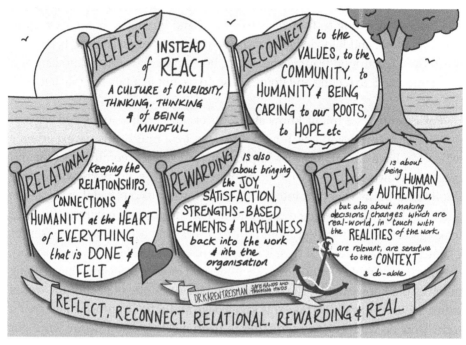

7.5. MORE R'S

In keeping with the R theme and building on the work by SAMHSA (2014), I have added some additional R's (of course there are plenty more we could add, and some of them overlap) which I hope may be helpful to you on your journey. These are: *reflect*, *reconnect*, *relational*, *rewarding*, and *real*.

7.12.1. Reflect

Reflect is about being in a culture of humility and curiosity, and truly trying to think, breathe, and reflect rather than purely reacting or acting. This can be hard when in fast-moving, unpredictable, and sometimes highly pressurized environments, and even more so in the context of stress, trauma, burnout, compassion fatigue, and organizational trauma (see Chapter 5). Reflecting is about being in our thinking mind instead of our survival mind and being mindful instead of having our mind full. It is about viewing things from multiple different angles, thinking creatively, and being expansive in our thinking: having meaningful thinking spaces, being curious instead of furious, stopping and pausing where possible, having access to meaningful supervision, and having a culture that supports and facilitates thinking and learning. This includes thinking around the day-to-day things, best practices, biases, and disparities (Chapter 6), the overall vision and mission, and more.

Sometimes we need to sit with not knowing, which can be tricky, and have the humility and openness to continue to learn, reflect, listen, and be curious. It is so important to have a growth mindset and to be continually evolving and, where helpful, re-calibrating. We are in the business of supporting others to potentially change and take on board new information and advice, and yet we can be rigid, fixed, and inflexible. And from an organizational lens, organizations are ever-growing, changing, and developing; they are not sitting still or fixed; therefore, we need to have ongoing reflection and realignment.

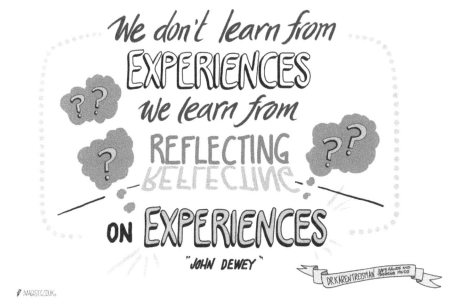

7.6. REFLECTING

7.12.2. Reconnect

This is about reconnecting to the values, to the community, to the caring and human part, to our roots, to hope, to our vision, to our mission. For example, why does our work exist? What are our values? Why do we do what we do? What brought us into the work in the first place and what keeps us in the work? What are our core and guiding values? What really matters and is important to us? How are we modelling and embodying our values? How are we not just dishing out advice but thinking and applying it to ourselves? What motivates and fuels us? How and where is the care in the caring profession? All this can sadly get lost in the context of organizational and system trauma, where systems are overstretched and underfunded, infused with blame and shame, or where there is a conveyer belt of feelings and pressures.

7.12.3. Relational

Relational is about keeping the relationships, connections, and humanity at the heart of what is done and felt. How would we want to be treated? How would we want our best friend or family member treated? How are we ensuring that the person isn't treated like a machine, robot, textbook, statistic, or experiment, but a unique individual? How are we holding on to the power of the relationship and how this can shape and influence interactions, trust, communication, and so much more? This also extends to how we are working together in a person-centred way with our team and colleagues (including team cohesion and collaboration), with other agencies, and with the community.

7.12.4. Rewarding

Rewarding is about bringing the joy, fun, satisfaction, hope, strengths-based elements, and playfulness back into the work and into the organization where possible. This might be things like celebrating and magnifying what is going well, noticing and sharing progress, the small wins, and best practice (not just serious case reviews or near misses). This also includes a culture of value, acknowledgement, and appreciation where the small things are the big things and people feel seen, heard, valued, and that they matter. It is about reconnecting to what pushes your professional reward buttons. What are some of the proud, refuelling, feel-good, or hopeful moments which you can marinate yourself in or hold on to? Are there opportunities to bring some humour, playfulness, and joy in (whether that is on away days, in the staff room, in team meetings, in informal interactions, in supervision, in the environment, etc.)? How do people convey and hold on to 'hope'? How do we also learn about and pay attention to aspects such as post-traumatic growth, adversity-activated development, vicarious resilience, compassion satisfaction, survivorship, healing and recovery possibilities, and so on?

7.12.5. Real

Real is about being human and authentic, but also about making decisions and changes that are in touch with the realities of the work, relevant, sensitive to the context, and doable. This is about translating theory into practice. For example, there is no point acting on recommendations which feel unachievable, add distress to people, or feel jarring with the setting. So, they need to respect and honour the context and realities of the work and the situation of the person or the team. It is also not about putting a silver lining or toxic positivity around things but really connecting with, acknowledging, naming, and thinking creatively about what it might be like, what is possible in the real world.

★ Take some time to look at each R (realize, recognize, resist, respond, reflect, reconnect, relational, rewarding, and real). What do these mean and look like to you, to your team, to the work, to the organization? Can you think of examples of them? How do they resonate with you and your work, or do they conflict and jar? Are there ones which should be in the forefront, and others which are less developed?

These will become clearer as we explore suggestions and examples in future chapters. These four R's will come to life when applied to a step-by-step approach in Chapter 9.

7.13. What are the core values of trauma-informed practice?

Having explored the four/nine R's, we will now take a closer look at trauma-informed values. The intention is that these values and ways of being will be meaningfully and intentionally integrated, modelled, embodied, and hardwired into the very fabric, culture, and feeling of an organization. This also means that they need to be more than just words on paper; they need to be recognizable and felt throughout the organization and the work. These will be briefly named with reflective questions in the box that follows. Then some real world and tangible examples of how these can be actioned or seen in the work are shared in Chapter 8. However, please note that this is intended as an introduction. For a more comprehensive guide to the values and to wider organizational areas, please see *A Treasure Box for Creating Trauma-Informed Organizations* (Treisman, 2021).

While we might know what the values are, it is also important to be able to name and evidence how they are felt and shown, what they mean, how they are embodied, why they matter, what happens if they are not present, how they align with you as a person, and so on. They can also be very helpful as a guide, or an anchor; for example, when in a new situation like the pandemic, or introducing a new practice, or reviewing a procedure, having values and the four R's can provide a helpful and grounding platform to return to.

7.14. How are these values linked to trauma and why?

These values evolve from our knowledge of needs around trauma. For example, some types of trauma can contribute to someone feeling 'done to', powerless, helpless, out of control, violated, unsafe, silenced, shamed, voiceless, dehumanized, and so forth. Therefore, it is vital to have services where people's safety and trust (a core value of trauma-informed) are prioritized, and danger and threat are reduced. A service where people feel seen, heard, that they matter, and feel not 'done to' is integral in avoiding mirroring, echoing, reinforcing, resurfacing, or activating these feelings and experiences. People need choice and a level of agency and control. They need transparency and clear communication, so that they avoid being marinated in secrecy and silence, or being lied to, deceived, betrayed, exploited. Services must not add to or be reminiscent or reinforcing of these experiences.

Another example is around the value of connection and integration. Trauma can pierce and wound; it can lead to disconnection. This might be disconnection of the mind from the body, from thoughts, from feelings, behaviours, and sensations, from the left and right and top and bottom of the brain, from the past, the present, and future. Trauma can come in disjointed, fragmented, and incoherent ways. Additionally, knowledge and theories can become disconnected and not integrated into practice or policies; people can become disconnected from the work or the values; and systems and teams can work in silos and be fragmented. So, connection and integration are crucial in creating more connected, cohesive, and communicating systems.

7.15. Some of the anchoring and guiding values

- Multi-layered safety and trust (psychological, emotional, relational, cultural, moral, internal, felt, and physical).

- Relational and relationship-focused approaches, including being humanizing.

- Voice, choice, agency, and mastery.

- Collaboration, communication, and transparency.

- Communication, curiosity, understanding, empathy, compassion, and reflection.

- Acknowledgement and celebration of strengths, survivorship, hope, and resilience.

- Cultural humility and responsiveness (see Chapter 6).

- Connection and integration.

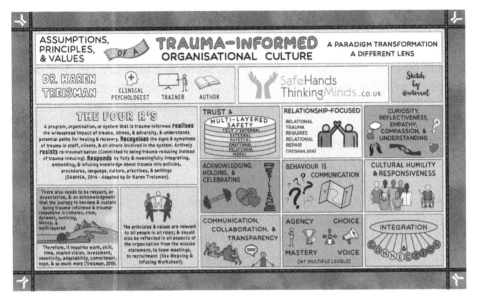

7.7. ASSUMPTIONS, PRINCIPLES, AND VALUES OF A TRAUMA-
INFORMED ORGANIZATIONAL CULTURE

For a poem I wrote and read around trauma-informed and reducing organizations, please see https://m.youtube.com/watch?v=LRJ9w3jIvow.

Box 7.1.

Some reflective questions and considerations around trauma-informed values

When reviewing our teams, organizations, and systems, we want to consider how some of the values are infused and what they might mean and look like. However, naturally, they need to be tailored to the specific service, as there is no one size fits all. Some broad aspects to consider are described below, intended, not as an exhaustive list, but as a springboard for further discussion and reflection. More tangible examples of bringing these values alive in practice are offered throughout this book but also more specifically in Chapter 8. Please note that questions around the value of cultural humility are not shared here as Chapter 6 covers this area.

Please take your time individually, with a team, or in a working group to go through them, break them down, reflect on them, expand on them, and revisit them. It can be very helpful to visually represent your responses in a drawing, chart, or graph. It is also very useful to explore what the responses are like at different times and from different perspectives. Some values will of course overlap and be interwoven with other values. Some will be more relevant or possible, depending on the context, and inevitably won't be able to be practised all the time. These are not meant to be rules.

Safety and trust (psychological, emotional, relational, environmental, physical, ideological, moral, cultural, felt)

★ What might facilitate, hinder, increase, or decrease people's trust and safety from the start to the end of their visit/day/ engagement with the service or when working in the service? (This is where a narrative walk-through approach of the detail of the service, from first contact to last contact, can be extremely useful. The more people who use and work in the service from a range of perspectives do this, the richer it is likely to be. See worksheet 9.1 in Chapter 9 to support you in doing this.)

★ What might increase people's feelings of danger, dysregulation, stress, and threat? What might be potentially re-traumatizing, activating, trauma-inducing, or 're-triggering'? This includes viewing 'triggers' and hotspots as multi-layered (e.g. autobiographical, sensory (including smells, sounds, sights, feelings, sensations), emotional, relational, cognitive, and physical; see Chapters 3, 4, 5, and 9 on re-traumatizing and trauma-inducing experiences for lots more examples and information around this). What are you/the organization doing to support people who work in the service and who access the service to feel emotionally, relationally, and psychologically safe, supported, and secure?

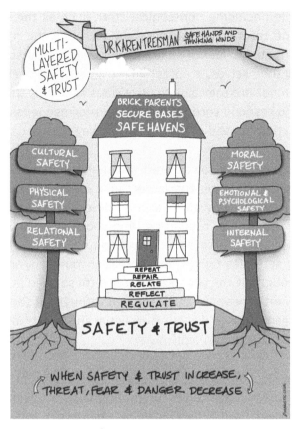

7.8. SAFETY AND TRUST

★ Are people able to respect and recognize that people coming into services, such as a GP surgery, a dentist, a hospital, might already be 'triggered' and already in survival/crisis mode, and that this can filter into their responses and interactions to the services which are being offered and experienced?

★ Is attention given to things that can make people feel physically safer and more comfortable, and which might be activating, such as lighting, room temperature, seating, noise, signage, smells, sounds, small spaces, the type of artwork displayed, fire alarms, certain words on materials and signs, locks on doors, darkened corridors? (See Chapters 3 and 4 on activating experiences and body-based 'triggers', and Chapter 9 on thinking about the physical environment.)

★ Are people (including non-clinical staff, such as the security guard, the caretakers, business support, and the reception desk staff) able to identify and recognize signs that someone, including themselves, is potentially 'triggered', activated, and dysregulated? Are they able to be curious as to why this might be, and to respond through a trauma-informed lens and in a co-regulating instead of co-escalating way?

★ Is training available for all staff (including non-clinical staff) around understanding the importance of safety and recognizing 'triggers', as well as around de-escalation skills and creating containing, regulating, and soothing environments and experiences? Are regulating, coping, grounding, and soothing activities taught, promoted, encouraged, and modelled throughout the organization? Are these used at regular and relevant times? Are these infused throughout the culture of the organization and seen as essential and beneficial, rather than as a luxury or an add-on?

★ Is there a recognition that the services, structures, processes, and systems in place can be unintentionally re-traumatizing, 're-triggering', and activating? (See Chapters 3, 4, 5, and 6.) Are there processes in place to minimize and improve these? Is there an intentional effort and action around evaluating these, reflecting on them, and actively trying to find ways to improve, develop, and problem-solve around them (e.g. staff's facial expressions, language and communication styles, how consent is gained, restraint, certain assessment measures, type of environment and room, lack of choice)?

★ How does the organization recognize, understand, and respond to people and teams in distress and in conflict? How is the impact, nature, and complexity of the work acknowledged and supported? Is there training and ongoing work around this?

★ Do people have a space/forum where they can reflect on the work itself, and the impact of the work, such as reflective practice or supervision (or a menu of support options)? Does this space feel safe, containing, supportive? Is the impact of the work acknowledged formally and informally? Are there informal and formal processes for debriefing and checking-in with each other (e.g. after an incident, a difficult decision, a change in situation)?

★ How are things such as assaults, threats, substance use, and self-harm responded to in a way that promotes multi-layered safety and trust? How can people learn from these events and reduce them?

★ How are things like bullying, microaggressions, discrimination, and harassment acknowledged and responded to? How is ethical practice ensured, and how is unethical practice responded to?

★ Is there a culture of shame and blame, fear, panic, and threat, or of openness and transparency? (Of course, this may vary depending on a range of factors.) Are there permissive messages about being human and learning from 'mistakes'? Are mistakes normalized and de-stigmatized? This includes feeling able to show and share some of the emotion and impact of the work. Is there an emphasis on being a learning culture and having a growth mindset? Being able to reflect and review?

★ Do people generally feel that they are listened to, valued, heard, and seen? How are people's values and principles acknowledged, honoured, and respected (in a way that also keeps the balance of the organization's needs)?

★ Are people shown qualities such as compassion, respect, empathy, curiosity, reflectivity, containment, and understanding by leaders and colleagues?

★ Do people feel able to share when they feel they are struggling or are feeling stuck? Are discourses about being 'weak' or 'not tough skinned enough' actively addressed?

★ How safe do people feel to speak up, to whistleblow, and to call things out? What are the discourses and messages around this? How are disagreement and conflict responded to? Is there fear of retribution?

★ If necessary and needed, are meaningful apologies made and suitable ownership and accountability taken?

★ How are people's dignity and integrity held in mind and respected? This is crucial given that trauma often dehumanizes people and is a violation of their dignity and integrity. Is respect for people's personal space, privacy, and boundaries prioritized? Are rooms soundproofed, or efforts made to minimize distraction and maximize confidentiality? Is there thought around other elements of privacy, such as drapings over windows, or reducing the feeling of other people looking in, or consent around medical students being present, and so on? If something needs to be done, for example, during a medical examination, or when someone is being checked in on for safety reasons, is it done in as thoughtful, compassionate, and safe way as possible?

★ Are areas such as informed consent, information sharing, and confidentiality considered carefully? This includes issues around accessibility, language, and transparency.

★ Is there lone working, sickness, and joint working policies in place which are monitored and adhered to? Do people have access to a mobile phone when out in the community?

★ Are the fire, smoking, and health and safety policies and procedures up to date, meaningful, and reviewed? Are these communicated with all staff?

★ Is there careful thought around things like locked doors, keys, cupboards, and exit routes? (This includes their accessibility, the feeling they convey, the communication around them, the need for them.) The actual and narrative walk-through exercise in worksheet 9.1 in Chapter 9 can really support this process.

★ Have the safety elements of areas such as car parks, bathrooms, exits, entries, common areas, corridors, therapy rooms, and waiting rooms been considered? Are there specific safe walking routes or procedures in place for potentially more 'risky' situations or visits? Are there security systems and people in place? Do people know about these and feel comfortable and able to use them? Are these done in the most non-invasive, thoughtful way possible? Are these reviewed and communicated?

★ Are there safety, wellness, and risk assessment plans in place, and are these meaningfully reviewed and used? Are they accessible and evaluated? Are possible scenarios practised and discussed? Are incidents and near misses reviewed and learned from, and this learning actioned?

★ Is there clear signage and maps, so that people feel oriented, guided, and welcomed? These should also consider cultural, communication, and language differences (see Chapter 9). Even better, are people welcomed, greeted, and guided by the person whom they are meeting?

★ Is there an effort, where possible, to increase space so that people don't feel cramped or trapped, and to make spaces appear more welcoming and supportive?

★ Do people have accurate and working contact numbers, sign-posting service lists, signals for help, and communication systems with peers and support?

★ Is careful thought given, through a trauma lens, to procedures such as admission, restraint, exclusion, and seclusion? This should include when, how, and why these take place, and what needs to happen before, during, and after (short and long term).

★ Is there a clear plan for responding to internal emergencies and crises, which is regularly reviewed?

Relationships and personalized services

★ Is there understanding and acknowledgement of the importance of relationships and trust within the work, for the people being served, and for the organization? (This includes everyone in all roles, from how business support answer phones and greet people, to how the maintenance team respond to property damage, to how the communication team sends emails, to how assessments are undertaken.)

★ How do you want people to feel when working in your organization and using the services provided? What implicit and explicit messages do you want them to read, feel, hear, notice, and learn from? How is this aligned with your values and principles?

★ How are the services humanized and relational? How would you want to be treated, interacted with, and written about? How would you want someone you loved to be treated, interacted with, and written about? Would you want to be treated or supported within the service that you work? Or a loved one? How would you feel if you or a family member/close friend had to use the service you work in? Would you recommend it?

★ Does this extend to relationships and connections between services and agencies and to relationships between different roles? For example, how connected is a senior leader to people in other parts of the organization? How present and available are they? How connected are different teams with each other?

★ How are breaches in relationships responded to, like abuse of power or conflict, bullying, harassment, discrimination, traumatic re-enactments?

★ Are wider relationships considered and supported, such as key adults in a person's life, the wider family, the relationship with a worker or someone in the community?

★ What is done in teams to support staff cohesion, morale, connection, and relationships? Do people feel able to contact other people or reach out in times of need? Is the team providing a safe space, a secure base, and a safe haven? How does the team respond and interact with each other when there is a celebration, when there is a conflict, when there is a loss, when there is change?

Curiosity, empathy, compassion, understanding, reflection, and viewing behaviour as communication

★ What are you bringing into the situation yourself, as a team, as an organization? What lens, bias, kaleidoscope, discourses, and frameworks are you looking at things through? How might this also be influenced by your own power, privilege, access, and status? What has influenced your decision about…? What was your thinking around…? What might this be like from another perspective? (See Chapter 6.)

★ What implicit and explicit assumptions, beliefs, attitudes, expectations, biases, prejudices, and judgements might there be at an individual, family, team, organizational, and societal level?

★ What can you do better? What can you learn, improve on, do differently? What can you learn from other people? What are you missing?

★ Is there space and time to reflect on and acknowledge the complexity and impact of the work? Are the rationale, benefits, and need for reflection acknowledged and prioritized? Are there spaces to be reflective, to think, to expand on your understanding, to try to increase meaning-making? Is there space to be able to reflect on some of the advantages and disadvantages of the work, of your role, of the decision-making, of the environment, of the wider context, and so on (e.g. supervision, team meetings and reflective practice, away days, formulation spaces, development days, reflective journals, therapy)?

★ Are there opportunities to link theory with practice, and expand on areas of knowledge, certain skills, certain models, different approaches, a wider lens, and so on? (This might include training, reading, shared learning opportunities, and supervision.) Is there access to resources, such as books, documents, podcasts, webinars, and papers, to expand knowledge? Is there a supportive culture around learning and development? Does this include learning from other systems, organizations, and countries about best and innovative practice?

★ Are there opportunities to formulate and share ideas, and learn from multiple voices and perspectives?

★ How are ways of being and skills like empathy, compassion, reflectiveness, and understanding interwoven throughout the organization (e.g. in interactions, from HR processes through to assessments)? How are they modelled, felt, and embodied?

★ How can you gain a better understanding of a person, team, system, organization? What might be happening? What is the behaviour or action communicating? What is its purpose, function, need, history? Is there a sense of being curious and thinking about what has happened to someone and why, as opposed to what is wrong with them? How can you be curious instead of furious (e.g. with those you are supporting, yourself, your colleagues). How can you be 'mindful' instead of having your 'mind full'?

★ How are you putting yourself in the shoes of others through perspective-taking and empathy? What does something mean from another person's perspective, words, and experiences? Do you hold in mind that each person is unique ('same storm different boat', from Chapter 1)?

★ What is the meaning-making behind their behaviour, signal, comment, and so on? What is the meaning-making about their life, experiences, identity, needs, and so on? What has influenced these? How are you considering who the person is within the wider context and within the landscape of their experiences (including aspects such as societal discourses, culture, power)?

★ How are you exploring who the person is? What are their stories, journeys, and experiences? What matters and is important to the person, and the people around them? What are their hopes, worries, expectations, wants, and needs?

★ How are you thinking about a holistic formulation which is ongoing, evolving, and collaborative? Is there a starting position held that says people are trying their best?

Strengths, hope, and best practice

★ Is there time to reflect on, be curious about, acknowledge, and magnify the things, situations, and feelings that people, teams, and organizations have survived, navigated, overcome, and developed from? Where do these qualities come from and why (e.g. honesty, grit, compassion, assertiveness)? What have they learned from this survivorship? What can they draw on in future situations? How can this help them to support others to have hope?

★ How often and in what ways do you, your team, and your organization recognize, enrich, celebrate, and discuss your colleagues, the people you work with, the teams, the organization's strengths, skills, qualities, resources, progress, and so on?

★ How are people's passions, motivators, ambitions, strengths, and so on explored and acknowledged?

★ What 'small wins', steps, moves in the right direction, and progress have you already made? What building blocks are already in place? What journey have you already been on? What footsteps have you already taken?

★ What do you feel is going well and what are you pleased about? Are there opportunities to highlight and share things that people are proud of, grateful for, and which are going well? What makes a day a good day for someone, what are someone's sparkle moments in their job, what do they appreciate in their colleagues and in the work?

★ What do you feel you, your team, or your organization is already doing which is helpful and aligned with the ideas and values of adversity, culturally, and trauma-informed practice?

★ What are you most proud of and grateful for as an individual, team, or organization? What have been some of the sparkle, turnaround, lightbulb, treasured moments and achievements so far? What can you anchor on to, use as a memory bank, soak in, and be inspired by in difficult times?

★ How are conversations of 'hope' encouraged and made room for? When people are feeling in a place of little hope, what tools, resources, and strategies are there to support them? Are there people from whom they can borrow some hope, wisdom, strength? How can hope be invited to be people's constant travel companion? What inspires and motivates you and others?

★ Who are people's inspirers, cheerleaders, and motivators?

★ What parts of the work give you the most satisfaction, motivation, enjoyment, and joy? What part of the work is aligned with your values and what is important to you? What pushes your reward buttons? What refuels you and others around you?

★ Are there multi-sensory, creative, and expressive ways of displaying, enriching, and embedding individual, family, team, and organizational strengths, skills, and resources? For example, a tower or skyscraper of team strengths, a team tree of progress, a team patchwork of positives and possibilities, team murals, shields, or crests, a sparkle moments jar, board, or wall, a snakes and ladders picture of the distance travelled.

★ Where appropriate, do interventions and assessments attempt to see the whole person, family, and context, and widen the frame and picture? Can you see the person behind the diagnosis, crisis, label?

★ Are problem-saturated language and negative discourses and labels avoided? Is consideration given to the choice and impact of the words used in meetings, reports, letters, signs, texts, materials, the website, daily logs, interactions, and so on? How balanced are they?

★ Is there an emphasis on hope, moving forward, and future thinking? Are strengths and resources acknowledged and identified verbally, non-verbally, and creatively? Is there time to acknowledge and appreciate what is going well?

★ How strengths-based and balanced are the intake forms, measures, assessment tools, reviews, agreements, plans, and meetings? For example, if someone is asking about trauma, are there also discussions and measures around protective factors, power resources, and strengths? How are opportunities for progress maximized and increased? How are protective factors magnified and supported? If there has been an incident, is there also a focus on all the other days and moments when there was not an incident? Or when a 'problem' or difficulty is absent or reduced? In Narrative Therapy, this is often referred to as finding the unique exception.

★ Are there opportunities for people's voices to be heard, honoured, and respected? How is everyone seen as an expert of their own experience?

★ How are people's skills supported and elevated? Are there opportunities to learn from each other and to develop? Is development encouraged and supported?

★ Are there opportunities to explore, enrich, and reflect on future thinking and opportunities and around wishes, hopes, and visions?

★ What messages of hope, inspiration, positivity, and strengths are displayed and shared around the building and in other forms of communication, such as on the walls, in posters, on blogs, in magazines, in events, in plays, in the names of the rooms? (Be mindful of toxic positivity, as explored below.)

★ Does the environment help people to feel more nurtured, supported, and connected? Does it increase people's feeling of being valued? (See Chapter 9.) This might include having wellbeing rooms, calming corners, nurturing nests, Zen zones, sensory rooms, and nurturing staff spaces.

★ How are stories of hope, strengths, best practice, and survivorship shared and heard?

★ What is done to bring play, connection, fun, and humour into the work, the team meetings, and the organization?

★ What is done to support community and team cohesion, connection, morale, and team spirit?

★ How are people recruited, inducted, and welcomed? This can be 'small' things like having welcome packs, mugs, and cards for new starters, and includes how people are made to feel about the role during recruitment and induction.

★ How are people celebrated (if they wish to be)? Is there a culture of value, appreciation, and thanking people and letting them know that they matter in your team/organization? How are people thanked, valued, invested in, elevated, acknowledged, and shown to be appreciated by each other, the team, and the organization? For example, this could be saying good morning, hello, thank you, well done; smiling; sending a thank you message or card; managers giving shout-outs; giving someone a hug if they need and want it; looking up from one's computer screen; offering a drink; checking-in with each other; making time for each other; being interested in each other. Within this, small things can make a big difference, for example little token gestures, such as a mug with some treats inside, or a post-it note with a treat on someone's desk saying 'thanks for all the hard work', or a regular supply of biscuits, snacks, drinks.

Co-production, voice, choice, agency, and mastery

★ How inclusive is the organization? How are people at all levels included and their opinion meaningfully asked and listened to? Who is given prominence and privileged? Who is silenced, ignored, neglected? What do you think the people using your services would say about their involvement, voice, choice, power, and partnership? How is the service 'doing with', and not 'doing to'? Is there an understanding as to why this is so important?

★ How does the organization support growth and skill development? How does it elevate and celebrate people? How does it support progression and sharing of skills? How do you feel your team and organization support reciprocity, meaningful feedback, power-sharing, partnership, and relational collaboration?

★ How are power, status, and privilege reflected on, acknowledged, and responded to?

★ What training and support are there around understanding participation and co-production? What messages are given around this and it prioritized?

★ How are 'experts of experience/people with direct experience' included as partners, or involved and consulted with at all levels in meaningful, non-tokenistic ways? Do they have opportunities to design, shape, and drive services? Are they represented on boards, in leadership roles, in interview panels? How are the people who have used services and who have lived experience placed at the heart of the service?

★ How much ownership, voice, and choice do people have in the support they receive? (It can be helpful to go through worksheet 9.1 in Chapter 9 to reflect on the different areas and processes within the service.)

★ Do people have clear and accessible messages about their rights? Are these accessible and communicated? This might include complaints procedures, feedback mechanisms, access to an advocate, access to a lawyer.

★ Within reason, how much choice do employees have within their role (e.g. flexible working, diversity of workload, personal development opportunities)?

★ What mechanisms and processes does the organization have in place for obtaining and integrating regular and meaningful input and feedback from the people who are using and working in the services? (This includes research, feedback boxes, focus groups, informal feedback, during inspections, surveys.) How is this feedback responded to and any decisions then implemented? How are the outcomes, decisions, and rationale, including changes made, communicated to people to show that they have been listened to and heard? How is the organization (and you) addressing adverse or concerned feedback in a timely, sensitive, and thoughtful manner?

★ How well do those processes and forms of feedback address whether or not the organization has tried to be culturally responsive, and trauma-informed? How are the values and commitments of the organization being felt and embodied?

Communication, collaboration, and transparency expanded
Communication

★ How are changes, restructures, decision-making processes, and things happening in the organization communicated from a trauma-informed lens? How is this done in a way that acknowledges how difficult change can be, with opportunities for people to be involved and feed back, and with intention around the language and timing?

★ Is consultation about change done in a clear, real, and transparent way (e.g. not feeling as if the decision has already been made and it is a tick-box exercise)?

★ How well do the organization and team communicate and ask for meaningful feedback? How effective are these communication styles? To what extent do people feel in the loop and part of things?

★ How creative and multi-modal are the communication styles that are used? This might include infographics, animations, podcasts, videos, and presentations.

★ How is communicating via technology done in a way that works, is effective, and supports people to feel connected?

★ How is communication thought about in the wider sense, such as brochures, materials, the website, letters, signs, online forums, posters, and newsletters? If you reviewed them through a trauma-informed lens, are they suitable? Is there anything that could be done to improve them? Have they been collaboratively created?

★ What mechanisms and processes does your organization have in place for obtaining and integrating regular input and feedback from the people who are using and working in services?

★ How accessible, visible, creative, reciprocal, meaningful, and effective are these? Do people know about them? How are you responding to and implementing the changes suggested, and communicating to people they have been heard and listened to?

★ How are the changes and actions communicated? For example, 'You said, and we listened…'

★ Are there clear contact details at the bottom of emails and letterheads?

★ Can people contact the organization without getting endless voice-operated messages? Does this allow for people who need adaptations, such as those who are deaf or blind or who don't have access to a mobile phone? If there is a voice message, is this regularly listened to?

★ What methods does the organization use to connect with people, and share information, concerns, and best practice? How useful and effective are these? Do they model the model? Do they reflect the values of trauma-informed practice?

★ How is communication done in a relational, respectful, and human way?

★ How are conflicts and disagreements responded to?

★ How are strengths, progress, positive news, and best practice examples communicated and celebrated?

★ How is attention paid to non-verbal forms of communication, such as body language, body positioning, eye contact, facial expressions, and so on? (Hold in mind some of the cultural and societal nuances and differences within these.)

In considering the power of language and storying – thinking consciously and deliberately about the language used and the words chosen when communicating from an adversity, culturally, and trauma-informed lens:

★ Is it descriptive or opinion language? Is it, where appropriate, person-first language? Is the language respectful to the person's choice and meaning-making? Is the language balanced, including strengths? Is the language judgemental/pejorative? Is the language clear, using everyday words, or does it use jargon or clinical language? How might someone hearing themselves described in this way feel? Is the language sensitive of people's culture and areas of difference? Are acronyms needed and necessary? How accessible are they? How well are they explained to people who may be less familiar with them? What might the acronym represent? (See Chapters 6 and 7.)

★ How are people's communication and language needs considered and supported? What adaptations are made to support these needs (e.g. those for whom English is not their first language, those with visual or hearing needs, learning needs, speech and language difficulties, executive function difficulties)? Are there creative and multi-modal ways of communicating to optimize learning?

In communicating clearly goals, objectives, procedures, values, role definitions, tasks, expectations, and so on:

★ How clear and defined are the goals, objectives, tasks, expectations, roles?

★ Do people working for the organization have a clear way of articulating what they do, what the organization does, what the values are, and so on?

★ Is there a sense of a shared identity and language?

★ Is there transparency, for example about the requirements of the role?

★ How effectively are people communicating about clinical work with the team around the person? How is the support joined up?

★ Is there clear communication before, during, and after assessments and interventions?

In considering how information is shared between agencies, during referrals, transitions, and through meetings, and so on:

★ Is the information handwritten? How clear are the notes?

★ Are issues of confidentiality and consent kept at the forefront?

★ Will another agency understand them, including acronyms used?

★ Are they clearly marked with the date, time, and name of the person recording them?

★ Are thought, care, and attention given to the language and tone used?

★ How would someone reading their notes feel? Would you write about yourself or your family member/loved one in that way?

★ Would the notes stand up in a court room?

Collaboration

We need to work together in as integrated, connected, and cohesive way as possible; in a multidisciplinary way, with access to a range of professionals so that we can draw on their expertise. Ideally, we want to create communities of minds, hearts, innovators, and inspirers. We want to draw on a range of perspectives and disciplines, and make sure we are working in a joined-up way.

★ How collaboratively does the team work together? How connected, integrated, and cohesive are they?

★ How are people working in a multidisciplinary way? What efforts are made to ensure that this is as effective as possible?

★ Where possible, how are collaborative problem-solving and decision-making being supported?

★ Are there efforts to join up and ensure that people are not re-inventing the wheel or repeating work already done, but are instead drawing on existing resources and each other's expertise?

★ How inclusive is the organization? How are people being communicated and collaborated with? Who is being heard and prioritized? Whose voices are not represented (e.g. birth parents, fathers, foster carers, a particular service)?

★ How is the organization meaningfully, genuinely, and authentically collaborating with those on multiple levels, with multiple perspectives, including community leaders and those with direct experiences? This might also include people such as community healers, elders, and spiritual leaders.

★ What opportunities are there to collaborate, disseminate, share, and connect with the community and other agencies doing similar and complementary work?

★ Are there opportunities to share best practice and to have things like learning circles, learning collaboratives, shared conferences, joint meetings, and cross-agency shadowing opportunities?

★ How is information shared, and how are transitions, pathway plans, and referrals done?

★ Are there opportunities to learn about the local context and to do shared and cross-learning (e.g. shadowing opportunities, shared panels)?

Transparency

In trauma experiences, there is often a sense of secrecy and avoidance. This can also be mirrored at a community level where things can be brushed under the carpet. Organizations can also echo this, and there can be a sense of mistrust, and a general lack of openness and transparency. This can also feed into people feeling 'done to', out of the loop, devalued, or excluded. There may be confusion, frustration, and an array of other ripple effects. Therefore, decisions and processes, where possible, should be done in a transparent and honest way.

★ How transparent and communicative are things around what might happen, what is happening and why, and what might happen next and why? This might include sensitively naming the elephant in the room, as well as sharing with people the thinking behind a decision and the context and journey which has surrounded it. It might include things like funding, and wider contextual pressures.

★ Are the aims, goals, function, purpose, mission, vision, funding, and policies of the organization clearly communicated and transparent?

★ Are people's diaries and workloads accessible for those who need to see them?

★ Is there discussion and transparency around some of the limitations, tensions, and challenges of the organization, and of tasks, projects, and so on, as well as some of the progress, hopes, and strengths?

★ Are there opportunities to be open to honest and to provide productive feedback, through formal and informal processes?

★ Is there an attempt by people to communicate in a transparent and sensitive way? For example, in a cross-agency meeting, being honest about some of the dilemmas and pitfalls, as well as lessons learned.

★ Are processes for complaints, concerns, and disciplinary actions as transparent as possible? Is there a working or development group and ethics panel to ensure and develop these?

★ Are there processes around people being able to access their notes, records, and files?

CHAPTER 8

Making the Difference: Infusing Trauma-Informed Values into Practice

8.1. What will be covered in this chapter

- Empathy, compassion, curiosity, listening, and how we make people feel

- Some feelings, feedback, experiences, quotes, stories, and memories shared about difficult health experiences

- Limbic whisperers – our own regulation systems

- Communication and actions before, during, and after an appointment or interaction – some key tips and examples

- After the intervention

There are many different ideas, suggestions, and changes shared in this chapter, and inevitably these vary depending on the context, purpose of the service, and various other factors. Each service has its own personality, culture, aims, history, and purpose. Some will resonate and fit with you, and others will not; however, it is for you to reflect and think about what you are already doing and what could be tweaked, adapted, changed, or added to your practice. So, in essence, take the information and embed it where appropriate. It is acknowledged that many of these ideas may be already in use, which is wonderful. Moreover, the aim is not to shame or blame people or services where these things are not happening, as we know there are many reasons why this might be the case. Additionally, they are not intended to be an exhaustive or prescriptive list, but rather offer food for thought and some practical, real-world examples of how small things can make a difference – 'every interaction is an intervention' (Treisman, 2017a).

These examples come from informal and formal feedback from hundreds of people who use or have used health services, from a wide range of practition-ers who work within services, and from the extant literature. They are not a replacement for wider systemic and organizational changes as listed at the end of Chapter 5, nor for addressing some of the organizational and system stress and workplace culture as described in Chapter 6. However, they are in line with the values of trauma-informed practice, as well as having a trauma lens, and anchoring on to the four R's of trauma-informed practice: realize, recognize, resist, and respond.

There will also be a series of boxes at the end of the chapter, with some stories, tangible examples, and contributions from people which offer some new ideas and expand on the ones shared. Your own procedures, practice, and setting can be reviewed and reflected on using some of the questions shared in Chapter 7 and the step-by-step worksheet in Chapter 9, and of course through other avenues such as seeing a trauma consultant.

8.2. Empathy, compassion, curiosity, listening, and how we make people feel

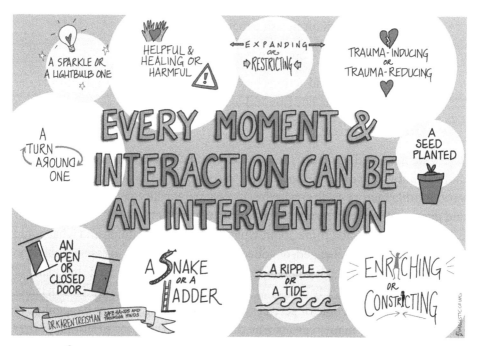

8.1. EVERY MOMENT AND INTERACTION CAN BE AN INTERVENTION

One of the most important parts of relational, person-centred, and trauma-in-formed health care is how we make people feel. This does not mean that there won't be times when we must make painful decisions, or add physical pain to someone through a procedure, or deliver difficult news. However, how this is done is the crucial bit. We are our greatest tool and strategy, and so often it is how the message is delivered – as Maya Angelou says, it is how we make people feel which stays, lingers, and leaves a mark. We know that this delivery style and the way we make people feel can make a massive difference, for example when someone calls customer services to say their internet is not working, or they have a leak in a pipe. The response can either be co-regulating and helpful or co-escalating and stress-inducing; it may add to an already annoying or stressful situation, and influence how the person feels and what they say about that company.

In this situation, we are not just representing ourselves, but potentially the hospital, clinic, team, our profession, the organization itself, and our own relationship to 'help'. So, it is important to think about how our interactions represent this and what messages we want to convey. We can open doors or close doors, be healing and helpful, or be harmful or unhelpful. It is that whole sense as Dr Sandy Bloom says around, say what you mean without being mean saying it. So, it is important to think about how our interactions represent this and what messages we want to convey and how every interaction is an intervention (Treisman, 2017).

For example, you might be explaining a procedure, or delivering news, or asking personal questions. For you it is business as usual, you might have done it numerous times, sometimes on a daily basis; so you might go into autopilot, or in your head, know why you are doing it or asking that question. But it is important to remember that to the other person it may be unfamiliar, life-changing, scary, confusing, overwhelming, anxiety-provoking, shocking. It might be their first time hearing that news or those terms, or undergoing that procedure. That person might be one of 20 people you are seeing that day but they might have been waiting for that appointment for a year, or it has come after years of trying to see someone or to get answers, or they have taken time off work or travelled a long way for the appointment.

How they might feel can be entangled with that person's past and previous experiences with health professionals, hospitals, their body, feeling heard, feeling powerless, and so on. They may have had past medical and health-related stress and trauma, experienced abuse of power, been silenced and oppressed, discriminated against, and so on.

It is so important to think about what this might be like from their perspective. Of course, we do not know, as we are not mind readers and we do not have emotional or life x-rays. So, it is crucial to be curious, to ask, hold in mind multiple possibilities, and have humility. *How would you feel if it were you, your parents, partner, child, loved one? Would you recommend you as a practitioner or your team/service to others?* How we come across extends not just to our words and choice of language, but to our facial expressions, tone of voice, positioning, body language, whether we talk over them, rush them, look disinterested, roll our eyes, stare at the computer screen, imply that we aren't present or interested.

Of course, it varies from situation to situation, but having someone truly listen, be curious, be compassionate, and empathize, validate, and acknowledge one's experience can make a profound difference (see Chapter 3). We need to think and ask about what matters to the person, what this is like on a daily basis for them, how this impacts their life, and to let them know that we hear how painful, stressful, or difficult it is. Having someone genuinely saying things like 'What I hear you saying is.../I am so sorry you are experiencing that/I can't imagine what that must be like/I am not in your shoes, but I wonder.../Thanks for sharing...' can go a long way.

We also know, particularly in the context of trauma, that people have often felt invalidated, silenced, their pain ignored, minimized, dismissed, and so on. Therefore, in addition to expressions and actions of empathy and acknowledgement, we also need to avoid statements which can minimize, patronize, invalidate, and shut down conversations, as well as position people in unhelpful and potentially reinforcing and activating places. This can feed into toxic positivity, trying to put a silver line around something that is distressing to that person. Avoid statements such as 'It could be much worse', 'It is only mild discomfort', 'Oh bless you, you are an anxious one', and 'I know exactly how you feel'. Likewise, minimizing statements using 'at least' are unhelpful: 'At least you got pregnant', after someone has had a miscarriage. We should not be telling someone how they feel or how they should feel, but supporting their own meaning-making. Although there may be common themes and these can be helpful to normalize and to validate, remember that each person will still have their own unique experience.

Moreover, we also know there are some very practical implications. For example, if someone is feeling tense or in a heightened state, it might be harder for them to undertake procedures, and they may require sedation or additional staff, have higher blood pressure, and be more likely to have conflicts and strained relationships with staff. Likewise, when someone is worried or feels judged, shamed, or hurt, they might be less likely to share concerns, ask questions, or make disclosures, and be reluctant to come for further appointments or check-ups, such as blood tests, mammograms, and cervical screenings. For some people, this can mean that when support is sought, their problems are more severe or even at a critical stage.

The way we make people feel can impact how much a person trusts, feels safe, or respects the person they are seeing. This can make a difference to how someone might engage, whether they listen to and follow advice, and what they might say to others about the centre or hospital or person. This has both reputational risk but also ripple effects on societal and public health and organizational messaging (e.g. apprehensions around vaccinations).

Take the example of a child who is scared of blood tests and who has a chronic condition. If they are held down, or forced, or have a more distressing experience of blood tests on that occasion, not only will they likely tense up and move, making the procedure harder, but their distress will inevitably have an impact on their future blood tests, appointments, and investigations. This experience will also impact their relationship with staff; it is likely to require more staff and more time, not just in this moment but for future appointments. It will also be upsetting for the staff and the parents, and for the other people receiving care nearby, who will witness the distress.

In another example, I was in a very busy and overstretched A&E. There was a man, for whom English was his second language, sitting at the front by the doors. I could see he had been crying and he was gently moving around and appeared restless. I heard him respectfully and quietly go up to the person at the front desk and ask her for an update on his wife. He explained that he had been there for hours without news and the last time he had seen her she was not breathing and was in an ambulance, and he didn't know what was happening or what to tell his children. Clearly, he had asked several times before. The woman was minimizing and dismissive, and ushered him off. Each time the doors opened and a nurse, doctor, or janitor or whoever came in, he would go and politely ask them the same question. He was repeatedly told they didn't know, were not the right person to ask, he needed to wait his turn, asking wasn't going to make it any quicker, and he was ushered off. I could see he had no water, and the machine was empty, it was freezing cold, and he had clearly rushed out the house in a short-sleeved shirt. There was no food, and there were no chargers or available plugs, so his phone had run out of battery. As the hours went on, he continued asking, understandably each time his tone slightly raised and his urgency increasing. Eventually, he stood up and shouted, 'Where is my wife? What is going on?' Within minutes, security was called, and he was escorted out of the building. There are so many things that were happening here, but the accumulation of missed opportunities just escalated instead of regulating the situation, and it was dehumanizing and minimizing for the husband. It made an already difficult situation far worse and the ripples were far-reaching, with people witnessing his distress, the messages being given, and with the time taken repeatedly to speak to him.

Similar scenarios can be found throughout the literature. For example, Havig (2008) reported several provider-centred inhibitors of disclosure, such as embarrassment, judgement, scrutiny, expressions of pity or repulsion, avoidance, or displays of disinterest in the response. Moreover, the quality of the therapeutic relationship and alliance has repeatedly been found to be a significant predictor of 'outcomes' and as a crucial vehicle and anchor for change, regardless of the modality of treatment and the interventions offered (Baldwin *et al.*, 2007; Barber *et al.*, 2009; Castonguay *et al.*, 2006; Hill, 2009; Lutz *et al.*, 2007; Priebe & McCabe, 2006).

While it can be hard as a practitioner to feel deskilled, and unhelpful, or to be in a place of uncertainty – and this can jar with training expectations of having the answers, fears of being seen as incompetent, and with one's rescue valency and of wanting to make a difference – it is important, where possible, to hold on to safe uncertainty (Mason, 1993). Just because we can't see something or can't identify it or it doesn't fit with what a journal or academic textbook says, it does not mean it is not there, is not being experienced, and is not valid. It is okay to not know or to validate some of the frustrations around this, and to acknowledge someone's experience and remember that they are the expert of their own experience. It's okay to question whether there was something we should have done that we didn't, or whether something was missing from the picture, or to admit that we wish we had the answers, or knew more, or are sorry that something is happening.

How we make people feel is so much more than just words, non-verbal cues, and body language; it is also in things like the maintenance of the physical environment, and the posters on the wall (see Chapters 7 and 9). It is also in the wider experiences, such as having certain items accessible (discussed in sections which follow in this chapter), or having corridor conversations which can be overheard. Of course, these are sometimes necessary, but we need to be mindful of how confidential information can be said within earshot of others; for example, having an HIV status loudly announced in front of other people, as well as seeing staff point and then hearing them whisper loudly so others can hear about it.

Graphic details are sometimes shared, which can be shocking or distressing to others hearing who are not used to being exposed to the sorts of situations staff might be. Some people have mentioned hearing staff talk about their fun weekend and hysterically laughing, while they themselves were in agony and having to wait to be seen in A&E for five hours. Others have spoken about corridor conversations which seemed to be mocking, joking about, or sharing details of patients, and how inappropriate this felt, but also made them wonder how they would be spoken about. Similarly, conversations can be overheard about patients being 'a pain in the bum', 'difficult', 'a waste of time', and so on.

See Chapters 3 and 4 for some examples of how people have felt within health settings and how we can use this feedback to shape and influence our practice and put more emphasis on how we make people feel.

8.3. Limbic whisperers – our own regulation systems

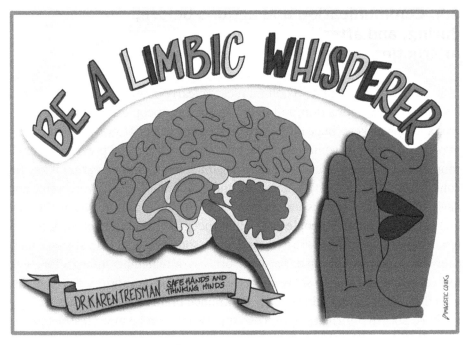

8.2. LIMBIC WHISPERER

While thinking about how we make people feel, it is important that we become more aware of our own autonomic states and how to be our own and other people's limbic whisperers. This fits with Stephen Porges' polyvagal theory, and how we need to find ways to activate people's social engagement and safety systems. This is about how someone's voice, tone, facial expressions, gestures, touch, way of listening, proximity, and much more can convey important cues of safety to the other person's autonomic nervous system. Porges calls the process of automatically and continually scanning our environment for features of danger or safety neuroception. In neuroception, our defence systems are dampened down and our social engagement system comes online (Porges, 2007). It is like being on a plane, and looking at the air hostesses to see if they seem calm or unsure and panicked. We want people to feel they are in safe hands, thinking minds, and regulated bodies. This emotional contagion and emotional holding can set the scene and lead to a whole ripple effect of responses, including mutually escalating arousal. It is about how we make people feel at a somatic, embodied, and felt level. This is why our own ability to be grounded, thoughtful, and containing is crucial; and why we need to be mindful and prioritize our own wellbeing (Chapter 6).

8.4. Communication and actions before, during, and after an appointment or interaction – some key tips and examples

It is extremely important to communicate clearly before, during, and after a visit, procedure, interaction, and so on. Again, some people are excellent in this area and this makes a huge difference on so many levels. However, for a variety of reasons, including some system factors, staff burnout, and pressurized environments (Chapter 6), this can be lacking for some. Communication is key for consent, building rapport, establishing and maintaining trust, overcoming and navigating through barriers and concerns, and much more. Moreover, in the context of trauma, so often people have felt silenced, powerless, shocked, deceived, ignored, not believed, mistreated. And when someone is in fear, stress, shock, overwhelm, and pain, it can be harder to process or remember information, or to feel confident and able to share concerns or question 'authority'. This is in line with the concept that brains in pain, or strained brains can sometimes struggle to think, absorb information, process, etc. People can be more distracted and struggle with paying attention or concentrating, only taking in small portions of what they hear. This isn't helped by the medical jargon that is sometimes used, which might be familiar and everyday language to the practitioner but for others can seem like a foreign language. This can be further exacerbated if someone has speech and language difficulties, additional learning or cognitive needs, if English is a second language, if someone is blind or deaf, has dementia, a head injury, cannot read or write, and so on. So, they might need repetition, and for the information to be conveyed in multi-modal ways.

8.4.1. Before an appointment or interaction

First impressions count and set the tone for future interactions. Clear information can also support people to feel more prepared, as well as minimizing confusion and additional questions. For example, it can help to think about what information is provided or sent out to people before they attend their appointment, whether by email, text, letter, in brochures, videos, or on the website. This should ideally include clear information about what to expect and what might happen before, during, and after the interaction. Practical information including timing (important for people to be able to plan around work, childcare, other caring duties, food, etc.) and what to bring is essential.

It is also important to address frequently asked questions and explain jargon, and avoid using acronyms. Advice from practitioners and from other people who have gone through the procedure and can offer helpful advice (co-produced and engaging ideally) is also useful. This might include common worries, feelings, questions, hopes, expectations. It is also helpful to consider how this information might be understood or could be adapted to be more inclusive, for example if the person has previous trauma, concerns about the test or outcome, or health anxiety; if English is a second language; if they are deaf or blind; if they are in a wheelchair; if they have additional learning needs; if this is their first time undergoing this procedure, and so on. See Chapter 6 for more on health disparities and biases.

As a psychologist, I find it useful to have an introduction video and written information about me and the service. Where possible and appropriate, I also share information about the building and sometimes make a short video, for example about the room or the space or directions or showing the journey to get there. I also have some friendly personalized ways of introducing myself as seen in the images below; and a series of images about how people might feel coming to see me, and their frequently asked questions. It is helpful to consider if there are multiple ways of presenting this information for different needs and learning styles (e.g. a brochure, video, poster, infographic, comic, diagram), and to consider whether there are aspects which can be added to increase accessibility, such as captions, subtitles, different colours.

It is also important to have clear information about where to find the building, with ideally a video, a map, clear instructions, parking and public transport information, and directions. Key contact information is vital too. Sometimes, these systems are tricky to navigate, which can add to confusion, mistrust, and frustration before someone even attends, especially if they have additional needs like speech and language difficulties, or do not speak much English. So, think about other options such as email, text, or voice recording and whether someone needs an interpreter or an allocated parking space.

Consider any forms that need to be filled in – how useful and relevant are they, especially if they ask for potentially distressing or personal information, and how accessible are they? Where appropriate, some services can send an optional form for people to choose to complete around their wellbeing or needs.

This is highly recommended and can make a real difference to some people. It acknowledges that the service appreciates that the appointment might be stressful or activating for some people for a variety of reasons. Depending on the service and aims, it might include questions on how they are feeling about coming to an appointment; this can have tick boxes beside feeling words or pictures, as well as space to any not included. It might give options for people to tick, circle images, or share aspects which might be activating for them or which might add stress to them, such as noises, being made to lie down, certain types of touch, body positions, certain phrases, certain smells. There should be space for them to expand these if they wish to. It might ask for suggestions of things that might help someone to feel more supported and cared for or which might make a difference to them. Some forms might list things which could be provided and people circle or add to these. For example, some people might require more pain relief, extra time factored in for a procedure, or creative solutions for swallowing tablets, having injections, and so on. Although this might all seem quite time consuming, it is likely to reduce harm, distress, and complaints, and have an impact on future interactions.

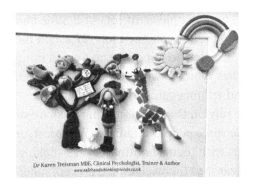

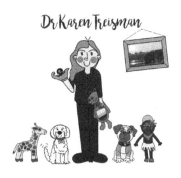

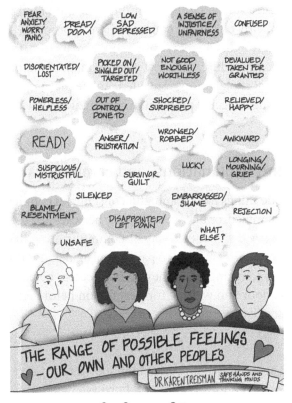

8.3, 8.4, AND 8.5.

8.4.2. During an appointment or interaction

Keeping a person's dignity and integrity at the forefront of your mind is important, especially in the context of trauma, where someone has often felt dehumanized and objectified, and their dignity and integrity may have been violated.
Be clear, transparent, and compassionate during the meeting and interactions,
sharing what is happening and why. Remember to check-in and acknowledge

people's differences and preferences – some people want lots of details and want to see the procedure, be part of it if possible, see the tools, or watch the screen; others want very little information. It is also important to hold in mind that we do not have emotional or life x-rays, which is why a universal approach is important (see Chapter 7). Stress and trauma can show themselves in so many different ways, and we should not rely on the person having to share or disclose their feelings. Be aware that while some people's trauma, discomfort, or distress might be more easily identifiable, with them shouting, crying, shaking, trembling, or fainting, others might retreat into themselves and go very quiet. Others might make jokes, nod their heads, and smile.

With communication and integrity at the forefront of our practice, it is also important to explicitly talk about consent where appropriate, and to listen and respond accordingly – this might require more explanation, more strategies, or even stopping the procedure. Ask how you can make them more comfortable, and offer additional explanations if needed. As the playwright George Bernard Shaw said, 'The single biggest problem in communication is the illusion that it has taken place.'

8.4.3. Consent, explanations, and communication

This might include things like meaningful consent and communication around being touched, examined, or uncovered. It may be necessary to stop a procedure, and to have an agreed signal or a way of communicating like a card or hand gesture that the person wants you to pause. It also includes things like drawing curtains, covering someone when they do not need to be naked or exposed, or knocking on the door and waiting for permission before entering. Here is an example to illustrate this.

> When I had severe burns, I was taken into a room and undressed. I was naked and in a lot of pain. The burn was 40cm plus in area, so it covered a large portion of my body. The nurse needed some equipment and medication and so she left me standing naked in the room in front of the door; I was unable to move due to the positioning and pain. However, she forgot to close the door as she left and took about ten minutes before returning. Not only was I left wondering what was happening, where she was, and if she was coming back, but I was also naked and unable to move. I felt utterly embarrassed, vulnerable, and exposed. Numerous people walked past the room,

peering in, including other people receiving services and their family and friends visiting, other doctors and nurses, and other staff such as domestic staff. I found this very uncomfortable, and I can only imagine what this might have felt like to others who might have gone down a memory time hole (e.g. around feeling exposed, lack of integrity, being peered at or watched).

Introducing yourself, and clearly explaining your role and what is going to happen, is essential. This might seem like an obvious one, but in highly pressurized environments it can be forgotten. Introducing yourself is also important for building trust and rapport, but bear in mind that for some people, especially if you are wearing a mask and there are several people in the area, this can be confusing. So having clearly identifiable ID badges is important. If someone is a specialist or has a role that might be less obvious, it is important to share this. This is particularly the case for those who might be new to the setting, have learning needs or dementia, or whose country of origin might have very different systems.

Someone had just had a baby by caesarean; the baby was premature but generally seemed healthy and was doing well. About two hours after the baby's arrival the baby was sleeping in the hospital crib besides her mother. A woman unknown to the mother of the baby walked in, picked up the baby, turned around, and proceeded to walk out of the ward. The mum felt confused, shocked, and worried. She was still dazed and sleepy from the medication and birth; she couldn't walk from the epidural and caesarean section and was still processing having a new baby. Thankfully, her sister was in the ward visiting and saw the panic cross her sister's face. She ran after the woman saying, 'Excuse me, excuse me, excuse me.' The woman did not hear or respond and so her sister had to raise her voice even louder to get her attention: 'EXCUSE ME.' Eventually the woman turned around and looked surprised and a bit irritated. The sister explained that the woman had come into the space, not introduced herself, not shown her ID, and had taken her niece without explaining who she was, where she was taking her, what they would be doing or looking for, and when she would be bringing her back. The woman looked shocked and apologized and explained that she was on autopilot and was so busy that she hadn't thought about it. This can often happen, especially in busy settings and when juggling a lot. This mum had had three babies and was relatively comfortable in a hospital setting but understandably still felt worried by this encounter. Imagine if this had been someone who had a past medical trauma, or who had previously experienced the loss of a baby, or been hurt or abused by a stranger. Similarly, this could have been someone who didn't have her sister there, or who didn't understand due to having a learning disability or English as a second language.

When explaining what will happen or describing a concept or a procedure, it is important to use multi-sensory, jargon-free, and accessible explanations; for example, employing props, visual aids, diagrams, or videos. This is often done more with children or those we know have additional learning needs, head injuries, or dementia. However, most people benefit from having information explained in different ways and often we aren't aware of someone's learning style, speech and language needs, or the impact of fear on them. When I explain parts of brain development, I generally use three different brief explanations, one using Lego or Jenga blocks, one using an animal picture (and sometimes animal miniatures or puppets), and one with a diagram, such as Bruce Perry's pyramid image from his neurosequential model.[1] If people are still struggling, I might use something like the brain architecture game from Harvard University's Center on the Developing Child,[2] or a video featuring Dan Siegel's brain hand model.[3] Usually this is helpful to explain the concept, but people do report that having the information presented in two to four different ways enables it to become embedded. We also know that when someone is about to have a procedure sometimes it can be helpful to visit the place beforehand, practise the journey, and play with the equipment. Play specialists in hospitals do fantastic jobs with this, but also it is important to remember that it is not just children who might benefit from a more stepped approach.

During the intervention, it is vital to communicate what is happening for the person, who might be feeling very scared and alone. For example, during an MRI scan, this would involve explaining the process as it takes place, giving

---

1   www.bdperry.com/clincal-work.
2   https://developingchild.harvard.edu/resources/the-brain-architecture-game.
3   https://drdansiegel.com/hand-model-of-the-brain.

count-downs, offering words of comfort, and so on. It's important to be aware of the physical environment and things that might distress or 'trigger' people and decrease their sense of safety and trust; for example, the wording or images on posters, banging and slamming doors, loud music, people peering in through glass slots on the window, and the use of statements such as 'Spread your legs', 'Stop being silly', and 'Calm down'. (Numerous examples of 'triggers' and stressful medical experiences are shared in Chapters 1, 3, and 4, and some ideas about the physical environment are given in Chapter 9.)

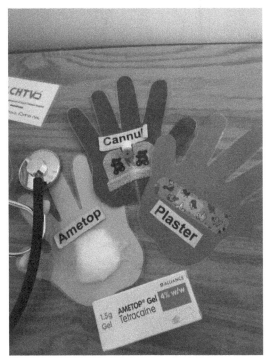

8.6. MULTI-SENSORY AND CREATIVE WAYS TO EXPLAIN PROCEDURES (IMAGE SHARED BY SUSAN MARSHALL, A SENIOR REGISTERED HEALTH CARE PLAY SPECIALIST)

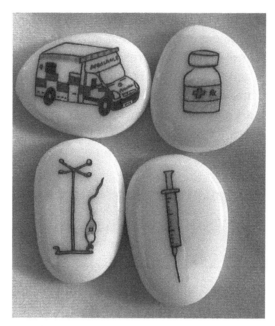

8.7. SOME MEDICALLY THEMED STONES

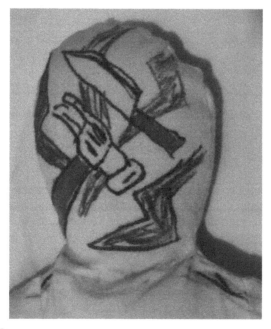

8.8. IMAGE DRAWN BY A MAN SEEKING ASYLUM WHO WAS
STRUGGLING TO CAPTURE THE SEVERITY OF HIS HEADACHES

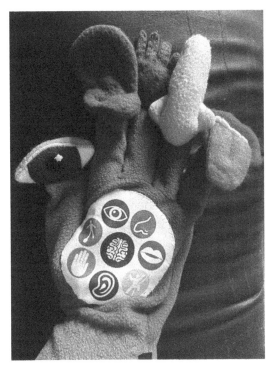

8.9. A PUPPET USED TO EXPLORE DIFFERENT MULTI-SENSORY EXPERIENCES

8.4.4. Students being present and consent

Sometimes students are present during an intervention. While students do need to observe and learn, especially in teaching settings, it should not be at the detriment of the person receiving care. Sometimes, medical students walk in without consent, or consent is asked for when they are already present and it can be difficult for the person to say no in front of them. Some people are happy for students to observe, but others may feel like a specimen or a case study, and find being spoken about like a textbook potentially dehumanizing. In addition, having more people – strangers – in the room than needed can feel embarrassing, overwhelming, and impersonal.

A ten-year-old girl had a diagnosis of lichen sclerosus. It was a rare form, and so she was seen as 'exciting' and a 'great learning opportunity' for students. The main site of the lichen sclerosus was in her vagina. She was just starting to go through puberty and to develop pubic hair and more of an awareness of her body. She had never been seen naked by a boy or a man, apart from her dad years previously, when she was little. So to be lying on a hospital bed with her legs spread apart and multiple young male students peering down at her and asking questions was embarrassing and humiliating. She teared up but no one noticed or acknowledged her discomfort, probably because they were focused on the lichen sclerosus rather than on her. After about 15 minutes, her mum, who couldn't really see her face among the crowd of people, said that it was inappropriate and unnecessary, and that people should leave. This experience not only was uncomfortable but scarred her emotionally, as she did not want to go to future appointments and either avoided them or found them distressing. When she was older and needed smear tests, she would find them activating or would avoid them altogether.

Occasionally, students, trainees, or newly qualified staff might boast to others or on social media about their first ever surgery or putting someone on a ventilator. It is understandable to be proud or excited about such things, but it is important to remember that, for the patient, it might have been their worst day ever, or they might be writing about someone's friend, parent, or child. People are not experiments or pin cushions. There are ways to share things in a respectful, thoughtful way and consider how it might be interpreted by other people.

8.4.5. Meaningful interaction and the use of names

Although it may not always be easy, it can make such a difference when the practitioner is prepared, makes the appointment as meaningful as possible, and values the person's time. For example, some people can wait months to see a doctor and then on arrival find that the doctor has not read their notes, and the whole appointment is taken up by the doctor reading the notes, flicking through files, and repeating what has already been said or done previously.

It may seem a small thing, but it is important to ask how someone would like to be addressed. Whether this is about abbreviations, chosen names, formal titles, pronouns, or pronunciation, it is essential to respect a person's wishes. This also includes anyone accompanying the person and, for example, not assuming they are the mum when they could be the foster carer, grandma, sister, family friend, or social worker. It takes seconds to ask about this but can make a huge difference to the interaction and how someone feels.

8.4.6. Scaling questions during appointments

Scaling questions are often used and can be extremely helpful to gather information, increase awareness, and track progress. However, these questions can be reductionist, and can lead to further confusion and lack meaning. For example, if someone is asked where, on a scale from 0 to 5, they would position their pain today (0 being the worst and 5 being the best), and they answer 3, often the practitioner will nod and move on. Do they understand what that means or looks like? This lacks meaning and is generally not useful. One person's 3 might be amazing and positive to them as they are usually at a 0, 1, or 2; another person's 3 might be terrible to them as they are usually a 4; another person's 3 might be awful to them but interpreted as 'good' by the practitioner. Some people tend to be 'positive' or want to appear 'strong' or don't want to worry or burden the doctor, or they are worried about the consequences if they say it is bad or worse.

Therefore, when scaling questions are used, for them to be meaningful it is important to explore and be curious. For example, you might ask questions depending on the context, such as if someone says 3: 'Describe 3 to me', 'What does 3 mean or look like?', 'What made you choose 3?', 'What is keeping you from being a 0, 1, or 2?' (this helps to identify their protective factors), 'What might support you to move to a 3.5 or 4?', 'What might other people say if they were in a similar situation or about you?', 'Where is the norm/typical/baseline for you and what factors contribute to this?', 'How might this change on a good day/bad day?', 'Where would you like to be?', 'What would be different?'

It is also important to remember that scaling might take some people down a time hole to feeling that there is a right or a wrong answer, to maths at school, or to other assessments where they have felt judged or restricted. Also, some people, depending on their age, speech and language, and cognitive ability, can struggle to say a number and it can feel abstract. So, they might benefit from being told that they can change their minds, that there is no right or wrong answer, and questions could be framed in multi-sensory ways, which can also be less abstract, more tactile, more playful, and more regulating for some.

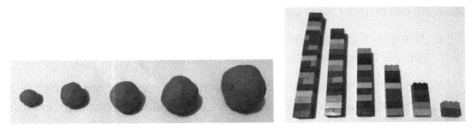

8.10 AND 8.11. SCALING QUESTIONS USING PLAY-DOH AND LEGO

8.4.7. 'Every interaction is an intervention' – one word can make a difference

The language we use in interventions can have a profound and powerful impact, and it is free! Using the right sort of language rarely takes more time, and can save lots of missed opportunities and miscommunication, and yet has such ripple effects. Language can shape our attitudes, expectations, beliefs, feelings, perspectives, and so much more. Language can help us make sense of the world, our experiences, and ourselves. It is also one of the main ways in which we communicate and connect with the people around us, and with ourselves (e.g. our self-talk and narratives). Language can fuel connection or contribute to disconnection and misunderstanding. Language is *so* powerful; it can hold so much weight, and it can be like a tattoo or a shadow that travels with you. Like a weapon, it can wound and leave a lasting impact. Language can restrict people and reduce them to boxes and labels. Language can contribute to people having tunnel vision, seeing only the word, or the label, not the person or the bigger picture.

A study by Loftus and Palmer (1974) demonstrated the power of words, and of a single word (numerous other studies have taken place in recent years). In this study, one group of people watched a video of a car accident and were then asked to estimate the speed the cars were travelling when they smashed into each other. There was also a control group; for them everything was exactly the same – the room, the person, the tone of voice – but one small word was changed. The control group were told that the cars bumped into each other, as opposed to 'smashed'. A week later they were all then asked if they saw blood or broken glass in the video of the car accident. The smashed group were significantly more likely to see blood and broken glass, even though there was no blood or broken glass! And the estimated speed also depended on whether the verb bumped or smashed was used. The associations with the word smashed had primed people to see things differently. This illustrated how a single word can shape what comes next and what people might assume, expect, remember, and do, and how being conscious of how language is used is crucial. Here are some other examples which illustrate how powerful words and slight changes in words can be (take some time to reflect on each of them):

- Using the word 'case', as in 'caseload' or 'my case', instead of 'the person', 'people I work with or support', or their name.

- Referring to someone's baby as a foetus or describing miscarriage as a 'pregnancy failure' or 'foetal demise', or due to an 'incompetent cervix'; or referring to a 40-year-old who is pregnant as 'geriatric'.

- Saying, 'What did you get yourself into today?', which can lead to people assuming that the practitioner blames them for their own injury or situation, rather than saying, 'I am sorry this happened to you. Can you tell me how it happened?'

- Saying someone is 'attention-seeking' instead of talking about how they might be 'attention-needing and connection-seeking'. See a person differently and you see a different person. See a behaviour differently and you see a different behaviour.

- Commenting on someone's weight and diet without knowing the person's history and relationship to food and their weight and body image. Some comments, assumptions, and judgements around this can cause people to feel shamed, blamed, and judged, which can impact future interactions.

- Telling someone, 'You look so well', 'You don't look sick', 'Well, it can't be that bad if you managed to work or socialize.' These sort of statements are loaded, they make a lot of assumptions, and can also make people feel minimized, silenced, and misunderstood. Moreover, they can be inaccurate as the reasons behind the person's appearance can be multi-faceted.

- Describing someone as 'resistant' or 'refusing' advice or a treatment suggestion, as opposed to 'cautious', 'hesitant', 'unsure', 'curious', 'apprehensive', 'protective'.

- Using 'at least' in a minimizing way, for example when someone has a miscarriage, saying, 'At least you got pregnant.'

- Using the words 'trigger' or 'discharge' for military personel and police can be unhelpful. Or telling someone to 'relax' during an intervention, when they were told to 'be quiet and relax' or 'stay still, relax' by the men who trafficked and raped them.

Always try to consider a person's context and be curious about the best use of language to support their unique situation.

8.4.8. Confirmation and attentional biases with relation to language

We know that certain biases can influence and shape people's beliefs and behaviours. For example, with *attentional bias*, the more you look for something and pay attention to it, the more you can see and notice it. This is like taking your brain to the gym repeatedly – you strengthen a particular area or focus. When you buy a new car, you might be more likely to see that type of car on the road, or when you are pregnant, or trying to get pregnant, or have just had a miscarriage, you might be more likely to see babies, bumps, and prams everywhere. When you look for the negative or problems, you are more likely to see them; or when you are looking for the strengths and hope, you are more likely to see them. Similarly, if you have been primed for someone being anxious, you are more likely to interpret their actions in that way.

This can be interwoven with *confirmation bias*, where there is a tendency to search for, interpret, and recall information in a way that affirms or supports your prior beliefs or hypotheses. For example, having a diagnosis can helpfully or unhelpfully frame what people see and interpret. This also raises interesting questions about context. Language can create a magnifying glass where we only see the things which a word or phrase has primed us to see. So if someone is described as a 'hypochondriac', 'anxious', 'aggressive', 'emotional', or an 'attention-seeker', everything they do, which there might be various other reasons for, is assumed to give weight to the original theory. Other possibilities are ignored, and the person is reduced to a label. Moreover, they might be discredited, disbelieved, judged, and so forth.

If someone is described as 'angry' or 'aggressive', you are more likely to interpret their body language as a potential sign of intimidation, anger, and aggression because you are paying more attention to those cues. There are further biases within this, such as people being more likely to see or describe people who are Black or have a loud voice or who are living on the streets as aggressive (see Chapter 6).

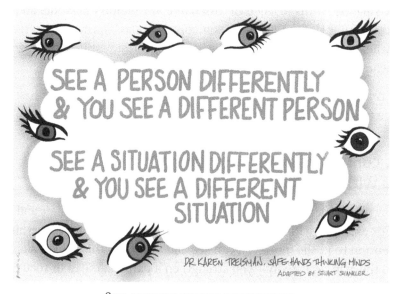

8.12. VIEWING THINGS DIFFERENTLY

Someone with a diagnosis of 'personality disorder' or 'anxiety' or 'schizophrenia' might have everything they do or say explained or reduced to this often-inaccurate label; and people might only see the label or diagnosis, not the person and their needs. Language can be so powerful because it can be stigmatizing and controversial and add additional difficulties because of the negative associations with it. The diagnostic term 'personality disorder' can add further stigma and barriers, as the person is more likely to be seen as a problem, a deficit, a maladaptive behaviour, or labelled as being 'manipulative', rather than seen as coping and protective in the context of their lived and living experiences.

As the saying goes, see a person differently and you see a different person; see a situation differently, and you see a different situation; see a behaviour differently and you see a different behaviour (Stuart Shankler, adapted and expanded by Karen Treisman).

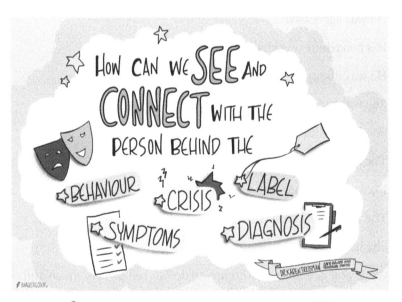

8.13. SEEING THE PERSON BEHIND THE DIAGNOSIS

Diagnostic overshadowing occurs when there is an assumption that the behaviour of a person with disabilities is part of their disability. For example, someone can have a diagnosis of Down syndrome and also be struggling with low mood, or be trying to communicate their sexual needs, or also might have been abused, but this will be overlooked because of their disability.

Context and perception play such a huge role. For example, in one context someone working 100 hours a week would be deemed impressive and hardworking, a candidate for promotion, but in another context it would be seen as problematic, with the person labelled as a workaholic, or manic, or showing signs of burnout. In one context, a social worker might arrive late and be met with understanding as they have been to court or had to attend to an emergency, but if a parent whose child is on the child protection register and they are known to social services turns up late, they might be described as chaotic and unreliable.

8.4.9. Vague and generalized descriptions

Another important consideration in interventions concerns the use of vague and unclear descriptions which often appear in letters, logs, reports, handover notes, and other written documents, as well as being used in meetings, supervision, and in court. These can lead to misinterpretations, with misinformation being passed on, and assumptions and generalizations being made. Here are some examples:

- She has been engaging in sexualized behaviour.

- He was aggressive.

- His behaviour was challenging.

- He was disruptive.

- She was rude.

- She has additional needs.

- The relationship is volatile.

- He was unkempt.

- The house was messy.

- She has sleep issues.

These vague and generalized statements do not tell us very much and can lead to all sorts of assumptions and confusion. For example, my version of someone being 'aggressive' or 'threatening' due to my background in prison work and youth violence might be coming at me with a knife or gun, while for someone working in a private school setting, the term 'threatening or aggressive' might involve a person raising their voice or swearing. There will be differing family, professional, and cultural concepts of what 'aggression' means.

Similarly, when talking about 'sexualized behaviour', one person might mean touching their penis once, another might mean sexual assault, another might be referring to a four-year-old child, and another to a 75-year-old with a diagnosis of dementia. This vague description does not shed any light and is very easily misunderstood. Or, for example, what one person classes as 'challenging' or 'difficult' might hugely vary but is completely subjective.

Moreover, when we make vague statements about things like 'sleep issues', what does this mean? Someone sleeps too much, sleeps too little, doesn't have access to a bed, is having nightmares, is scared of the dark, struggles to fall asleep or stay asleep, sleepwalks, wets the bed? How often do 'sleep issues' occur and what do they look like? This is the same for vast umbrella statements like 'behavioural issues', 'parenting issues', and 'mental health issues'.

These vague terms can feed into confirmation and attentional bias, as shared earlier. Moreover, how will these statements be understood in a few months or in several years' time by other professionals, or by the person whom they are written about (their notes belong to them)?

So, where possible and particularly for reports, it is important to state the facts and include actual description, and to be specific and not assume the other person is a mind reader and knows what we mean. If an opinion is being given, then this should be clearly stated as such. For example, 'Some professionals might consider...', 'It is debatable...', 'This needs to be interpreted with caution...', 'In my opinion...'

8.4.10. Person-first language

Person-first language refers to the importance of using words to avoid reducing someone to a label, a box, or a behaviour. Of course, it does not fit every situation or person (many people do not feel it is suitable when discussing neurodiversity and deafness), and we need to be respectful and ask, and be open to adjusting our language. If we just see someone as their behaviour, we reduce them to this, we close opportunities down for other parts of them, we restrict people to a label, and we feed into a self-fulfilling prophecy and confirmation bias. People cannot and should not be summed up in a single word. They are not their behaviour or a problem. Their behaviour or symptoms do not define who they are.

★ How can we see the person behind the behaviour/the crisis/the label? How would you feel if you were defined and reduced to a label or your most concerning behaviour?

Here are some examples of person-first language:

- A person is not an HIV patient, they are a person living with HIV; a baby is not an HIV exposed infant but rather a baby or child exposed to HIV.

- A person is not a drug addict, they are a person, with a name and with lots of other parts of their identity, who also happens to use drugs. A person is not a drug abuser or addict, they are a person who uses or injects drugs.

- A person is not a diabetic adult, they are a person with a diagnosis of diabetes. A child is not an epileptic child, but a child with a diagnosis of epilepsy.

- A person is not an offender, they are a person first, with a name, with lots of other parts of their personality, who also happens to have carried out an offence or multiple offences.

- A person is not a self-harmer, they are someone with a name, age, hobbies, interests, and different parts of their personality, and they might happen to occasionally cut their arms.

- A person is not a 'bed wetter', they are someone who wets the bed.

- A person is not bipolar, they are someone who has been given a diagnosis of bipolar. This is the same for statements about schizophrenia.

Would you describe someone by saying 'she's cancer' or 'he's HIV'? People might read that and be a bit shocked and confused. So why do we so often say things like 'he's ADHD' (attention deficit hyperactivity disorder), as if 'ADHD' is all the person is, as if this is their whole identity? Would they greet you with 'Hi, nice to meet you, I'm ADHD'? Why would we reduce someone to a socially constructed label? A diagnosis or what happened to someone is not their master or their main identity. That person is a person first – with lots of different parts to their identity and personality, who might also happen to have a diagnosis of ADHD, a term given by other people to that person. If they do have a diagnosis and this is something that is helpful for them, then it is still different to say 'Bob is 13 years old, he loves football and dogs; he is funny, kind, and sporty, and he also has been given a diagnosis of ADHD' rather than 'He's ADHD'.

Sometimes people use definitive terms to describe people or to reduce them, such as 'He is always rude' and 'He's never on time'. We need to leave more room for change, and use 'sometimes' or 'occasionally', or be more accurate and factual ('five times out of seven in the last week he has been late').

8.4.11. Choice and options

Choice isn't always possible for a variety of reasons but, where possible, being mindful of offering options is important, especially when people have felt powerless and without a voice. Here are just a few areas where we could offer choice in our practice:

- Name and/or pronoun or how they would like to be addressed and referred to.

- Their meaning-making of their experience and/or diagnosis.

- Language, terms, and words.

- Seating or body positioning, including standing, sitting on the floor, or moving around, and so on.

- Practitioner; for example, a woman requesting a woman, particularly for observations, one-to-one appointments, internal examinations, and so on.

- A chaperone, or someone to come or stay with them.

- Treatment, decisions, or interventions.

- Appointment times, location, and how contact is made (e.g. phone, email, text).

- Virtual or face-to-face appointments, consultations, and so on.

- Food and drink.

- Activities, materials used in an activity, opting out or passing on an activity or intervention.

- The goals and focus of the work.

What else would you add that fits your context?

8.4.12. Having access to items which might make a difference, including food and drink and a multi-sensory lens

Again, this will vary as of course what one needs in a dentist clinic will be different from a GP surgery, or a psychological therapy centre from an inpatient ward or an A&E department. It can also vary due to Covid and other health and safety protocols. However, small things can make a big difference to people, including how they feel, how they interact with staff, and what they request or need. Items might be purchased or donated. Here are some suggestions, but think about what you would include.

- Multiple plug points for phone, iPad, and laptop chargers.

- Access to some spare and most popular phone-charging cables. When people are waiting in A&E or are admitted to hospital, they are often less stressed or bored if they can play with or watch things on their phone, give updates, and communicate with family. Friends and family also feel more connected and don't have to rely on the ward staff or hospital phones.

- Vibrating or other communication systems (instead of beeps), noise-cancelling headphones, or ear plugs. Certain environments for people working in and using the services can be very loud, which can be distracting, annoying, and stressful. This can also impact people's ability to hear information and to sleep. It can be even harder for some people who have more of a sensory sensitivity, additional learning needs, are hypervigilant, and so on. For some people, noises and sounds can be activating and associated with other difficult experiences. Some environments will inevitably be noisy and this cannot be completely alleviated; however, in addition to the items listed here, it can help if staff are mindful of their voice levels, including not shouting people's names, being careful not to slam doors, keys jangling, and so on. When music is played, for example during labour or an MRI scan, it helps if people are given a choice in the type and volume. Other things such as soft vinyl flooring and sound-absorbing ceilings can also be helpful.

- Extra blankets, heated cushions, fans, and cooling pads. Temperatures can vary hugely in health settings, as well as people's temperature related to their health.

- Board games, crosswords, books, magazines, activity books or items, and fidget regulating items. These can make a big difference, as well as giving a message we care. Some wards or settings have 'take what you need tokens', 'take what you need trolleys', activity boxes, Zen zones, sensory corners, pampering kits, and welcome or wellbeing packs or boxes (e.g. for new parents or people on a long-term ward).

- Gowns that are not see through and have Velcro that is not worn.

Of course, all this will vary depending on the context, such as in A&E, versus an inpatient setting. However, access to food and drink is important. Not only is it a basic need but we know the difference it makes to some people's mood, health, and wellbeing when they do not have access to food. They may feel faint or dizzy, have low blood sugar, and so on. If food and drink are not readily available, it can make people feel uncared for or deprived, particularly those who have not had access to food or have been starved or malnourished, restricted around food, or have an eating disorder, and so on.

Therefore, access to regular meals, whether that be working machines, cafés which are open long hours, food provided, regularly present food trolleys, or snack buckets, is important. Within this, care should be taken over dietary requirements, whether this be cultural diets, health-related diets, allergies, and so on. Here is an example taken from my personal experience.

Recently, I broke my ribs and had to go to A&E. My blood pressure was all over the place and my thyroid levels were high, so I was feeling weak and shaky. This was in addition to the multiple unsuccessful attempts to insert a cannula. I had been unexpectedly sent from the GP to A&E before I was able to eat and then waited for over seven hours to be seen. There was no café, no shop, no trolley, no vending machines, and no access to food. Eventually, after I'd fainted, the nurse kindly offered her own sandwich, which I wouldn't accept as she needed it, but also because I am coeliac and can't eat sandwiches. In addition to there being no food, the water machine was empty, so there also was no access to water. Staff were super busy and seemed annoyed at the request for water, however politely framed.

In Chapters 2, 3, and 4 we explored how trauma and stress can be multi-sensory and therefore can have a multi-sensory impact and require multi-sensory approaches. A lot of this is shared in Chapter 9, where we look more closely at the physical environment; however, some other ways to consider this are shared here. Remember, of course, nothing works for everyone. Some people might like to have low-level music playing in the background or access to other things that help them to regulate, like a certain smell sprayed, around or put on their wrist, on an item like a stress ball, or under their nose (different people will have different preferences, allergies, memories, or possible 'triggers' around smells but our olfactory sense can be a powerful way of shifting someone's affect and arousal levels). Other people might like something they can touch, feel, or do, like a stress ball, a glitter stick, a Rubik's cube, a stretchy, a piece of material, a grounding stone, a game, something to colour in.

This multi-sensory approach is not just for the people receiving care but also for staff. Having access to wellbeing plans and wellbeing items, Zen zones, and calming corners can work well for staff. Brain breaks in meetings, or during handovers or debriefings, can also be helpful, as well as integrating rituals for wellbeing into their daily routines. Sometimes, it is also about how we interweave the multi-sensory ways of being more playful. For example, I might bring an elephant puppet or item into a team meeting or supervision and talk about the elephant in the room; or have a Rubik's cube and talk about problem-solving. Moreover, when thinking about things like policies, we know they are often collecting dust on a shelf, are skimmed through, or not read. If these can be conveyed in multi-sensory ways using images, videos, graphics, and so on, they become more engaging and accessible.

8.5. After the intervention

At the end of the intervention, appointment, and so on, it is important that the person knows what happened and what the next steps are – for example, when they will hear about the next appointment, what to do if they are concerned, what to expect next. Many people find that even if the hospital care is very good, when they get home they experience numerous symptoms and difficulties they don't feel prepared for and are surprised, shocked, confused, and worried about these. Not only can this cause additional stress but also means more time-consuming requests to services as people have to call to get answers. While people can be told what to look out for in the first few days after a procedure, they may not know what to expect in the weeks or months after. It can be helpful to have some of the physical symptoms listed, as well as information on when to seek help or be concerned.

Some people find it confusing and stressful to have to chase up news or information, not knowing whether a referral has been made or when they might get results of tests and so on. So being clear on timeframes and what to do and expect can save a lot of time for the person receiving the care and the people delivering it.

Sometimes, the letters or information provided contain jargon and people have to resort to google or ask medical friends to translate the language. A lot of services have made amazing progress in this area, for example writing directly to the person, as it is about and for them, and imagining them without a medical background reading the information. When information for fellow colleagues is needed, it is helpful to also have a jargon-free summarizing paragraph so that the person can easily understand the information.

Use of jargon and acronyms can lead to miscommunication and confusion, to people feeling lost or stupid, and some feeling unable to check or ask. If people introduce themselves as from, for example, the PQI or the JGU team, and assume that the person understands what this means, it can be very othering and excluding. This is particularly the case for people new to systems, where English is a second language, those with additional learning, speech, language, or communication needs, and those who are struggling to hear or process information for a range of reasons. Acronyms can mean different things in different contexts; for example, DV to someone in child protection might be domestic violence, but to a nurse it might mean diarrhoea and vomiting. DNR to one person might mean did not return, but to another, do not resuscitate. SLT to one person might mean speech and language therapy/therapist, and to another, senior leadership team. The list is endless. In addition, some of these terms sound confusing when they are said out loud; for example, in the UK within child protection, children are sometimes referred to as CIN, children in need, but when said out loud this sounds like sin, so often people are shouting across offices, 'He's a sin', 'We have a sin meeting.'

When delivering results or difficult news, particularly in letter form, it is important to think about the impact of this on the person – will they read it alone, will the person understand it, what questions might they have, what follow-up is offered?

Remember that most people see multiple practitioners, often using different systems, and that doctors often see numerous people and so do not remember each person or the details or there are months or years in between appointments. Writing clear summary, referral, and handover notes is therefore crucial, so that if that doctor is not there, leaves, does not remember, or another person is reading, they have the key information.

Some services, depending on the setting, also include ways to give feedback about the users' experience – to express concerns, complaints, and ideas for improvement, as well as positive experiences and compliments.

Box 8.1.

Trauma-informed care in pain management

By Dr Deepak Ravindran, NHS consultant

I work full time in a very busy district general hospital, leading the complex pain service in secondary care and providing consultant support to the community pain services for my county. Trauma-informed practice has been a game-changer for my pain practice in terms of a patient-centred approach that fosters trust and shared decision-making. It has really revolutionized my clinical work in every aspect, including patient communication, consultation, assessment, investigation, and treatment. *The Body Keeps the Score* by Bessel Van der Kolk (2014) was a very important book that started me on the trauma-informed journey. It highlighted the role of adverse childhood experiences in amplifying chronic pain and various physical and 'mental health' conditions. I realized how traumatic stress that is persistent can cause a cascade of biochemical reactions that can adversely impact the developing immune, hormone, and nervous systems (see Chapters 2 and 3). This can then present downstream as physical and mental health conditions that we recognize as distinct entities in our mainstream medical practice.

I was interested to see what the prevalence of adverse childhood experiences would be in my pain clinic, so in 2018, for a ten-week period, I conducted a survey among all patients seen in the clinic. Analysis of the data showed that more than 40% of patients referred had significant ACE scores (>4/10). I realized that the four R's of trauma-informed care - realization, recognition, response, and preventing re-traumatization - were not being offered to our patients. We know that patients with trauma histories can interact with the health care system very differently and this can range from medication or treatment adherence to the hospital/health care environment where they can either feel safe or unsafe. And the data now exists to suggest that those with traumatic stress and high ACEs have three times more risk of chronic pain and might be high users of health care provision locally.

Once I realized and started to recognize traumatic histories, I worked to raise awareness among my department and hospital colleagues. I have encouraged my team to understand the principles and embed trauma-informed care in our care of inpatients and outpatients. In 2020, I organized the county's first ever trauma-informed pain study day, which was very well attended. I have given numerous presentations over the last few years to a wide variety of health care professionals, ranging from hospital doctors/consultants to perioperative physicians and primary care practitioners, to social workers/social prescribers and patients. This has been on the intersection between trauma, its impact on the immune and nervous systems, and the resultant conditions like chronic pain, mental health issues, and even physical conditions like diabetes, asthma, obesity, hypertension, and autoimmune conditions.

Bearing in mind the likely high prevalence of trauma, stress, and adversity (we support this with a screening tool), we have learned to try and implement the trauma-informed values such as safety, trustworthiness, choice, collaboration, and empowerment (see

Chapter 7). These principles help us to pay attention not only to the consulting room and physical environment but also to patient preferences, using things like motivational interviewing techniques, and to specific facilitators or barriers to their care. It helps us move the dialogue from 'Why are they like this?' to 'What has or might have happened to this person?'

It is noteworthy that we haven't had a single complaint from our patients in the last few years related to communication, which attests to our ability to be empathetic and compassionate in a trauma-informed manner. We have had generally longer consultation times for chronic pain patients in community and secondary care, so adopting a trauma-informed approach hasn't increased our time spent in our consultations and it has made it more valuable to the patient and to the clinician in terms of outcomes and strategies moving forward.

Trauma-informed care means that we exercise greater caution when thinking about stronger or potentially dependence-inducing pain medications or even interventions for pain relief. Patients who have a high ACE score are likely to have a more sensitized and hypervigilant neuro-immune system. As the risk of dependence or addiction could be higher as well as the failure rate of interventions, screening for ACEs (when done sensitively and thoughtfully and in unison with other information-gathering approaches) can have a major implication on clinical practice. Conversations are more tailored to the patient's needs, and once trust is established, they may be more open to exploring other non-injection or non-drug options for pain management.

The challenge of introducing trauma-informed care into the mainstream is that there are not many professionals right now who can support such patients and offer help on an ongoing basis. This needs to change, and more funding needs to be made available as this truly can be transformative. More research is needed within a pain clinic perspective to see how our existing treatment regimens can be modified or adapted to include trauma-specific and trauma-informed interventions. We are working with the University of Reading to explore these options.

We understand that not all chronic pain patients have a history of childhood trauma, and many can experience traumatic episodes during adulthood; therefore it makes sense that treating all chronic pain patients as if they do have a possible history of trauma is holistic and comprehensive. As we understand more about the neu-ro-immune overlap in conditions like chronic pain, mental health disorders, autoimmune conditions, and various long-term conditions, trauma-informed care becomes the ultimate foundation and the future of clinical patient-centred holistic care.

For more on this please see our paper on the influence of ACEs in main management (Tidmarsh et al., 2022).

Box 8.2.

Why does dentistry need to be trauma-informed?

By Christina Worle, general dental practitioner, and clinical lecturer at Bristol Dental School

Many people experience fear over visiting the dentist, but for some this can be severe, even leading to dental treatment being totally inaccessible. This may mean that people miss out on a vital health care service. Dental fear may be caused by previous negative dental or health care experiences, or previous traumatic life experiences, or often elements of both.

Traumatic past dental experiences may have involved a dentist who didn't stop when the patient asked or didn't listen when they said they were in pain. My experience is that more than the pain itself, the dentist's perceived lack of concern for the patient's pain and a refusal to stop are the factors leading to a complete loss of trust, and subsequent fear of future appointments.

A trauma-informed approach to dental practice is vital when working with people who have experienced other types of trau-mas. There are many 'triggers' that exist in a dental setting (see Karen's image 3.9 in Chapter 3), but fairly common are those caused by previous physical or sexual abuse. This can make lying down in the dental chair and experiencing close contact around the head and neck very difficult. The power imbalance inherent in health care settings can also mirror abuse dynamics and make people feel unbearably vulnerable.

Sadly, when patients avoid dental care for a long time and only attend for emergency treatment, extraction can be the only option left. That emergency dental appointment with an unknown clinician in order to have a tooth out can be a traumatic event, which may further perpetuate the cycle of dental fear and avoidance.

People may have experienced feeling judged and discriminated against because of the (sometimes poor) appearance of their teeth. This can be casual and unknowing discrimination by health services, including dentists. The tremendous shame and fear of judgement that people can feel is another huge barrier to their seeking treatment, in which they are trapped in an endless cycle of fear, shame, and avoidance.

A trauma-informed approach can be helpful to enable everyone to access dentistry, no matter what their past experiences. It is very much not a one-size-fits-all approach, and it is imperative to listen, and problem-solve with each patient as an individual. Nevertheless, the following considerations may be helpful when working in a trauma-informed way.

Considerations for dental teams
General:

- Seek out trauma-informed training to learn more; it does not need to be dental-specific to begin. You may find you are already incorporating some elements of trauma-informed practice into your work but have not heard it called this, especially if you work within community and special care dentistry. New resources are emerging to develop your practice. An easy-to-access resource with a range of useful information is the Dental Fear Central website (www.dentalfearcentral. org/tips/trauma-informed-care).

- Trauma-informed training is for the whole dental team (clinical and non-clinical) and should also include organizational leaders. It should be authentic and come from the top down as well as the bottom up, so all team members feel supported.

- Nowhere is whole-team trauma-informed training more vital than for frontline administrative and reception staff. They are the first team members that will welcome people entering the dental practice, and also the first to take the brunt of any fear-induced 'aggression' from patients. It is imperative they are supported to feel safe de-escalating these situations while maintaining empathy. They will need support to help

them with any negative experiences and also to remain compassionate, open, and curious.

- Prioritizing your own wellbeing and wellness is vital.

Before the appointment:

- Where certain groups are excluded from dentistry, it is helpful
  to collaborate closely with this group and support organizations that already have a good relationship with them in
  the community. This can help to promote a positive attitude
  to dentistry and the value of oral health. It could take many
  forms, including listening to and working alongside those with
  various lived experiences, or partnering with local organizations. This can bring dentistry to 'where people are', begin
  to break down barriers, and challenge the perception that
  dentistry is always a scary experience. Even if only organizations are reached and not service users, this positive attitude
  can trickle down via support workers to patients, reducing
  anxiety.

- Those who have a support or key worker can support a patient
  by beginning a conversation with the dentist that the patient
  may not feel able to do at that time. This can start to allay
  fears and allow the patient and dentist to work towards
  arranging a consultation, while making the dentist aware of
  any particular issues or boundaries.

- Collaboration is a two-way street! You will have the opportunity to learn huge amounts about the challenges that different groups of people face, and also to gain feedback on your
  approach and how to make it even better.

- Phone or virtual consultations before the first in-person
  appointment can be a vital step in making a patient begin to
  feel safe engaging with dentistry. Fears can be discussed, and
  problem-solving to mitigate these fears can begin, ready for
  the first face-to-face appointment.

- Always encourage patients to bring a trusted person with
  them to appointments if they would find this helpful. This
  could be a family member, friend, or a support worker. A
  trusted person can help with anything a patient may find

difficult during what could be a daunting experience, such as form filling, waiting for the appointment, and explaining 'triggers' to the dentist. Having a trusted advocate in the room can also help empower patients to ask questions about their treatment, and helps to balance power dynamics.

During the appointment:

- Small things can make a huge difference. Dentists could consider greeting and introducing themselves to patients in the waiting room, especially for the first appointment. An informal introduction, warm greeting, and some small talk go a long way.

- If feasible, patients may want to chat in a private non-clinical area initially, or at least while not sat in the dental chair. This may be all that happens in the first appointment.

- The whole team should use a non-judgemental and compassionate approach.

- While you should be open to explore patients' previous experiences in the context of what 'triggers' them about dentistry, remember that people may not want to discuss this, especially at the initial appointments. In my experience, there is always a valid and understandable reason for a fear of something. Respect this and move to problem solving. Often, people can tell you exactly what they need you to do to help them cope with the dental treatment, and this is often fairly simple to follow.

- During treatment, it is useful to establish a stop sign and *stick* to it. Empower anyone in the dental treatment room (e.g. your dental nurse and anyone supporting the patient in surgery) to stop treatment if they feel they need to. Take any expression of pain seriously and have a low threshold for topping up local anaesthetic.

- It is important to explain everything you do as you do it (unless the patient has said they don't want you to do this). This includes asking consent to touch them and start procedures.

- For more difficult dental treatments (e.g. some oral surgery procedures or full dental clearances) referrals for sedation or even general anaesthesia can be valuable tools if indicated. Additionally, depending on previous trauma suffered, the influence of sedation may feel unacceptable to certain patients as the sedative effect can make people feel out of control and vulnerable. Where possible, it is in the interest of a person's long-term dental health for them to build up to receiving dental treatment under local anaesthetic alone.

- The most important factors are your relationship with the patient, and the trust between you. Expect to have to earn people's trust, and not be granted it automatically. Few people enjoy having dental treatment, but if you have built a trusting relationship with someone and they feel you are doing all you can to help them and make it as comfortable as possible, then it is something they can manage.

- Clearly from the above, longer appointments will be required. However, I have found that although initially appointments may take longer, once you have built a good relationship with patients, appointment times return to average.

System/leadership considerations

- This type of dentistry is intensely meaningful and rewarding but does not easily fit into, for example, the current UK NHS general dental system due to the additional time needed with patients (at least at first). I remain hopeful for change and there are several promising new NHS initiatives being developed. However, sometimes you may not be able to take as long with a patient as you would like. You should tell the patient that this isn't their fault, that they are not the problem, but the system is. We must not blame patients for the failings of the system we work in.

- Please use your voice to advocate for trauma-informed dentistry. I feel an important element of dental leadership is to advocate for groups who may struggle to access dentistry and invite people into forums where their voices can be heard, and changes can be made.

- Management of cancelled and non-attended appointments is difficult; there has to be a balance between maintaining the viability of a service, and empathy for what the patient is going through. Avoid shaming language in 'did not attend' letters at all costs; this is about more than just laziness or a lack of caring.

Considerations for other health care professions

- Freedom from pain and a restored smile are important to help someone let go of shame and build self-esteem.

- Tooth-brushing and looking after your smile is a valuable form of self-care.

- If you are a health care system professional working with people who would benefit from a more caring approach, please ask and advocate for trauma-informed dentistry and help us change the system so this can be an option for those who need it.

- If you are a health care professional working with a dentist then reach out! Dentists do not get professional supervision, and although they may seek this privately, I have found the support and friendship of members of different organizations I have worked with professionally and personally invaluable.

Box 8.3.

Working in paediatric mental health liaison teams

By Dr Carlotta Raby, clinical psychologist

Through my work in paediatric mental health liaison teams, I have witnessed how unsafe it can feel for some children and young people (CYP) to come to an A&E department for help. They might have recently experienced a traumatic event; they may have had historic experiences with adult caregivers (including medical and mental health professionals) that could make seeking help (especially in crisis) extremely frightening; and they could be presenting in acute mental distress.

The environment can be overwhelming to the senses. For example, there are often bright lights, people moving fast, other patients in pain or behaving unpredictably, the sound of alarms, the presence of security staff, and strong smells (such as disinfectant), to name just a few! Many CYP admitted to A&E will have concurring medical needs, so they may also be in significant physical discomfort.

Being in such an environment can 'trigger' traumatic memories for some people and will likely be a particularly difficult place for anyone who is hypersensitive to sensory information. CYP may also experience a lack of control if they decide to leave but are not able to for any reason (e.g. if a Mental Health Act assessment is thought to be required, or there is not a safe place yet identified to discharge them to). This can further increase their perception of threat.

Trauma-informed practice is essential in A&E. It is important for staff to remember that, in crisis, absorbing and retaining information can be more difficult than usual. Patiently, repeatedly, and consistently reminding CYP in simple language and in writing of where they are, why they are there, and what actions staff are doing to ensure they get their needs met can help (social stories can be useful). Listening to (and validating) how the young person is feeling, involving them (wherever possible) to increase their sense of control and safety, and reminding them that staff are there to assist them can be reassuring. Where there is uncertainty, it can be containing if this is named and the process of getting answers from credible sources to move to a place of increased certainty is explained.

CYP should be told how long a mental health assessment might take. They could be supported to co-create a care plan to engage effectively with staff while in A&E, and manage the sensory environment (e.g. being in a slightly quieter space, having noise-cancelling headphones, using fiddle toys and distraction activities). They should be supported to identify their goals (even if this is just to get out), and staff actions could be set against these goals clearly. This could be written down and left with them to revisit, if needed.

When the mental health assessment begins, CYP should be helped to understand the role of professionals involved (as they may have seen many different health professionals by this point). They should be informed of the likely timescale of the assessment, the limitations of confidentiality, and the process of decision-making. This can help CYP to understand staff's duty of care to them and staff's responsibility to act in their best interests. Teams should try to ensure that messages are clear and consistent. If there are miscommunications, time should be taken to understand these and consequently repair any relational rupture, where possible.

Creating a 'safe enough' relational and physical environment and stating an overt interest in CYP sharing their narrative (as the experts of themselves) so that staff can meet their needs and help them to achieve their admission goals can lead to detailed co-created formulations (including detailed risk assessments) on which co-created safety plans can be developed.

When actions that may need to be taken to increase safety feel frightening or frustrating, it is important to take time to listen and understand this, and to offer as much control as possible (e.g. perhaps they can help to agree on wording if information is to be shared with another agency).

If effective care plans have been co-developed with CYP while in A&E to increase environmental and relational safety and lower distress, these could be turned into a hospital passport to be shared with paediatric colleagues and other hospitals, so that if they are admitted in the future this could be a more comfortable experience.

If it is more difficult for CYP to engage, despite the above actions, this could be understood within their wider formulation and compassionately responded to. Whether a young person is discharged or admitted to another ward, endings are important and staff should take time to say 'goodbye' and to wish them luck with the next steps of their journey. They should be asked for feedback on their care to help inform teams of anything that could be done to improve their experience and to understand what was helpful.

Working in a trauma-informed way in A&E goes some way to mitigate the potentially iatrogenic impact of crisis admissions. It is founded on children's rights principles (particularly Articles 12 & 13 of the United Nations Convention on the Rights of the Child) and involves CYP as experts of their situation and as decision-making partners with control and choice, despite the acuity of their situation, wherever this is possible.

Within a framework of relational respect and care, CYP are likely to be more able to openly share the root cause for their distress, allow staff to co-formulate with them, share risk more openly, safety plan effectively, and consider how best to help them to get their needs met. Building epistemic trust in a crisis setting can increase overall trust in health care professionals, and bridge into more successful engagement in well-matched treatment pathways later on.

Box 8.4.

Trauma-informed care and maternity services

By Claire Spencer, infant feeding midwife, Guy's and St Thomas' NHS Foundation Trust, London & Maternity Clinical and Care Professional Leader, Lambeth Together, and LEAP Health Team member

Maternity services are in a unique position, being there to change the course of an adult's life and experience of health care, as well as at a baby's start in life.

My training with Dr Karen Treisman enabled me to explore how the principles of trauma-informed care could be applied to maternity services. It helped me to see the barriers our system has in being able to value interpersonal relationships. Importantly, understanding organizational culture from a trauma-informed perspective has been a vital part of ensuring that the burden of responsibility is not laid with individuals (health professionals or those in our care). A whole-system, universal offer is crucial to apply the four R's (realize, recognize, resist, and respond - see Chapter 7), especially when we want to avoid any further trauma across the life course of women and their families.

How to achieve positive change for parents and babies is a continued learning experience for me. The complex nature of relationships, mixed with our complicated traditional medical model health care system, means delving below the surface of physical care provided to pregnant women. This can seem challenging at times!

I was fortunate to be able to attend trauma-informed training through a seconded role with Lambeth Early Action Partnership (LEAP).* As an infant feeding midwife, my appetite for understanding more about the impact of interpersonal experiences stemmed from the UNICEF Baby Friendly Initiative standards of comfort, closeness, and relationship building for parents-to-be and their babies.

Moreover, if trauma-informed care was ever needed in maternity care, it is now. Each damning report into maternity services in England (Independent Maternity Review, 2022a, 2022b) and successive MBRACCE reports for the UK and Ireland (Knight et al., 2019, 2020, 2021, 2022) illuminate the urgent need for an authentic focus on the role of relational care.

Building a network of allies who align their practice to the trauma-informed care model involves talking about trauma-informed care at most (*all*) times and finding a safe group to do this with. Putting trauma-informed training into practice is most definitely a team event! I have found that being a member of our anti-racism working group is an avenue where trauma-informed care has a significant role as they are entirely aligned and interconnected. Using a trauma-informed lens to view this highly emotive subject provides a framework for understanding the complexity and impact of racism. It ensures that cultural humility is present in our discussions and training of staff.

I found an ally in our safeguarding lead midwife. She can 'see' the need for knowledge, especially for minoritized groups. For our annual safeguarding training I developed a micro-introduction training for all maternity staff. This by itself can't change organizational culture nor can it cover everything in the short time available. However, it has opened up so many conversations locally and nationally about the benefits of developing a more strategic approach long term for trauma-informed training for all staff. Useful resources like the Safe Hands and Thinking Minds website, NHS England's guide to trauma-informed care in the perinatal period (NHS England, 2021), and *Nurturing Maternity Staff* (Smith, 2021) provide a platform for further discussions.

Being a visible champion, 'modelling the model' in my interactions with families and my colleagues is essential to provide hope, compassion, and empathy in a potentially traumatized system. It has been useful to link trauma-informed care and principles to current workstreams and strategies in the unit and wider NHS Trust (e.g. linking to the wellbeing and wellness for staff widely promoted during the Covid-19 pandemic). There is positive benefit in reframing the language used in maternity services, for example in training, policies, and clinical handovers - rather than 'ineffective latch', use 'deeper attachment' for effective breastfeeding, and describe women as connection-needing or seeking rather than attention-seeking if they present with high needs.

Now that my eyes have been firmly opened to the trauma-informed space, I feel it is vital that service planning and implementation have trauma-informed approaches to achieve high-quality woman-led and personalized maternity care. Clinical leadership at all levels is a key target for integrated care roll-out in England. As the Clinical and Care Professional Leader with Lambeth Together for Maternity, my trauma-informed care training and perspective will enable me to influence the changes that are needed in our system in the commissioning and planning of service delivery. I hope to be able to spread the knowledge and support other leaders to take a trauma-informed view. This must be central to the co-production and implementation of any future maternity transformation plans.

On a personal level, through a trauma-informed lens, my long-standing frustrations with the NHS system are less difficult to maintain. I feel more hopeful that the system can change and, importantly, that I can be a positive change agent in my frontline role. I am now more genuinely present for emotional regulation when shifts are hard; so, colleagues and students are heard and valued.

My professional and personal boundary setting, with compassion and empathy for myself and others, enables colleagues to see another way is possible while maintaining psychological safety and not compromising on delivering high-quality care. A trauma-informed view can be seen and felt by colleagues as a novel approach to care, inducing some cynicism. It takes consistency to reassure and build confidence in being relationally present and clinically effective.

Despite my enthusiasm, energy, and passion for relational care through a trauma-informed lens, I have learned it takes time. Changing the juggernaut of our maternity system will be slow but not impossible, so don't lose confidence at the pace of change. It is crucial to use your trauma-informed 'eyes' to shine the spotlight for others to see. Fear and nervousness of opening wounds can overshadow the narrative, and this is where knowledge, training, and evidence become a key factor in bringing about positive change. I see my role as arming myself with evidence-based knowledge, modelling the trauma-informed care model, and, ultimately, challenging the system to realize where trauma-informed principles and guidelines can be a force for real, authentic change.

* LEAP's mission is to give thousands of children in the LEAP area aged 0-3 years a better start in life and to use learning and evidence to positively influence early years services across Lambeth and beyond. It aims to demonstrate how to improve children's life chances through investing in early years provision and connecting local services together. LEAP is funded by the National Lottery Community Fund as part of the national A Better Start programme, which funds local partnerships in five areas across England to test new ways of making support and services for families stronger, so that children can have the best start in life.

Box 8.5.

Perinatal loss

By Dr Samantha Day, Consultant Clinical Psychologist and Clinical Lead, Maternal Mental Health Service, Birmingham and Solihull

Women are referred to our service following perinatal loss. It is often a time of acute distress, vulnerability, and disconnection from others around. Being referred to a mental health service can feel stigmatizing, confusing, and a step into the unknown. We know that information and preparation can support people to feel more confident in engaging in services which can feel intimidating. For this reason, shortly following a referral, our administrator phones the women to let them know we have received the referral, answer questions about the service, and give them a choice of appointments which they can book into for an assessment. In line with trauma-informed practice, we feel that choice is crucial, especially in the context of previously possibly feeling powerless and out of control.

In order to increase each person's comfort and trust in the service, and acknowledging how hard it might be for them to come and talk about their loss, we try to ensure that our website is as accessible and welcoming as possible, so it includes information about the service and short videos about the staff. We also have detailed leaflets which provide an explanation of the service, and information to reduce concerns and confusion. This also helps the women to feel more prepared and held in mind. The administrator, who has had some training in trauma-informed practice, also collects any information about what the women need in order to feel more comfortable in assessments. The women are given a phone number so that they can call our administrator before the appointment if they have any questions.

Box 8.6.

Supporting those who have experienced pregnancy loss through their current maternity journey

By Sophie Garcia, specialist midwife, perinatal mental health services

Pregnancy after the loss of a baby can be an extremely anxious time for most parents. Many women and their partners are expected to cope while navigating a similar journey which they did with their previous pregnancy, with certain routine practices such as scans now possible trauma 'triggers' for these families. Understandably, they often are misunderstood and struggle to navigate through the maternity process.

The 20-week ultrasound scan can be a trauma 'trigger' and a key milestone in this pregnancy. For many, this scan was the point where a problem was detected, or where their baby was found to have died. By unpicking the worry that this scan brings and relating this back to their previous experience, women can understand their anxiety and normalize their intense feelings. By identifying 'triggers', such as being in the waiting room or the silence of the sonographer as soon as the scan commences, we can discuss how to cope in these situations or how we can support them to make it easier. For example, they might listen to an audio or their relaxing playlist, use up breathing or square breathing, or smell essential oils, such as lavender. I also work to see whether there can be adaptations to care, such as a separate area where someone can wait for appointments, or alternative routes to avoid 'trigger' areas, or a supportive staff member to accompany them to appointments.

When working with women who are terrified of childbirth due to previous traumatic experiences, I personalize each woman's care using psychoeducation and coping skills. We learn ways of relaxing to manage highly stressful situations in pregnancy and labour. With every woman, we develop a personalized self-soothing kit of items that induce a sense of safety (e.g. photos, music, objects which can be added to throughout pregnancy and brought into labour).

We also create a birth 'blueprint' - my version of a birth plan - which gives us the chance to talk about all the possibilities that can occur during birth, what this may look like, when, and why they may be appropriate. We can then use the skill of 'cope ahead' (from dialectical behaviour therapy) to see how it may feel for this change to come about, what may be needed and how we could adapt, and what coping mechanisms might be helpful. A birth blueprint enables the woman and her partner to express their preferences but also be in control of what coping mechanisms they might utilize in case of change. It can open lines of communication between them and their midwife so that she can acknowledge their wishes and realistically support them. The birth blueprint also includes 'trigger' mechanisms that the women have practised and used to help them to cope, which staff can utilize when supporting them.

Box 8.7.

How to conduct 'check-ins' in team meetings in a more creative, relational, and trauma-informed way

By Dr Karen Treisman

Check-ins have become a popular and commonly used tool, particularly in team meetings, but also in a range of other forums. However, often they can feel patronizing, awkward, and tokenistic, and be stress-inducing. If you just say to someone 'How do you feel today?' they might think or feel:

- This is just a tick-box exercise.

- I don't know how I feel and/or I don't want or feel able to share.

- If I say I am not okay, it might be weaponized or used against me.

- The person or people don't actually care.

- Last time I said I wasn't okay, I felt it wasn't acknowledged and validated. I was left feeling exposed and unsupported, and no one checked-in on me later.

- We don't have time, so either it is rushed or for me it isn't the priority at this moment.

- You just want me to say 'I am fine' so we can move on - or 'I am good' (which can feed into toxic positivity).

- I don't feel comfortable or safe in groups, or in this space.

- Great, I can talk the whole time (and then one person speaks for a large period of time and other people trail off).

- I've already replied to this three times today.

What else would you add to the list, as there are many more responses?

Of course, this varies depending on the meeting, the relationships, the psychological safety, and so on, and there is no right or wrong way to conduct check-ins. Here are some suggestions for considering check-ins which focus on the four R's of a trauma-informed approach and integrate aspects such as choice and voice.

- What is the rationale behind 'check-ins' – why do we have them?

- What are your team's concerns and apprehensions around check-ins?

- Are check-ins felt to be useful and relevant, for example for collaborative problem-solving, reflecting on past experiences?

- Is there another 'ice-breaker' or connecting, grounding, playful, or regulating activity people might prefer?

- Is the term 'check-in' helpful? Does it reflect the purpose? Would you prefer a different phrase or name? The term used can often guide the activity.

- When is it appropriate to do a check-in and when will it not be done? If it isn't done because of other pressing things, for example, how can this be acknowledged, and the team directed to another available time or forum?

- What is it for and not for? Agree some shared parameters.

If it is agreed to go ahead with check-ins where appropriate, then here are some ways to facilitate them (again, this will vary depending on the context and discussions agreed by the team):

- Everyone in the meeting 'checks-in' in turn, and there is choice around how to express themselves; for example, people might verbally say how they are doing or feeling with words, or they might use feelings/sentence-completion cards to identify this, or instead choose a hashtag, a meme/gif, a YouTube clip, a song, a puppet, a doodle, and so on. This is about being more multi-sensory and creative, bringing playfulness in, but also allowing and encouraging options and choice.

- People also have the choice to pass and opt out, and this is honoured and appreciated.

- If someone shares something or if they have said they are not okay, this will be heard and validated, and they will be thanked for sharing. There will be discussion about what they might need and how this can be appropriately followed up.

- If someone does not want to opt out but also doesn't want to discuss their feelings, they can share something else, such as something that happened or something they are proud of.

- Then the process will be reviewed, reflected on, and evaluated to decide whether it is helpful or needs tweaking or changing. Again, this might not be done every time, but if not, it is important that this is named and acknowledged, and people are aware of other forums or formal and informal places they can feel seen and heard. These concepts can be adapted to other exercises.

Box 8.8.

Applying trauma-informed care as a paediatrician

By Sarah Boutros, Paediatric Consultant, Barts Health (London)

Applying trauma-informed care in practice has helped me improve my daily practice as a paediatrician. I feel more empowered to work with complex and traumatized young people. It has become so important to my daily practice that I regularly teach colleagues about it.

Understanding trauma-informed care principles and the background of trauma science has helped me recognize trauma responses in distressed children and young people. I have been able to educate children and their families about what this means for them, helping reframe the narrative. This helped a 13-year-old who was admitted to the ward with self-harm. She had experienced sexual abuse and past emotional abuse when younger. She described how she fought back and lashed out when others annoyed her at school. I explained that fighting back has been her survival mechanism learned from previous trauma and that with time and therapy she could find new ways to express her emotions and react to perceived danger. I noticed a feeling of relief in her following this explanation. Explaining trauma responses to parents/carers and other professionals involved in the care of children can also really help change the narrative and the language used around these children, moving from blaming and negative language around behaviours to that of understanding and recognition of traumas experienced.

When faced with acutely distressed young people I have been able to apply trauma-informed care principles to manage the situation. Recently, I was working in a paediatric emergency department when a 14-year-old boy, who was likely involved in transporting illegal drugs, was brought in after being stabbed. In the chaos of the resuscitation area, I stayed with him, talking to him and explaining what was happening, paying attention to things that 'triggered' him and led to agitation, and working to reduce those 'triggers' (e.g. asking people to leave the room when there were too many people). I went at his pace when asking what had happened, and I ensured that his pain was being controlled. I knew that he was unlikely to disclose what was going on. I respected his boundaries and did not push him to answer questions he did not want to answer, while being honest and clear with him about who would need to get involved to try and keep him safe. When I had to leave to see another patient, I told him I would be back to see him at the end of my shift – when I came back to see him he was visibly surprised I had followed through with my promise. He thanked me for looking after him.

Box 8.9.

A trauma-informed lens on human trafficking

By Sarah Boutros, Paediatric Consultant, Barts Health (London)

Human trafficking is a serious crime and human rights violation, committed across the globe, in which victims are exploited for someone else's gain (United Nations, 2000). Adults and children of all nationalities, ages, and genders are at risk of exploitation and many may become exploited in multiple ways, either concurrently or in succession (Wood, 2020). Those exposed to early adversity, such as the loss of a parent, familial dysfunction, and other forms of inter-personal violence (domestic abuse, child maltreatment, and sexual abuse), are at higher risk of exploitation. People who face economic hardship are also at higher risk of exploitation as traffickers exploit those in precarious situations with promises of a better life (Wood, 2020). Victims of human trafficking often experience many layers of trauma, before, during, and after their exploitation.

Research tells us that victims and survivors of human trafficking often access health care but may not disclose their experiences (Ross et al., 2015). There are many complex reasons for this, including genuine fear of repercussions on themselves and others, mistrust of professionals, previous negative experiences within health care, and shame and stigma. The complex and multi-layered trauma faced by survivors means that using trauma-informed care is incredibly important to support the long road to recovery.

In 2020, I conducted qualitative research on trauma-informed care for children and young people (CYP) who had been trafficked and what this would look like in practice. From interviews with professionals working with CYP who had been trafficked, I found that trauma-informed care starts with a holistic understanding of human trauma. It is from that place of understanding that providers are then able to be more empathetic, non-judgemental, and compassionate towards trafficked CYP. I found that trauma-informed care is primarily a relational care model built on safety, trust, choice, collaboration, and time taken with CYP. This relationship aims to empower CYP, providing them with the tools and language to regain control of their lives. Building genuine connections can facilitate CYP to make important disclosures and enable access to specialized services. However, the findings support that relationships with CYP may still be positive and beneficial for CYP even when disclosures do not occur. This suggests that establishing a robust relationship between provider and the young person is a supportive intervention in itself, regardless of whether the young person chooses to disclose. This is consistent with research indicating that relationships between CYP and trusted adults promote resilience in young people.

Understanding the value of a trusting, safe, and collaborative relationship with my patients has dramatically changed my practice and approach to distressed or traumatized children and young people. I now know that giving time, providing young people with choices, allowing them to take control, and collaborating are all more important than obtaining a disclosure or getting the full medical history. As health care professionals, we want to be told what the problem is so that we can fix it. Practising with trauma-informed care in mind means accepting that we often do not get the whole story but that our interactions with traumatized people can still be therapeutic. I now teach this to all my colleagues.

Box 8.10.

Trauma-informed consultations in a sexual assault centre setting: the 'unsuccessful' examination, followed by finding hope

By Dr Michelle Cutland, consultant paediatrician

Much of what health professionals do in their day-to-day role is 'task', 'process', and 'outcome' focused and occurs within time constraints. For example, 'This person has come to me with x problem. I need to ask a, b, and c questions and test for condition d and e to decide if this treatment or outcome is indicated and make sure I do it within xx minutes as that is my clinic appointment slot/ward round time.'

To insert trauma-informed principles into the care we offer in our setting we have had to change this thinking by removing time constraints (we are lucky we have the luxury of this and acknowledge that not everyone can, but some middle ground is hoped to be possible) and proactively inserting more choice into the consultation. One of the ways we crudely measure this is by the number of young people who *do not* want a physical examination in our setting following recent sexual abuse (it's around 8-10%).

If a young person does not want an intimate or any physical examination in the context of recent sexual abuse, then rather than feeling that we (the health professional) have failed in our 'task', we take it as a measure of success of a truly collaborative trauma-informed consultation. We have had to educate staff by explaining that if they don't manage to complete an examination because of fully informed patient choice, then that isn't a failure of their 'task' but instead they have given the young person choice over their bodies and about what we do for/to them (after a situation when they were not given choice in that). It also means that they feel empowered and given voice to express that choice, which when having a consultation with a health professional can be difficult due to the natural power imbalances in that relationship. It also means that the choices they make have been listened to, heard, and ultimately respected. We also positively reinforce the decision-making that they did.

By reframing 'the unsuccessful examination (task)' as something to measure as a success in choice and empowerment, it also means we can be more creative about involving them in what we can do instead. For example, maybe they want an examination, but they want a particular person with them, so choose a different day or time; or perhaps they want forensic samples but not an examination and then we can try self-taken samples; or perhaps they aren't sure if they want a particular vaccination, so we can offer time and more information and then follow-up with a phone call at an agreed time some days later.

Finding the 'hope' when writing child protection medical safeguarding reports

Medical assessment/examinations are commonplace following alleged or suspected harm and are undertaken by experienced clinicians. These are broad and holistic evaluations of that child's health and wellbeing that explore what life is like for that child as well as looking for physical and behavioural signs which may support the concerns or allegations of harm.

After a medical assessment, the clinician writes a comprehensive medical report that is shared with other agencies, such as police, children's social care, and the child's general practitioner. These documents are often referred to in child protection case conferences and form part of material that may be used in family or criminal court settings.

In our setting, we see children in the context of suspected or alleged sexual abuse. Research suggests that children and young people want to be seen as a whole person in this context and not an identity defined by victimhood, and that hope and optimism are key for recovery (Warrington et al., 2016).

We encourage these two principles to be central to our report writing by asking our clinical staff to consider two things when writing these reports:

1. How might the young person reading this report feel about themselves? Would they feel known? Would they feel heard? Are they described as a whole rather than in the context of abuse? Would they feel judged by any language used?

2. Where is the hope? What are the strengths in this child's life? What are their ambitions for the future? What makes them happy? Who do they feel safe with?

We have found that this process brings warmth to the reports that we write as well as a critical lens through which to view and address the language we sometimes use. We have also reflected that highlighting the 'hope' is a process that benefits clinicians to reduce vicarious trauma.

An example extract from a fictional safeguarding medical report of a 15-year-old abused by an uncle might read like this:

Albie reports that he has dyslexia but this doesn't affect him much at school and he has extra time in exams. His favourite subject is art, especially anime style and graphics, and he would like to be a tattooist when he leaves school.

There is no history of self-harm and no suicidal thoughts. Gaming with friends makes him happy. He describes feelings of anxiety in groups and feels less anxious online. After thinking about it, he identified his older sister as the person he would talk to with any worries, but not his mum as he doesn't like to see her upset. He said he doesn't often talk about 'stuff' though, and keeps thoughts inside. We commended and thanked him for feeling able to chat about this with us today.

Albie was a wonderful young person to meet. He reports a number of recent adverse experiences, including abuse by a trusted adult. Albie and his whole family require holistic support moving forward.

CHAPTER 9

The Physical Environment

9.1. What will be covered in this chapter

- An introduction to the importance of the physical space
- An opportunity to give messages and a feeling through the building
- Signage, posters, visual images, the entrance, and orientation
- Multi-sensory 'triggers' and environment
- Colours, furniture, regulating elements, and access to nature
- Cultural and learning differences
- How to incorporate these ideas for your own physical space
- Expanding on the step-by-step worksheet using the example of a waiting room or reception area

9.2. An introduction to the importance of the physical space

Please be mindful that the suggestions in this chapter are not about making physical changes in isolation but as part of a bigger and more integrated process. We know that you can have the most beautiful and well-designed building, but if the feel and people don't match, then any interventions will lack weight and impact. Similarly, you can have a building which is outdated, but if the people make you feel welcomed, heard, and connected, the building is less relevant. So, getting the physical environment right is a combination of the outer and inner elements. Of course, any changes to the physical environment need to be balanced with health and safety guidelines and requirements (which can sometimes jar with what we want to do, particularly with some of the changes

297

due to Covid) and other important factors, but it is hoped that each person can use the ideas here as an inspiration and then apply them to their context in whatever way is possible. This will inevitably vary hugely; for example, what is possible and needed in a GP building will differ from an A&E department, or what a dentist's office requires will not be the same as what's needed in a psychiatric ward.

This said, the physical environment can make a big difference to people's mood, feelings, and the overall ambience. Not only can it shape how people feel, it can also convey important messages about the services that someone might receive, and about the energy and care of the staff and organization. The physical environment is generally the first thing people see and notice, so it really does count. A building can either increase or decrease levels of stress and arousal; it can make people feel calm, welcomed, looked after, and safe, or tense, anxious, disoriented, and so on. This applies to how we feel when we enter a nursing home, school, a hospital, a GP surgery, someone's home, and even more generally when we are choosing a restaurant, hotel, or café.

The physical environment is an easier and more tangible thing for people and organizations to change or tweak, compared to some of the other more complex aspects of adversity, culturally, and trauma-informed, infused, and responsive transformation. Due to funding and other factors, most organizations won't have the privilege of designing a new purpose-built building and won't be able to make large structural changes; however, small changes, such as decoration, signage, temperature, and lighting, can make a huge difference.

People tend to be attuned and sensitive to their environment, and those who have experienced trauma and feel 'triggered', dysregulated, stressed, and hyper-vigilant are often more likely to notice and zoom in on the environment which surrounds them. Ideally (of course this will vary depending on the function of each unique service), a building such as a hospital or a residential home should support people to feel contained, warm, and calm, and work towards spaces being healing, nurturing, and reparative, rather than trauma and stress-inducing. Henry Rey (1994) said that buildings should be like a 'brick mother' (I prefer a 'brick parent'). In relation to attachment theory, I think this gives a sense of a building being both a secure base and safe haven, someone's roots, and their wings.

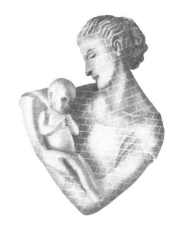

9.1. THE BRICK PARENT

9.3. An opportunity to give messages and a feeling through the building

The building also is an opportunity to model the model and to embody and communicate care. For example, if the building is unclean and not maintained, it can convey messages of not caring, and people might wonder how it could possibly be an attentive and caring environment for them. This can also be conveyed through small things, such as having puzzles with pieces missing, the water tank being empty, or the magazines in the waiting rooms or on the wards being torn and old. On the flip side, think about the difference it can make when you go into a toilet and there are free supplies to use, such as tissues, sanitary pads, condoms, or deodorant; or when there is a replenished fruit bowl on the table, or water in the tank, with cups available.

★ It is useful to ask if the building could talk, what would it say? And to narrow this down even more, if the waiting room/entrance/therapy rooms/sensory room/intervention rooms and so on could talk, what would they say? If you could describe the feelings of the building (and the spaces within it) or its personality, what would you say? What messages and feelings do people receive from the building?

★ What is the purpose of the building and services and is this clearly felt? Does this consider the history of the building, and its positioning and associations within the community? What messages does it convey from the outside to the community, to visitors, and to family? (Think about murals, mosaics, stained glass windows, welcoming art, sculptures, etc.)

★ How are the values of adversity, culturally, and trauma-informed practice embodied and paid attention to in the environment (e.g. multi-layered safety and trust, relational and humanizing, collaborative, connecting and integrating, considering cultural humility, responding to and understanding behaviour as communication, increasing agency and mastery, being transparent and communicative)?

★ How is the building and space cared for? Is the building maintained and cleaned? How do people respond and leave people feeling inside the building? This might be security people, the person at the entrance or reception, the domestic staff, the maintenance staff, the catering staff, the porters, the health practitioners.

★ How are the maintenance, caretaking, and property teams included and involved? For example, how does a maintenance person respond to a person in a nursing home who has set the fire alarm off, or soiled a sofa, wet a bed, or broken a TV? How quickly are repairs done?

★ Is there attention to the 'small' details? This might include updating the magazines, having water available, having all the pieces of puzzles in the boxes, having access to tissues or toiletries, taking down outdated information on display boards, having enough toilet paper in the toilets, providing a choice of books and activities.

★ Is there access to items that people might enjoy, find useful, or need (led by the person)? This might include crosswords, magazines, books, fidget items, colouring items, art and craft items, phone chargers, ear plugs.

9.4. Signage, posters, visual images, the entrance, and orientation

The entrance is people's first impression and experience of the building, so it is an important area to think about in terms of feelings, values, accessibility, and safety conveyed. This includes how people are greeted and welcomed, how accessible the building is, the feeling and look of the doors, the sound of any buzzers, bells, and alarms, the signs and posters outside, and so on. Bear in mind also that many people entering might already be feeling worried, in pain, overwhelmed, 'triggered', and so on. This might be someone who:

- is coming to spend time with a parent who doesn't remember who they are because of dementia
- is in physical pain
- has previously had a miscarriage, stillborn baby, or a traumatic birth
- has a fear of hospitals, needles, and so on
- is coming to get a potential life-changing diagnosis
- is undergoing a procedure which they are worried about
- is being checked and examined following a rape or disclosure of abuse

- has been waiting 18 months for this appointment and has had a very long journey of difficult experiences.

- has never been to such an appointment before, for example with a dentist or an optician.

What else could you add to this list?

People may also enter and exit the building in the same place, so it is important to think about what they see when they leave, including the signs, the doors, the messages of hope. Clear signage extends to presenting important information, such as the opening and closing times, and out-of-hours/emergency contact numbers. Accessibility is an essential aspect to consider – are the brochures and materials fully accessible, and for someone with disabilities, is the reception desk too high up to see or reach?

9.4.1. Posters and signs and the messages they can give

Paying attention to the building can extend to what people might see, for example the bulletin board, the signs on the wall, the instruction posters, the plaques, the notices, and the brochures. The language, tone, colour, and images used can significantly affect how someone is made to feel. For example, one hospital I supported had several signs at the entrance of their building with bolded red words, such as ATTENTION, NO, STOP, and DON'T. These instantly felt unwelcoming and punitive, so we shifted this to clearer and more gentle messages.

Moreover, some messages have good intentions but for some people can be activating and resurfacing, such as graphic images of those hurt through domestic abuse, images of knives and guns, or images of burns.

It is helpful to think about the names of rooms. One organization I worked with changed the names of their rooms from 1, 2, and 3 to Hope, Inspire, and Believe. Small things can make a big difference. Do rooms have to be called 'treatment room', 'examination room', 'group room', and so on – could you think of some alternatives that would give a more positive message?

This also extends to displaying uplifting, hopeful, and inspiring messages. For example, some spaces have messages from past users of the services, sharing their journey and hopeful messages for those who have just arrived; others have things like a tree of wishes, or inspiring artwork. These kinds of messages can be supportive and hope-inducing, and make spaces feel less clinical and problem focused. However, there is a balance required, as these messages need to be mindful not to feed into toxic positivity, as detailed in Chapter 7.

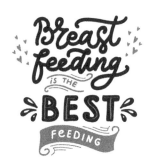

9.2. BREAST IS BEST POSTER

Take, for example, 'breastfeeding is best feeding' posters. These can be useful for many people and have some important messages, but imagine what it might be like for someone who has been told not to breastfeed because of HIV transmission, or for a foster carer/adopter/kinship carer/special guardian who doesn't have that option, or who has had a mastectomy?

9.4.2. Finding and navigating around the building

An important part of the physical environment (particularly in larger places like hospitals or day centres) is signage and helping people to find their way around. Struggling to find the right location and building, having to buzz four times to get in, being greeted in a non-enthusiastic unfriendly way, and then either having no instructions or being told to go to the left, then the second right, then up the stairs, and then to the third left is not a great start for anyone, let alone someone who is already in a place of dysregulation or stress. This means that they are likely to get to their appointment or job interview or to visit a friend/family member more distressed than when they started.

Compare this to receiving a clear map beforehand, with instructions for how to find the building/room (maybe even a link to a video showing where the building is); then if possible there is also clear parking (or details of where to park or public transport links), and clear signage (even better if this is in different languages and in Braille). This could mention any common confusions, such as it is not the first red door but the second one, making the correct location easy to find. Then where possible, you are welcomed by a friendly staff member as you enter, and someone is ready and waiting to take you to the place where you should be, or the person you are meeting comes to the entrance to greet you. The person at the reception or at the front is hugely important, they are the person's first impression and they set the tone. Again, these seemingly small things can make a big difference.

In some settings, it is helpful to have photos of staff members available for people to familiarize themselves with (including, where possible, agency staff and people in other roles such as domestic and maintenance staff). Some teams do this in fun and creative ways, for example creating a staff tree, having illustrated drawings, sculptures, Lego people. This can also extend to having some information about the service present on the wall – such as 'who we are, our values, our journey, our history, our promises to you'. It can be great when this is written or contributed to by people who use or have used the service, as it feels meaningful and co-produced.

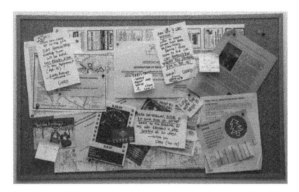

9.3. DISPLAY BOARD

Display boards are supposed to be places to display key messages and information, but they can be cramped, overcrowded, disorganized, and so on. There can be outdated messages from years previously and pieces of crumpled paper or those with tea and coffee stains. Not only does the information get lost but it can also create an impression of chaos and disorganization. (If the board could talk, what would it say or what messages or feel would it convey?)

★ How easy is your building to find? (Think about someone arriving for the first time, someone in pain, someone who doesn't know the area, someone who is stressed about being late or lost.) What information and directions (ideally written, pictures, and, if possible, a video) are people given to find it? How do these consider, for example, those who are in a wheelchair, those who use a Zimmer frame, those who are blind, and those who don't speak English?

★ Is there clear and accessible signage in and around the building? What messages does this convey?

★ How are people greeted and welcomed when entering the building or when staff arrive (including the person at reception, the security staff, the domestic staff, the person they are meeting, the person caring for them, visitors)? How are people supported to find where they are going? By a person or with very clear and accessible signage?

★ Are the reception desks, information, and brochures high-up so less accessible, or at a level all people can see and reach?

★ What signs and posters are on the walls? What messages and feelings do these convey? Do these think carefully about language, wording, and the images used? Do these consider the population being served and how representative and inclusive they are? Are these signs maintained, updated, and looked after (e.g. not crumpled pieces of paper with coffee marks)?

★ Are messages of hope, inspiration, and strength present? This can be in the images themselves, but also messages of hope from people who have used the service, inspirational quotes, shared artwork, and so on. These need to be thought about carefully, in terms of how different people may hear or feel about them.

★ How are the rooms and spaces labelled?

★ Is there clear information available, such as opening and closing times and emergency out-of-hours numbers?

★ Are there, where possible, photos of or information about key staff members and about the team's role, values, history, aims, and so on?

★ How are people's feelings of safety, regulation, and trust increased (e.g. clear name and ID badges, double glazing, fire safety, locking of doors, storage of medications or cleaning products, safety in the car park)?

9.5. Multi-sensory 'triggers' and environment

In the context of trauma, stress, pain, and dysregulation, people can experience multi-sensory overload and feel activated and 'triggered' (see Chapters 1–6).

Although everyone has different sensory profiles and preferences, we know, for example, that high levels of noise have been associated with a decrease in the ability to hear, comprehend, and retain information (Szalma & Hancock, 2011), and can contribute to cognitive load and diminish decision-making capacity. Sudden loud tones have also been associated with a heightened physiological startle response (Shalev *et al.*, 2000). This might include doors slamming, keys jangling or clanking, machines beeping, loud TV or music being played, clocks ticking, practice fire alarms going off without warning, raised and shouting voices, sirens sounding, seats squeaking when moved. Similarly, certain lighting, such as glare, bright, flicker, shadow, and reflection, can cause visual discomfort, with symptoms such as sore eyes, muscle aches, headaches, and migraines (Boyce, 2014). Also, aspects such as temperature (feeling too hot or too cold) can impact people's alertness, concentration, and mood. Therefore, these multi-sensory elements should be attended to in order to increase people's feeling of safety and decrease their feelings of danger and threat.

Moreover, other examples of sensory 'triggers' (see Chapter 3 for a more comprehensive discussion of this, as well as an experiential exercise around this) include things like smells (our olfactory sense), which can play an important role in people's arousal, mood, and comfort. Smells can also evoke a strong reaction and can be linked to a particular memory, moment, or person. So, strong smells, such as bleach or other cleaning products, alcohol on someone's breath, or a particular aftershave or perfume, can take someone down a time hole to the person who hurt them wearing that aftershave or perfume, or to a time when bleach was used to tidy up after an episode of domestic violence. It might also involve things like having crowded seats with chairs which don't allow for personal space, so people are in close proximity or touching each other. Stark, empty-looking walls might be reminiscent of relational poverty, seclusion, exclusion, or deprivation. Christmas songs and decorations might remind someone of how lonely they are or be reminiscent of loss or a time of violence.

9.6. Colours, furniture, regulating elements, and access to nature

We can try to incorporate in our buildings what we know about the psychology of colour, the positive benefits of nature, and what activities, shapes, patterns, and textures can be regulating (Britton, 2019; Leydecker, 2017; McCormick, 2017). Although every building will vary, and of course each person has their own unique profile and nothing will suit everyone, using elements of nature (e.g.

trees, leaves, shells, water, sky) and using neutral and nature colours, such as blues and greens, has been found to be more regulating. Be mindful, of course, of the need to be inclusive, and that some images and colours might feel quite 'gendered'.

Natural lighting, views of nature through windows to outdoor spaces, trees, greenery, and green spaces in general have been linked to improved positive health outcomes and social cohesion (Ekkel & de Vries, 2017), and associated with a sense of freedom, calmness, and openness (Ulrich *et al.*, 2008). Additionally, research findings generally associate blues and greens with improved mood and lowered arousal (Elliot & Maier, 2014; Jalil *et al.*, 2013). Blue's relaxing effects come from its association to nature – the sky, the sea, rivers, and lakes (Clarke & Costall, 2008; Eiseman, 2006; Mehta & Zhu, 2009). Similarly, the colour green also tends to evoke positive ambience due to its association with the natural realm, such as green foliage and vegetation. Green also has associations with the 'Go' signal which can be linked to a start and a new beginning. (Remember that there may also be negative connotations for some people; for example, blue may remind people of hospital gowns.)

It is also important to think about whether the furnishings leave people feeling safe, welcomed, and valued and can create a sense of privacy and comfort. Here are some points about regulating and calming elements that have been found to be helpful (remember to also consider health and safety needs):

- Where possible, it is helpful to reduce sharp edges and harsh lines, and integrate circular aspects such as round chairs, rugs, lamps, paintings, tables, cushions, and mirrors, or use furnishings to soften jarring corners.

- There should also be attention to things like the patterns, for example a wall being too busy and overstimulating, or creating associations for people with certain aspects of the pattern. Crosses and stripes might have religious or medical associations. While overly busy patterns can be a lot for some people, stark white walls can have associations with neglect, poverty, loneliness, seclusion, or other sterile settings. It's about finding a balance.

- Textures and fabrics can be important to think about as well, such as not having chairs that squeak, or cushions that feel itchy, and so forth. Ideal colours are often neutrals, blues, and greens. Of course, health and safety aspects need to be interwoven with choices for communal areas.

- Where possible, there should be some thought around windows/glass on the doors to support privacy; for example, having a drape as well as a positively worded sign to let people know the room or space is in use.

It's great to have natural light, but there needs to be thought about what the person can see, and if others can see in. This extends to staff, where being in a glass room to have confidential conversations can feel unsafe and exposing for some.

- Where possible, have space between furniture, so that people don't feel too much social pressure to talk, or have to touch each other. This reduces the feeling of being crowded or squashed, which can make people feel uncomfortable, overwhelmed, or trapped. This extends to having space in narrow corridors, which can be crowded and make people feel trapped, and also creates access, for those in wheelchairs, for example.

- Seating needs to feel regulating and comfortable. Of course, there is variation within this between different settings and it depends on people's physical needs (and might require an occupational therapy assessment). Chairs that rock or spin, armchairs that feel cocooning, or bean bags can be comforting. Other rooms may have things like dens, Zen zones, and calming corners.

- It is important not to make spaces too cluttered or chaotic. Remember the messages and feelings the building is trying to create. This can include things like display and notice boards. Labelled boxes and storage can be important here as well, to support people to feel organized and orientated.

- Noise should be kept to a minimal. This is very difficult in busy hospital settings, so, of course, it will vary, but it is also important given that noises can be distracting, overwhelming, and, for some, 'triggering'. In terms of safety and privacy, it is important to feel that, where possible, there is confidentiality. This can be optimized by things like soundproof headphones, ear plugs, soft vinyl flooring, sound-absorbing ceilings, white noise, and vibrating systems. It is also important to be mindful of corridor conversations and to be respectful when people are sleeping or trying to have quiet time. Staff need to be aware of the volume of their voice, and of things like banging doors. Thought should be given to the choice and volume of music played. Of course, this varies, and for some people certain noises might be reassuring or comforting, particularly those who find silence eerie, unnerving, or 'triggering'.

- Regulating elements which draw on sensory integration and processing ideas and concepts are useful. This might include having things like rocking chairs, dens, beanbags, water movement, as in an aquarium, access to fidget items, having equipment like balance boards, weighted items, and yoga balls, sensory gardens, sensory rooms, nature elements, TV with calming images, colouring-in walls, textured walls, and a maze or labyrinth which stimulates movement as well as creating left-right brain integration and activation. Items such as hand gel, shampoo, and conditioner can create different responses – there might be a neutral, and then one that is either up-regulating, alerting, and invigorating, or down-regulating and calming for that person (e.g. potentially lavender for calming and citrus for invigorating).

- Calming music spaces or Zen zones can be very regulating. This could be specific rooms or designated areas, such as the corner of a room.

- Spaces where additional needs can be met are also useful. This includes prayer rooms, breastfeeding spaces, rooms for private conversations, spaces to connect and eat together, and spaces large enough to hold team meetings or training in. These spaces may be changeable, depending on the context; for example, on a neonatal intensive care unit, spaces where parents and carers can be close and interact comfortably with their babies will be needed.

- There should be easy access to things like water or other drinks, tissues, plasters, and snacks. Hooks for jackets or handbags should be plentiful, and numerous plug sockets are useful, as are spare and usable phone chargers.

- Communal spaces like the toilet need careful thought. A toilet is an important place in a lot of buildings. It is often where people go when they need some quiet time or when feeling overwhelmed or overstimulated, when they have an upset stomach, when they're anxious, and so on. Therefore, this might include things like thoughtful posters and messages on the toilet walls and doors, the decor being as calming as possible, and access to toiletries like sanitary pads, tampons, condoms, tissues, face wipes, and deodorant. Toilets also need to be well maintained.

The images that follow illustrate some ideas for trauma-informed changes to the physical environment.

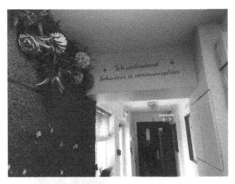

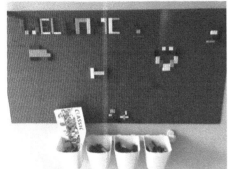 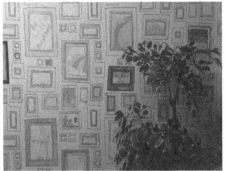

9.4, 9.5, AND 9.6. A TEXTURED GREEN GRASS WALL AND A QUOTE
ABOUT BEHAVIOUR BEING COMMUNICATION, AN INTERACTIVE
LEGO WALL, AND A COLOURING-IN WALLPAPER AND SOME PLANTS,
THREE STEPS RESIDENTIAL SERVICES IN NAVON, IRELAND

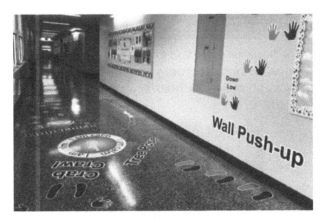

9.7. REGULATING MOVEMENT AND EXERCISES ON THE FLOOR AND WALL

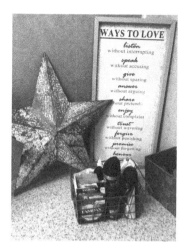

9.8. THE CALMING AND REGULATING SPACE CREATED BY DR KATE MARGARSON
IN THE YARBOROUGH ACADEMY TOILETS. THIS INCLUDES TOILETRIES TO
BE USED, PLANTS, INSPIRATIONAL QUOTES, AND CALMING BOOKS

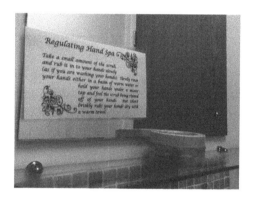

9.9. ADOPTIONPLUS IN MILTON KEYNES HAS THIS LOVELY SIGN IN
THEIR TOILETS, WHICH SUPPORTS PEOPLE TO HAVE A REGULATING
HAND SPA AND TO SAVOUR THEIR FEW MINUTES IN THE TOILET

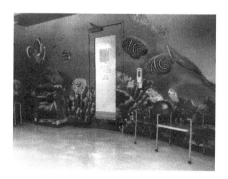

9.10. THE UNDER-THE-WATER THEMED WAITING ROOM
AT THE CHADWICK CENTER IN SAN DIEGO

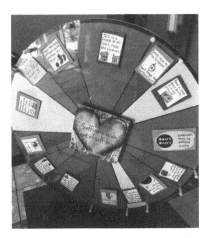

9.11. A SELF-CARE WHEEL WITH A FOCUS ON WELLBEING AND FEEL-GOOD MESSAGES,
WHICH WAS ACCOMPANIED BY A THERAPY DOG AND PLACED IN THE RECEPTION
AREA OF THE BEHAVIORAL HEALTH SERVICES BUILDING IN SAN FRANCISCO

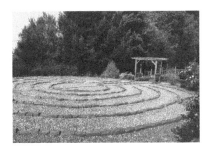

9.12. TRILLIUM RESIDENTIAL AND TREATMENT FACILITY (IN PORTLAND,
OREGON) HAS AN OUTDOOR MAZE AND MULTI-SENSORY GARDEN
WHICH HAVE TAKEN INTO CONSIDERATION IDEAS ABOUT LEFT-
RIGHT BRAIN ACTIVATION AND SENSORY ATTACHMENT

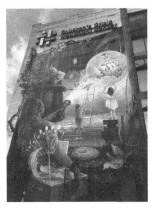

9.13. AN INSPIRATIONAL MURAL ON ONE OF THE WALLS AT THE CHILDREN'S
CRISIS TREATMENT CENTER, BASED IN PHILADELPHIA ARTS

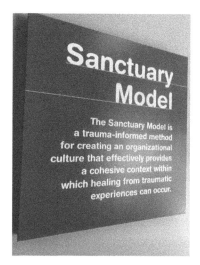

9.14. CLEAR SIGNAGE AND A VISIBLE PLAQUE ABOUT THE CHILDREN'S CRISIS
TREATMENT CENTER'S COMMITMENT TO TRAUMA-INFORMED PRACTICE

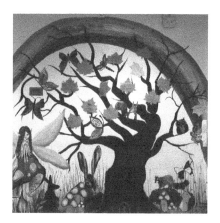

9.15. A DISCHARGE HOPEFUL MESSAGE TREE CREATED BY PEOPLE WHO USED THE
SERVICE ON OAK WARD, PART OF GREATER MANCHESTER MENTAL HEALTH TRUST

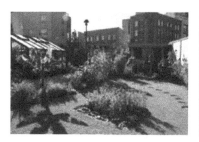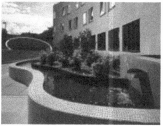

9.16 AND 9.17. A FREEDOM FROM TORTURE PURPOSE-BUILT SPACE IN
NORTH LONDON TO PROMOTE HEALING FOR SURVIVORS OF TORTURE. IT
WAS CO-DESIGNED BY THOSE WHO HAD EXPERIENCED TORTURE

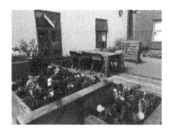

9.18. A GARDEN AND COMMUNAL SPACE IN AN INPATIENT FACILITY
ENCOURAGING INTERACTION WITH NATURE AND OUTDOOR GAMES

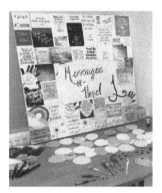

9.19. MESSAGES OF HOPE ON A WARD

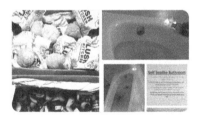

9.20. A SELF-SOOTHE BATHROOM ON OAK WARD IN
BOLTON, SHARED BY SIOBHAN BARLOW

The worksheet at the end of this chapter will help you to review and reflect on these questions:

★ Is attention given to environments which may be 'triggering' and dysregulating (e.g. smells, sounds, sights, textures, temperatures)? This might include stark walls, deprived environments, darkened corridors, boxed-in areas, uncleaned areas, chaotic, overstimulating environments, seating where people are having to be touching, doors banging, keys clinking, clocks ticking, Christmas songs playing, loud beeping, flickering lights.

★ Is attention given to things like cleaning and maintenance (e.g. smell of urine, full bins, blood, poo in the toilets)?

★ Are there things in the environment to help people to stay grounded, feel comfortable, and regulate (e.g. feature walls, fidget items, access to food and drink, ear plugs, phone chargers, blankets, fans)?

9.7. Cultural and learning differences

This needs to consider the practicalities of the service offered, as well as the safety elements, while also being mindful of people's intersection of identities. For example, if there is a paediatric ward, this needs to hold in mind how it might welcome and support both young children and adolescents, as well as their relatives. This might also extend to aspects such as how cultural differences are accommodated (e.g. religion, gender, sexuality, age, language, race), the types of magazines offered, and how accessible the building is for someone in a wheelchair or with other physical requirements. Thought could also be given to aspects such as having prayer rooms, or separate containers and apparatus in the kitchen for different dietary requirements, or having accessible toilets, and so on. Other considerations are around the location and accessibility of the building, both internally and externally (e.g. signage and systems for people who don't speak English, having signs in braille, wide corridors, being wheelchair friendly).

★ What is your environment like from different people's perspectives – from entry to exit? How does it feel? What messages are there (e.g. for someone who doesn't speak English, someone on the autism spectrum, different age groups, different genders, someone who is blind, someone in a wheelchair, someone from a particular religious background, someone who identifies as transgender)? (See Chapter 6.)

★ How is feedback from a range of people sought and incorporated?

★ How do you think about your environment in all aspects, from the signage to the things on the walls, to accessibility, to the choice of books/materials, to safety, to the toilets, to prayer spaces, and so on?

★ Is there thought about kitchen supplies, separate utensils if needed, and so on? What about different dietary needs (which might include having separate fridges or freezers, and how food is labelled, stored, and prepared)?

★ Do people have the things they might require for different parts of their identity (e.g. a prayer mat, a certain type of shampoo or skin product, a prayer book)?

★ Are there aspects like non-automatic doors, broken lifts, uneven ramps, narrow corridors, out-of-reach leaflets or brochures, and stand-only scales that could be changed?

Some questions and resources will be presented to support you in doing a walk-through, which can be a very powerful exercise in applying these ideas to your own environment.

9.8. How to incorporate these ideas for your own physical space

A narrative walk-through can be helpful, particularly as there may be parts of our environment that we do not see every day, when we are so focused on the task in hand, can be on autopilot, or have become desensitized. Spend some time using worksheet 9.1 to carry out a first imaginary walk-through of your environment. This can be optimized by breaking down the task, for example doing the reception/welcome area, a particular room, the hallways, the toilets, the staff room all separately – this allows you to zoom in on the bite-sized steps. Then if you want you can then do a whole imaginary walk-through. Try to attend to the above areas, as well as reflecting on the questions below.

Then as instructed in worksheet 9.1, after you have done your own imaginary walk-through, try and do one from a different perspective to your own, or even better from multiple different perspectives, including from a multi-sensory perspective. For example, a new starter, a person who is in distress, someone who doesn't speak English, someone in a wheelchair, someone who feels disoriented. What do you notice, feel, smell, hear, and see?

You can then do an actual physical walk-through and get other people to do the same, including those who use the service, as different people will see different things and it is important to hear from multiple voices and perspectives. It can be helpful to take photos or videos on your way through. This can also be positive when changes are made, so that you have before and after photos. It can also be useful to go and visit other similar spaces to learn from best practice and gain ideas and inspiration.

Worksheet 9.1. Steps to reflect on different aspects of the work of the organization from a trauma-informed lens

STEPS TO REFLECT ON DIFFERENT ASPECTS OF THE WORK & OF THE ORGANISATION FROM A TRAUMA INFORMED LENS

An exercise to support reflection, assessment, & to inform the development of action plans & ways forward

Take your time & go through the following questions (ideally with a few other people). You can write down, doodle, or sculpt your responses. You may want more space or a bigger piece of paper. You also may want to change the order of the steps or you may have additional areas to add. These steps are not exhaustive or prescriptive. It can be helpful to use the other supplied infographics & tables here.

 Choose an area which you would like to focus & reflect on & write it below (Start as small, specific, & as focused if possible).

 Do a backwards thought shower/brainstorm. This means reflecting on the **worst-case example or scenario**. For example, if you were doing this for team meetings, it would be reflecting on what the worst, most stressful, & trickiest team meeting would look like, feel like, be like?

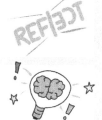

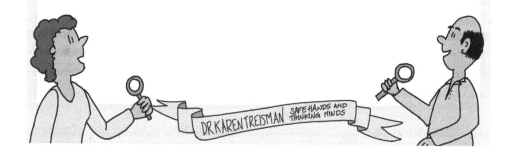

DR KAREN TREISMAN SAFE HANDS AND THINKING MINDS

STEPS TO REFLECT ON DIFFERENT ASPECTS OF THE WORK & OF THE ORGANISATION - FROM A TRAUMA INFORMED LENS

Now can you please do **an imaginary walk-through or take a narrative journey- Step-by-step (if possible, you might want to do an actual walk-through). It can be helpful to think about the before, during, & after of the process; or from the first contact through to the last. Think about what you see, notice, feel, observe, think etc.**

So, for example, for a team meeting, what does it look & feel like from before the team meeting, including the email about it, during the meeting, & after the meeting. Or another example, for a waiting room, what does it look like & feel like from entry to exit?

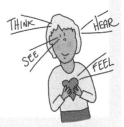

Now can you do an **imaginary walk-through or take a narrative journey- Step-by-step**; but this time from several other perspectives.

So, for example, from a new starter's perspective; or from a person who has experienced trauma e.g. By looking through a trauma-lens; or from a toddler/adolescent perspective; or from a parent in distress's perspective, or from someone who is disabled, or for someone who does not speak English, & so forth. Try & incorporate aspects such as **the multi-sensory experience**, what might people **see, hear, smell, feel, notice, taste.**

E.g. If looking at an aspect of your physical environment, such as a waiting room, what might this feel like, smell like, look like etc; think about everything from what you can hear, see on the walls, the type of chairs, the greeting of the staff, the signage etc; & how might this be different from different people's perspective including from trauma & cultural lens.

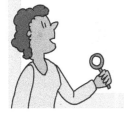

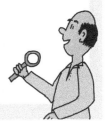

STEPS TO REFLECT ON DIFFERENT ASPECTS OF THE WORK & OF THE ORGANISATION FROM A TRAUMA INFORMED LENS

5 What are some of the things that are **going well already, that do feel helpful, & that do feel positive with the specific area of focus?** (Even if it is something tiny). What can be done to support, magnify, continue, & celebrate these things?

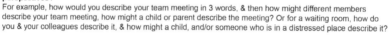

If you were going to describe the… in 3 words what would it be? How might this differ from other perspectives?
For example, how would you describe your team meeting in 3 words, & then how might different members describe your team meeting, how might a child or parent describe the meeting? Or for a waiting room, how do you & your colleagues describe it, & how might a child, and/or someone who is in a distressed place describe it?

6

 ①

 ②

③

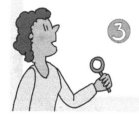

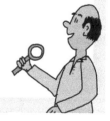

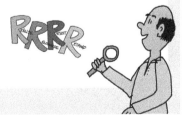

STEPS TO REFLECT ON DIFFERENT ASPECTS OF THE WORK & OF THE ORGANISATION FROM A TRAUMA INFORMED LENS

Where relevant & appropriate, how are the **values** of adversity, culturally, & trauma-informed & responsive practice **modelled, evident, & infused** in the area which you are discussing? (You may want to do this for the core organisational values as well. You can also use the values tables and sections to support you with this). An example of some aspects within the values would be, how emotionally safe do team meetings feel? What happens if someone is dysregulated or upset? How much choice do people have over the time, length agenda, set-up of the meeting? Whose voices are silenced, missing, privileged? How do people communicate within team meetings with each other, and how are things communicated with people who were not present in the meeting? How much space is there to share and discuss progress, proud moments, best practice? What is in the team meeting to support messages of hope and positivity? What is done to support people to feel connected to each other and the meeting? And so forth…

1. **Multi-layered safety & trust,**

2. **Choice, voice, agency, & mastery,**

3. **Collaboration, communication, & transparency,**

4. **Relational, relationship-focused, & humanised,**

5. **Curious, empathetic, understanding, kind, reflective, & compassionate,**

6. **Magnifying, noticing, & celebrating hope, strengths, & resilience,**

7. **Seeing behavior as communication & being curious around this,**

8. **Considering cultural humility & responsiveness**

9. **Integrating & connecting people, ideas, systems, the brain etc.**

How is this in line with the four R's? How does…. realise, recognise, resist, & respond?

STEPS TO REFLECT ON DIFFERENT ASPECTS OF THE WORK & OF THE ORGANISATION FROM A TRAUMA INFORMED LENS

8 What have you **noticed**, **learned**, & **reflected** on from doing this exercise and going through these steps? What might be your action plan, suggestions, or recommendations from this? It might be helpful to think about it as before, during, & after.

BEFORE

DURING

AFTER

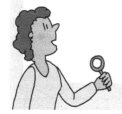

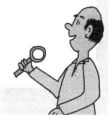

STEPS TO REFLECT ON DIFFERENT ASPECTS OF THE WORK & OF THE ORGANISATION FROM A TRAUMA INFORMED LENS

 Now you have some ideas, it is important to **widen your learning, to try & test it out, & to be collaborative**. For example, what does the literature say? What can you learn from other models or from best practice? What do wider networks & other people not present in these discussions think, feel, want to contribute etc.

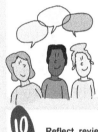
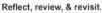

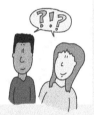

Reflect, review, & revisit.

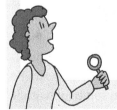
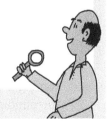

9.9. Expanding on the step-by-step worksheet using the example of a waiting room or reception area

Please note that these steps apply to any organizational or practice area, and I have also provided information on what these steps mean for a team meeting or assessment process.

1. *Take your time and enrich and expand – ongoing work in progress.* This exercise is far more meaningful if not rushed and really thought about, discussed, shared, and linked to the literature. The steps don't need to be followed like a recipe book – they are intended more as a guide. It is great to have multiple perspectives and, in this case, to bring in the trauma lens. It can be really helpful to draw or write your answers on paper or in some sort of visual output. It should also be a work in progress. Come back to it, add to it, test things out, ask other people. You might also want to draw on other chapters to go into certain aspects in more detail; for example, if thinking more about cultural humility, then check out Chapter 6.

2. *Narrow it down and be specific.* So, for example, thinking about your waiting room or reception area, go through the steps which are relevant. You may want to change the order or only choose a couple to work through and break them down into manageable sections. Similarly, you may like to do this as a whole team, or within a working group, or with others, for example a range of people who use the space. It is important to be specific and start small – it would be too vast and broad to do the whole physical environment, so while lessons can be learned and things hopefully applied, it is more manageable, less overwhelming, and more likely to be useful to start with, for example, the toilet or the waiting room. Similarly, if looking at team meetings or team spaces, it will be more useful to focus on a specific meeting, space, forum, or panel rather than trying to do them all at once.

3. *Worst-case scenario and backwards thought shower.* Once you have chosen, for example, the reception area or waiting room, you then can discuss using step two: what the worst/most tricky/stressful/distressing waiting room and entrance experience would be like. This is sometimes called a backwards thought shower. This might be anything – a rude and unwelcoming greeting at reception, big locked doors, inaccessible, dark, smelly surroundings, toxic positivity, hard to find, cold. Have some fun with it and use your imagination. This will naturally lead into people's experiences of and wishes for a lovely, calming, and welcoming entrance and

waiting area, and what this would look like, feel like, be. It can be useful for people to draw on past experiences of other buildings and spaces, as well as what they have seen and heard about. If looking at a backwards thought shower of a team meeting or an assessment, the step would be imagining the most trauma- or stress-inducing, ineffective, confusing, harmful, judgemental, boring team meeting or assessment.

4. *Personal narrative journey and walk-through.* This is where you do an imaginary walk-through or narrative journey from the beginning to end, from your perspective. For a waiting area, this might be from the street view and parking and arriving, through to getting in and being there, through to leaving after the appointment. What does it feel like? Look like? Smell like? Sound like? This includes the sensory experience. It can be helpful to think of three words you or your colleagues or people using the service would use to describe the entrance and waiting room space. How similar or different is this from how you or others would want to feel? If the walls could talk, what would they say? What messages are being conveyed? Sometimes, taking photos can aid this process and make it more fun.

5. *Multi-perspective, including a narrative journey and walk-through using your trauma lens.* Now you do the same, but this time from the perspective of other people in a place of stress or trauma or other situations, or from the perspective of other scenarios. For example, imagine walking in as a person who:

   - was assaulted or raped the night before
   - has had to get three buses to get there, has just had an eviction notice on their home, has no electricity or heating, and now has been told they are late and will have to wait two hours
   - has experienced domestic abuse that week
   - has experienced medical trauma and has a fear of hospitals
   - has just received a diagnosis of terminal cancer
   - last time they were there had a stillborn baby
   - is confused due to a diagnosis of dementia
   - is in agony and feels they are going to faint or die
   - is on the autism spectrum
   - identifies as transgender

◙ doesn't speak English and maybe has recently arrived in the country

◙ is homeless

◙ is in a wheelchair or using a Zimmer frame

◙ might have been hospitalized as a veteran

◙ has been previously sectioned

◙ has been tortured

◙ has had an injury

◙ is hearing voices.

And so on – there are so many other possibilities.

You can expand on this by doing a physical walk-through, and asking other people to do the same a few times. Sometimes, taking photos can aid this process and make it more fun. Similarly, if these steps are applied to reviewing an assessment process, you would think about the first contact to the last, from the letters or calls to inform about the assessment, through to the process itself, through to when someone leaves, gives feedback, and is referred on or discharged or informed of the outcome. And think about the detail of the steps, for example the wording in the letter, the room or virtual space, the questions asked, the seating. This includes considering what might the 'assessment' feel like in the above scenarios, such as if the person has been abused or is deaf and so on; or organizationally, what a team meeting feels like depending on the above and other scenarios.

6. *Strengths and proud parts.* Next, reflect on some of the aspects which you are happy about, proud of, enjoy, want to highlight, and so on, within the waiting space. This is the strengths-based lens and perspective. It might include, for example, the types of toys, the chairs, a particular sign, the carpet.

7. *The trauma-informed values and R's.* Apply the R's and trauma-informed values to the areas of focus (see Chapters 6 and 7).

So, for a waiting room, some brief questions follow (these are expanded on in each relevant chapter in this book).

★ Does the waiting room space *realize* and acknowledge that people arriving might be activated and in a place of stress/threat/danger/

dysregulation for a variety of reasons? (This includes ourselves, colleagues, visitors.) This might be as a result of past or current situations or experiences, as well as people's relationship to people, new places, health, their body, health care, and so on. If these steps are related to a screening or assessment process, it would be the same. Similarly, if doing these steps for a team meeting, what might team members be bringing in with them or experiencing personally and professionally? (See Chapter 5.)

★ Do staff *recognize* that people's distress, pain, or trauma might come out in different ways when in the waiting room? How are signs of distress (e.g. agitated, confused, clamming up, withdrawing, pacing, raising voice, seeking reassurance, being impatient) recognized and responded to by the staff, the security personnel, and practitioners in the building? And if these steps are being used in an assessment or team meeting, similarly, how might people's discomfort, distress, pain, and so on show itself or be communicated?

★ Is there care and thought within the waiting room space to *resist* adding distress or harm to people (e.g. unclear or no directions, the language and imagery on the posters, hard-to-find buildings, buzzers that don't work, flickering lights, water without cups, overcrowded seating, inaccessible counters, security guards that co-escalate instead of co-regulate, Christmas songs playing loudly, clocks ticking)? And if these steps are being used in an assessment or team meeting, similarly, what might add stress, discomfort, confusion, and harm – and what might reduce it? For example, team meetings might be tokenistic stress-inducing check-ins, or there is no agenda, times are not being stuck to, and people are being blamed or publicly shamed, or being sent endless paperwork to read, or feeling silenced or humiliated.

★ Is the knowledge of trauma and stress infused into the environment (*responding*)? For example, is there good signage, and multi-sensory and regulating elements?

★ In terms of some of the values (see Chapter 7), how is the waiting room increasing people's emotional, physical, moral, cultural, and relational safety and trust in the building and in the people within the building? How is it decreasing threat and danger? How is it aiming to be stress- and trauma-reducing instead of inducing? What is being done to make the environment as regulating and supportive as possible?

★ How is the space relational, welcome, connecting, and humanizing? What qualities are being modelled and embedded in the space? How are people left feeling? What messages are being conveyed?

★ How is the space conveying messages of hope and strengths?

★ How is the space thinking about supporting people's intersection of identity and cultural humility? This includes things like the toys, the materials, the accessibility, the signs, the imagery.

★ How is the space increasing people's choice, voice, ownership, and influence? How are there opportunities to feed back? Has there been some input, shared projects, and co-design of the space and functions within it?

★ How are people thinking about the language and wording, especially the signs, posters, materials, plaques, and so on?

There should then be time to reflect on areas not covered, on researching and reviewing the literature on physical environments and spaces, as well as drawing on other perspectives and thoughts, then trying to put this into an action plan which will be reviewed and tried.

Afterword

As we come to the end of this book, but not of the ongoing journey. I wanted to thank you for taking the time and energy to learn and reflect on this multi-layered and dynamic area. This book is a spotlight and it is a comma not a full stop, so I hope that it has planted some seeds of ideas, that it has been validating, reassuring, thought provoking, and that it has also given some food for thought, growth, and for some take home messages and golden nuggets. I hope it inspires further conversation, thinking spaces, exploring, connecting, and much more; and that we can think about the next steps, and how we can move (even if in tiny ways) from knowing to feeling, being, and doing. So much is about how we translate some of this into the real world and into a way that fits realistically for our role and our unique context. We know in the contexts which we work in and in the difficult times we are navigating through as health professionals it can feel overwhelming and like a mammoth task- sometimes, like pushing a boulder uphill. So, I hope that each of you will continue to recognise and celebrate what you and the people around you are already doing and what steps have already been taken; whilst also continuing to be hopeful disruptors, agents of change, and remembering that the small things can be the big things and that every interaction can be an intervention and can leave a heart print on ones journey.

Further Reading

Bellolio, M.F., Cabrera, D., & Sadosty, A.T. (2014). Compassion fatigue is similar in emergency medicine residents compared to other medical and surgical specialties. *Western Journal of Emergency Medicine*, 15, 629–635.

Belsky, J., Bakermans-Kranenburg, M.J., & van IJzendoorn, M.H. (2007). For better and worse: Differential susceptibility to environmental influences. *Current Directions in Psychological Science*, 16, 300–304.

Bloom, S.L. (2011). Trauma-Organized Systems and Parallel Process. In N. Tehrani (ed.), *Managing Trauma in the Workplace: Supporting Workers and Organizations* (pp.139–153). London: Routledge.

Bloom, S.L. (2013a). *Creating Sanctuary: Toward the Evolution of Sane Societies*, second edition. New York, NY: Routledge.

Bloom, S.L. (2013b). The Sanctuary Model: Changing Habits and Transforming the Organizational Operating System. In J.D. Ford & C.A. Courtois (eds), *Treating Complex Traumatic Stress Disorders in Childhood and Adolescence*. New York, NY: Guilford Press.

Bloom, S.L. (2013c). The Sanctuary Model: Rebooting the Organizational Operating System in Group Care Setting. In R. Reece, C. Hanson, & J. Sargeant (eds), *Treatment of Child Abuse: Common Ground for Mental Health, Medical, and Legal Practitioners*. Baltimore, MD: Johns Hopkins University Press.

Bober, T., Regehr, C., & Zhou, R. (2006). Development of the coping strategies inventory for trauma counselors. *Journal of Trauma and Loss*, 11, 71–83.

Bowlby, J. (1969). *Attachment and Loss, Vol. 1: Attachment*. New York, NY: Basic Books.

Burack, J.A., Flanagan, T., Peled, T., Sutton, H.M., Zygmuntowicz, C., & Manly, J.T. (2006). Social perspective-taking skills in maltreated children and adolescents. *Developmental Psychology*, 42, 207–217.

Danese, A. & Lewis, S.J. (2017). Psychoneuroimmunology of early-life stress: The hidden wounds of childhood trauma? *Neuropsychopharmacology*, 42, 99–114.

Danese, A. & Tan, M. (2013). Childhood maltreatment and obesity: Systematic review and meta-analysis. *Molecular Psychiatry*, 19, 544–554.

Dasan, S., Gohil, P., & Cornelius, V. (2015). Prevalence, causes and consequences of compassion satisfaction and compassion fatigue in emergency care: A mixed-methods study of UK NHS consultants. *Emergency Medicine Journal*, 32, 588–594.

De Bellis, M.D., Hooper, S.R., Spratt, E.G., & Woolley, D.P. (2009). Neuropsychological findings in childhood neglect and their relationships to pediatric PTSD. *Journal of the International Neuropsychological Society*, 15, 868–878.

DeCasper, A. & Prescott, P.A. (1984). Human newborns' perception of male voices: Preference, discrimination, and reinforcing value. *Developmental Psychobiology*, 17, 481–491.

DeCasper, A. & Sigafoos, A. (1983). The intrauterine heartbeat: A potent reinforcer for newborns. *Infant Behavior & Development*, 6, 19–25.

Dominguez-Gomez, E. & Rutledge, D.N. (2009). Prevalence of secondary traumatic stress among emergency nurses. *Journal of Emergency Nursing*, 35, 273–274.

Dong, M., Giles, W.H., Felitti, V.J., Dube, S.R., *et al.* (2004). Insights into causal pathways for ischemic heart disease: Adverse childhood experiences study. *Circulation*, 110, 13, 1761–1766.

Dube, S.R., Felitti, V.J., Dong, M., Chapman, D.P., Giles, W.H., & Anda, R.F. (2003). Childhood abuse, neglect, and household dysfunction and the risk of illicit drug use: The adverse childhood experiences study. *Pediatrics*, 111, 564–572.

Edwards, L. & Torcellini, P. (2002). *Literature review of the effects of natural light on building occupants*. Golden, CO: National Renewable Energy Lab.

Eigsti, I.M. & Cicchetti, D. (2004). The impact of child maltreatment on expressive syntax at 60 months. *Developmental Science*, 7, 88–102.

Esaki, N. & Larkin, H. (2013). Prevalence of adverse childhood experiences (ACEs). *Circulation*, 110, 13, 1761–1766.

Gee, G.C., Walsemann, K.M., & Brondolo, E. (2012). A life course perspective on how racism may be related to health inequities. *American Journal of Public Health*, 102, 967–974.

Giovino, G.A. (1999). Adverse childhood experiences and smoking during adolescence and adulthood. *Journal of the American Medical Association*, 282, 1652–1658.

Hamilton, S., Tran, V., & Jamieson, J. (2016). Compassion fatigue in emergency medicine: The cost of caring. *Emergency Medicine Australasia*, 28, 100–103.

Harnett, N.G., Wheelock, M.D., Wood, K.H., Goodman, A.M., *et al.* (2019). Negative life experiences contribute to racial differences in the neural response to threat. *Neuroimage*, 15, 202–205.

Harris, M. & Fallot, R.D. (2001a). Using trauma theory to design service systems. *New Directions for Mental Health Services*, 89.

Harris, M. & Fallot, R.D. (2001b). Envisioning a trauma-informed service system: A vital paradigm shift. *New Directions for Mental Health Services*, 89, 3–22.

Hui, A., Rennick-Egglestone, S., Franklin, D., Walcott, R., & Llewellyn-Beardsley, J.N. (2021). Institutional injustice: Implications for system transformation emerging from the mental health recovery narratives of people experiencing marginalisation. *PLoS One*, 16, 4, e0250367.

Juruena, M.F., Cleare, A.J., & Pariante, C.M. (2004). The hypothalamic pituitary adrenal axis, glucocorticoid receptor function and relevance to depression. *Revista Brasileira Psiquiatria*, 26, 189–201.

Kendall-Tackett, K. (2007). Violence against women and the perinatal period. *Trauma, Violence & Abuse*, 8, 344–353.

Kleinman, A. (1978). Concepts and a model for the comparison of medical systems as cultural systems. *Social Science and Medicine Part B: Medical Anthropology*, 12, 85–93.

Kleinman, A. & Good, B. (2004). Culture and depression. *New England Journal of Medicine*, 351, 951–952.

Leiter, M. & Maslach, C. (2004). Areas of Worklife: A Structural Approach to Organizational Predictors of Job Burnout. In P. Perrewe & D. Ganster (eds), *Research in Occupational Stress and Wellbeing: Vol. 3. Emotional and Physiological Processes and Positive Intervention Strategies* (pp.91–134). Oxford: JAI Press/Elsevier.

Magliano, L., Schioppa, G., Costanzo, R., Petrillo, M., & Read, J. (2017). The opinions of Italian psychology students about people diagnosed with depression and schizophrenia: A comparative study. *Journal of Psychosocial Rehabilitation and Mental Health*, 4, 147–157.

Marks, J.S. (1998). Relation of childhood abuse and household dysfunction to many of the leading causes of death in adults. The Adverse Childhood Experiences (ACE) Study. *American Journal of Preventive Medicine*, 14, 245–258.

Marsella, A.J. (2010). Ethnocultural aspects of PTSD: An overview of concepts, issues and treatments. *Traumatology*, 16, 17.

Marsella, A.J., Friedman, M.J., & Spain, E.H. (1996). *Ethnocultural aspects of posttraumatic stress disorder: Issues, research and clinical applications*. Washington, DC: American Psychological Association.

Ministry of Justice. (2011). *Statistics on Race and the Criminal Justice System 2010*. London: Ministry of Justice.

Perlman, S.B., Camras, L.A., & Pelphrey, K.A. (2008). Physiology and functioning: Parents' vagal tone, emotion socialization, and children's emotion knowledge. *Journal of Experimental Child Psychology*, 100, 308–315.

Perry, B. (2004). *Understanding Traumatized and Maltreated Children: The Core Concepts – Living and Working with Traumatized Children*. Houston, TX: The Child Trauma Academy.

Peters, D., Hodkinson, A., Riley, R., & Esmail, A. (2018). Association between physician burnout and patient safety, professionalism, and patient satisfaction: A systematic review and meta-analysis. *JAMA Internal Medicine*, 178, 10, 1317–1331.

Pollak, S.D., Nelson, C.A., Schlaak, M., Roeber, B., *et al.* (2010). Neurodevelopmental effects of early deprivation in post-institutionalized children. *Child Development*, 81, 224–236.

Pollard, R. Jr., Betts, W.R., Carroll, J.K., Waxmonsky, J.A., *et al.* (2014). Integrating primary care and behavioral health with four special populations: Children with special needs, people with serious mental illness, refugees, and deaf people. *The American Psychologist*, 69, 377–387.

Rauch, S.L., Van der Kolk, B., & Fisler, R.E. (1996). A symptom provocation study of posttraumatic stress disorder using positron emission tomography and script-driven imagery. *Archives of General Psychiatry*, 53, 380–387.

Saeri, A.K., Cruwys, T., Barlow, F.K., Stronge, S., & Sibley, C.G. (2018). Social connectedness improves public mental health: Investigating bidirectional relationships in the New Zealand attitudes and values survey. *Australian and New Zealand Journal of Psychiatry*, 52, 365–374.

Sangar, D. & Moore-Brown, B. (2001). Prevalence of language problems among adolescent delinquents. *Communication Disorders Quarterly*, 23, 17–26.

Sansone, R.A. & Sansone, L.A. (2012). Physician grief with patient death. *Innovations in Clinical Neuroscience*, 9, 22–26.

Shonkoff, J.P. & Garner, A.S. (2012). The lifelong effects of early childhood adversity and toxic stress. *Pediatrics*, 129, 232–246.

Sprang, G., Craig, C., & Clark, J. (2011). Secondary traumatic stress and burnout in child welfare workers: A comparative analysis of occupational distress across professional groups. *Child Welfare*, 90, 149–168.

Steinberg, A.G., Barnett, S., Meador, H.E., Wiggins, E.A., & Zazove, P. (2006). Health care system accessibility. Experiences and perceptions of deaf people. *Journal of General Internal Medicine*, 21, 260–266.

Streeck-Fischer, A. & Van der Kolk, B. (2000). Down come baby cradle and all: Diagnostic and therapeutic implications of chronic trauma in development. *Australian and New Zealand Journal of Psychiatry*, 896–918.

Sullivan, A.M., Lakoma, M.D., & Block, S.D. (2003). The status of medical education in end-of-life care: A national report. *Journal of General Internal Medicine*, 18, 685–695.

Sullivan, C.M. & Goodman, L. (2015). A guide for using the Trauma Informed Practices (TIP) Scales. Available at: www.dvevidenceproject.org/evaluation-tools.

Summerfield, D. (2001). The invention of post-traumatic stress disorder and the social usefulness of a psychiatric category. *British Medical Journal*, 322, 95–98.

Sylvestre, A. & Mérette, C. (2010). Language delay in severely neglected children: A cumulative or specific effect of risk factors? *Child Abuse and Neglect*, 34, 414–428.

Taylor, J.L. & Rew, L. (2011). A systematic review of the literature: Workplace violence in the emergency department. *Journal of Clinical Nursing*, 20, 1072–1085.

Teicher, M.H., Anderson, C.M., & Polcari, A. (2012). Childhood maltreatment is associated with reduced volume in the hippocampal subfields CA3, dentate gyrus, and subiculum. *Proceedings of the National Academy of Sciences of the USA*, 109, 563–572.

Vanthuyne, K., Meloni, F., Ruiz-Casares, M., Rousseau, C., & Ricard-Guay, A. (2013). Health workers' perceptions of access to care for children and pregnant women with precarious immigration status: Health as a right or privilege? *Social Science & Medicine*, 93, 78–85.

Williams, J., Paul, J., National Institute for Mental Health in England, & Royal College of Nursing and National Council of Nurses of the United Kingdom. (2008). *Informed Gender Practice: Mental Health Acute Care that Works for Women*. National Institute for Mental Health in England.

Zimmer, M.H. & Panko, L.M. (2006). Developmental status and service use among children in the child welfare system: A National Survey. *Archives of Pediatrics and Adolescent Medicine*, 160, 183–188.

References

Acevedo-Garcia, D., Noelke, C., McArdle, N., Sofer, N., & Hardy, E.F. (2020). Racial and ethnic inequities in children's neighborhoods: Evidence from the new Child Opportunity Index 2.0. *Health Affairs*, 39, 10, 1693–1640.

Addis, A., Moretti, M.E., & Syed, F.A. (2001). Foetal effects of cocaine: An updated meta-analysis. *Reproductive Toxicology*, 15, 341–369.

Afana, A.-H., Pedersen, D., Ronsbo, H., & Kirmayer, L.J. (2010). Endurance is to be shown at the first blow: Social representations and reactions to traumatic experiences in the Gaza Strip. *Traumatology: An International Journal*, 16, 4, 73–84.

Afari, N., Ahumada, S.M., & Wright, L.J. (2014). Psychological trauma and functional somatic syndromes: A systematic review and meta-analysis. *Psychosomatic Medicine*, 76, 2–11.

Afifi, T.O., MacMillan, H.L., Boyle, M., Cheung, K., *et al.* (2016). Child abuse and physical health in adulthood. *Health Reports*, 27, 3, 10–18.

Aldridge, D. & Somerville, C. (2014). *Your Services Your Say: LGBT People's Experiences of Public Services in Scotland*. Edinburgh: Stonewall Scotland.

Almuwaqqat, Z., Wittbrodt, M., Young, A., Lima, B.B., *et al.* (2020). Association of early-life trauma and risk of adverse cardiovascular outcomes in young and middle-aged individuals with a history of myocardial infarction. *JAMA Cardiology*, 13, 6, 1–5.

Amanullah, S. & Ramesh Shankar, R. (2020). The impact of COVID-19 on physician burnout globally: A review. *Healthcare* (Basel), 8, 4, 421.

Amaro, H., Chernoff, M., & Brown, V. (2007). Does integrated trauma-informed substance abuse treatment increase treatment retention? *Journal of Community Psychology*, 3, 57, 845–862.

American Nurses Foundation (ANF). (2021). *Mental health and wellness surveys 1 and 2: COVID-19 impact assessment series*. Author.

Anda, R.F., Felitti, V.J., & Bremner, J.D. (2006). The enduring effects of abuse and related adverse experiences in childhood: A convergence of evidence from neurobiology and epidemiology. *European Archives of Psychiatry and Clinical Neuroscience*, 256, 174–186.

Anderson, M.L., Leigh, I.W., & Samar, V.J. (2011). Intimate partner violence against Deaf women: A review. *Aggression and Violent Behavior*, 16, 200–206.

Anisman, H. & Kusnecov, A. (2022). *Cancer: How Lifestyles Impact Disease Development, Progression and Treatment*. London: Elsevier.

As-Sanie, S., Clevenger, L.A., Geisser, M.E., Williams, D.A., & Roth, R.S. (2014). History of abuse and its relationship to pain experience and depression in women with chronic pelvic pain. *American Journal of Obstetrics and Gynecology*, 4, 210–317.

Baek, M., Outrich, M.B., Barnett, K.S., & Reece, J. (2021). Neighborhood-level lead paint hazard for children under 6: A tool for proactive and equitable intervention. *International Journal of Environmental Research and Public Health*, 18, 5, 2471.

Baetz, C.L., Surko, M., Moaveni, M., McNair, F., *et al.* (2021). Impact of a trauma-informed intervention for youth and staff on rates of violence in juvenile detention settings. *Journal of Interpersonal Violence*, 36, 17–18.

Baibazarova, E., van de Beek, C., Cohen-Kettenis, P.T., Buitelaar, J., Shelton, K.H., & van Goozen, S.H. (2013). Influence of prenatal maternal stress, maternal plasma cortisol and cortisol in the amniotic fluid on birth outcomes and child temperament at 3 months. *Psychoneuroendocrinology*, 38, 907–915.

Bailey, Z.D., Krieger, N., Agénor, M., Graves, J., Linos, N., & Bassett, M.T. (2017). Structural racism and health inequities in the USA: Evidence and interventions. *The Lancet*, 389, 1453–1463.

Baker, C., Lund, P., Nyathi, R., & Taylor, J. (2010). The myths surrounding people with albinism in South Africa and Zimbabwe. *Journal of African Cultural Studies*, 22, 169–181.

Baldwin, J.R., Arseneault, L., Caspi, A., Fisher, H.L., *et al.* (2018). Childhood victimization and inflammation in young adulthood: A genetically sensitive cohort study. *Brain Behavior & Immunity*, 67, 211–217.

Baldwin, S.A., Wampold, B.E., & Imel, Z.E. (2007). Untangling the alliance-outcome correlation: Exploring the relative importance of therapist and patient variability in the alliance. *Journal of Consulting and Clinical Psychology*, 75, 842–852.

Bandstra, E.S., Morrow, C.E., Mansoor, E., & Accornero, V.H. (2010). Prenatal drug exposure: Infant and toddler outcomes. *Journal of Addictive Diseases*, 29, 245–258.

Barber, J.P., Connolly, M.B., Crits-Christoph, P., Gladis, L., & Siqueland, L. (2009). Alliance predicts patients' outcome beyond in-treatment change in symptoms. *Personality Disorders: Theory, Research, and Treatment*, 80–89.

Barello, S., Palamenghi, L., & Graffigna, G. (2020). Burnout and somatic symptoms among frontline healthcare professionals at the peak of the Italian COVID-19 pandemic. *Psychiatry Research*, 290, 113–129.

Barnes, J.H. & Chatterton, T.J. (2016). An environmental justice analysis of exposure to traffic-related pollutants in England and Wales. *WIT Transactions on Ecology and the Environment*. Penang, Malaysia, 431–442.

Barnett, E.R., Yackley, C.R., & Licht, E.S. (2018). Developing, implementing, and evaluating a trauma-informed care program within a youth residential treatment center and special needs school. *Residential Treatment for Children & Youth*, 35, 95–113.

Barsky, A. & Kaplan, S.A. (2007). If you feel bad, it's unfair: A quantitative synthesis of affect and organizational justice perceptions. *Journal of Applied Psychology*, 92, 286–295.

Bartlett, G., Blais, R., Tamblyn, R., Clermont, R.J., & MacGibbon, B. (2008). Impact of patient communication problems on the risk of preventable adverse events in acute care settings. *Canadian Medical Association Journal*, 3, 178, 1555–1562.

Baumeister, D., Akhtar, R., Ciufolini, S., Pariante, C.M., & Mondelli, V. (2016). Childhood trauma and adulthood inflammation: A meta-analysis of peripheral C-reactive protein, interleukin-6 and tumour necrosis factor-α. *Molecular Psychiatry*, 21, 642–649.

Bayram, K. & Erol, A. (2014). Childhood traumatic experiences, anxiety, and depression levels in fibromyalgia and rheumatoid arthritis. *Archives of Neuropsychiatry*, 51, 344–349.

Bécares, L., Nazroo, J., & Kelly, Y. (2015). A longitudinal examination of maternal, family, and area-level experiences of racism on children's socioemotional development: Patterns and possible explanations. *Social Science & Medicine*, 142, 128–135.

Bedwell, W.L., Ramsay, P.S., & Salas, E. (2012). Helping fluid teams work: A research agenda for effective team adaptation in healthcare. *Translational Behavioral Medicine*, 2, 504–509.

Belkacemi, L., Nelson, D.M., Desai, M., & Ross, M.G. (2010). Maternal undernutrition influences placental-fetal development. *Biology of Reproduction*, 83, 325–331.

Bell, S.T., Brown, S.G., Colaneri, A., & Outland, N. (2018). Team composition and the ABCs of teamwork. *American Psychologist*, 73, 4, 349–362.

Ben, J., Cormack, D., Harris, R., & Paradies, Y. (2017). Racism and health service utilisation: A systematic review and meta-analysis. *PLoS One*, 12, e0189900.

Ben-Zeev, T., Fein, S., & Inzlicht, M. (2005). Arousal and stereotype threat. *Journal of Experimental Social Psychology*, 41, 174–181.

Benjet, C., Bromet, E., Karam, E.G., Kessler, R.C., *et al.* (2016). The epidemiology of traumatic event exposure worldwide: Results from the World Mental Health Survey Consortium. *Psychological Medicine*, 46, 327–329.

Bennett, D., Bendersky, M., & Lewis, M. (2007). Preadolescent health risk behaviour as a function of prenatal cocaine exposure and gender. *Journal of Developmental and Behavioural Paediatrics*, 28, 467–472.

Bernardo, C.O., Bastos, J.L., González-Chica, D.A., Peres, M.A., & Paradies, Y.C. (2017). Interpersonal discrimination and markers of adiposity in longitudinal studies: A systematic review. *Obesity Reviews*, 18, 1040–1049.

Bhui, K., Nazroo, J., Francis, J., Rhodes, J., *et al.* (2018). The impact of racism on mental health. Available at: https://synergicollaborativecentre.co.uk/wp-content/uploads/2017/11/The-impact-of-racism-on-mental-health-briefing-paper-1.pdf.

Bisol, C.A., Sperb, T.M., Brewer, T.H., Kato, S.K., & Shor-Posner, G. (2008). HIV/AIDS knowledge and health-related attitudes and behaviors among deaf and hearing adolescents in southern Brazil. *American Annals of the Deaf*, 153, 349–356.

Blackburn, E.H. & Epel, E.S. (2012). Telomeres and adversity: Too toxic to ignore. *Nature*, 11, 490, 169–171.

Blacker, C.J. (2019). Medical student suicide rates: A systematic review of the historical and international literature. *Academic Medicine*, 94, 274–280.

Blair, E.W., Woolley, S., Szarek, B.L., Mucha, T.F., *et al.* (2017). Reduction of seclusion and restraint in an inpatient psychiatric setting: A pilot study. *Psychiatric Quarterly*, 88, 1–7.

Bloom, S. & Farragher, B. (2010). *Destroying Sanctuary: The Crisis in Human Service Delivery Systems*. New York, NY: Oxford University Press.

Borckardt, J.J., Madan, A., Grubaugh, A.L., Danielson, C.K., *et al.* (2011). Systematic investigation of initiatives to reduce seclusion and restraint in a state psychiatric hospital. *Psychiatric Services*, 62, 477–483.

Bourne, T., Shah, H., Falconieri, N., Timmerman, D., *et al.* (2019). Burnout, well-being and defensive medical practice among obstetricians and gynaecologists in the UK: Cross-sectional survey study. *BMJ Open*, 25, 9, 11, e030968.

Boyce, P.R. (2014). *Human Factors in Lighting*, third edition. Boca Raton, FL: CRC Press.

Boyd, B.A., Iruka, I.U., & Pierce, N.P. (2018). Strengthening Service Access for Children of Color with Autism Spectrum Disorders: A Proposed Conceptual Framework. In M.M. Burke (ed.), *International Review of Research in Developmental Disabilities, Vol. 54: Service Delivery Systems for Individuals with Intellectual and Developmental Disabilities and their Families Across the Lifespan* (pp.1–33). London: Elsevier.

Bramley, G. & Ftizpatrick, S., *et al.* (2015). *Hard Edges: Mapping severe and multiple disadvantage*. Lankelly Chase Foundation. Available at: http://lankellychase.org.uk/wp-content/uploads/2015/07/Hard-Edges-Mapping-SMD-2015.pdf.

Brave Heart, M.Y.H., Chase, J., Elkins, J., & Altschul, D.B. (2011). Historical trauma among Indigenous Peoples of the Americas: Concepts, research, and clinical considerations. *Journal of Psychoactive Drugs*, 43, 282–290.

Bride, B. (2007). Prevalence of secondary traumatic stress among social workers. *Social Work*, 25, 63–70.

Bridges, S. (2015). *Mental Health Problems. In Health Survey for England 2014.* London: Health & Social Care Information Centre.

British Medical Association. (2016). *Alcohol and Pregnancy: Preventing and Managing Fetal Alcohol Spectrum Disorders.* www.bma.org.uk/media/2082/fetal-alcohol-spectrum-disorders-report-feb2016.pdf.

Britton, E. (2019). Duchas: Being and Belonging on the Borderlands of Surfing, Senses and Self. In R. Foley, R. Kearns, T. Kistemann, & B. Wheeler (eds), *Blue Space, Health and Wellbeing: Hydrophilia Unbounded* (pp.95–116). London: Routledge.

Britton, R. (1994). *Re-enactment as an Unwitting Professional Response to Family Dynamics: Crisis at Adolescence.* London: Jason Aronson Inc.

Brockhouse, R., Msetfi, R.M., Cohen, K., & Joseph, S. (2011). Vicarious exposure to trauma and growth in therapists: The moderating effects of sense of coherence, organizational support, and empathy. *Journal of Traumatic Stress*, 24, 735–742.

Brody, G.H., Lei, M.K., Chen, E., & Miller, G.E. (2014). Neighborhood poverty and allostatic load in African American youth. *Pediatrics*, 134, 5, e1362–e1368.

Brooke, J. & Jackson, D. (2020). Older people and COVID-19: Isolation, risk and ageism. *Journal of Clinical Nursing*, 29, 2044–2046.

Broughton, S. & Thomson, K. (2000). Women with learning disabilities: Risk behaviours and experiences of the cervical smear test. *Journal of Advanced Nursing*, 32, 905–912.

Brown, L.S. (1994). *Subversive Dialogues: Theory in Feminist Therapy.* New York, NY: Basic Books.

Brown, S.M., Rodriguez, K.E., Smith, A.D., Ricker, A., & Williamson, A.A. (2022). Associations between childhood maltreatment and behavioral sleep disturbances across the lifespan: A systematic review. *Sleep Medicine Reviews*, 64, 101621.

Brunt, H., Barnes, J., Jones, S.J., Longhurst, J.W.S., Scally, G., & Hayes, E. (2016). Air pollution, deprivation and health: Understanding relationships to add value to local air quality management policy and practice in Wales, UK. *Journal of Public Health*, 39, 485–489.

Bryant-Davis, T. & Ocampo, C. (2005). Racist incident-based trauma. *The Counseling Psychologist*, 33, 479–500.

Bublitz, M.H. & Stroud, L.R. (2012). Maternal smoking during pregnancy and offspring brain structure and function: Review and agenda for future research. *Nicotine & Tobacco Research*, 14, 388–397.

Bucaro, S. (2010). A black market for magical bones: The current plight of East African Albinos. *Public Interest Law Reporter*, 15, 131–140.

Buhrich, N., Hodder, T., & Teesson, M. (2000). Lifetime prevalence of trauma among homeless people in Sydney. *Australian and New Zealand Journal of Psychiatry*, 34, 963–966.

Burke, S.E., Dovidio, J.F., Przedworski, J.M., Hardeman, R.R., Perry, S.P., & Phelan, S.M. (2015). Do contact and empathy mitigate bias against gay and lesbian people among heterosexual first-year medical students? A report from the medical student CHANGE study. *Academic Medicine*, 90, 645–651.

Burke Harris, N. (2018). *The Deepest Well: Healing the Long-Term Effects of Childhood Adversity.* Boston, MA: Houghton Mifflin Harcourt.

Burri, A. & Maercker, A. (2014). Differences in prevalence rates of PTSD in various European countries explained by war exposure, other trauma and cultural value orientation. *BMC Research Notes*, 7, 407.

Burstow, B. (2005). A critique of posttraumatic stress disorder and the DSM. *Journal of Humanistic Psychology*, 429–445.

Buss, C., Entringer, S., & Wadhwa, P.D. (2012). Fetal programming of brain development: Intrauterine stress and susceptibility to psychopathology. *Science Signaling*, 9, 5, 245.

Carpenter, L.L. (2007). Decreased adrenocorticotropic hormone and cortisol responses to stress in healthy adults reporting significant childhood maltreatment. *Biological Psychiatry*, 62, 1080–1087.

Carrion, V.G., Weems, C.F., Watson, C., Eliez, S., Menon, V., & Reiss, A.L. (2009). Converging evidence for abnormalities of the prefrontal cortex and evaluation of midsagittal structures in pediatric posttraumatic stress disorder: An MRI study. *Psychiatry Research*, 172, 226–234.

Carter, R.T. (2007). Racism and psychological and emotional injury: Recognizing and assessing race-based traumatic stress. *The Counseling Psychologist*, 35, 13–105.

Castonguay, L., Constantino, M., & Grosse Holtforth, M. (2006). The working alliance: Where are we and where should we go? *Psychotherapy: Theory, Research, Practice*, 43, 271–279.

Chandan, J.S., Okoth, K., Gokhale, K.M., Bandyopadhyay, S., Taylor, J., & Nirantharakumar, K. (2020). Increased cardiometabolic and mortality risk following childhood maltreatment in the United Kingdom. *Journal of the American Heart Association*, 18, 9–10.

Chasnoff, I. (2011). *The Mystery of Risk*. Portland, OR: NTI Upstream.

Chaveiro, N., Porto, C.C., & Barbosa, M.A. (2009). The relation between deaf patients and the doctor. *Brazilian Journal of Otorhinolaryngology*, 75, 147–150.

Child Poverty Action Group & Royal College of Paediatrics and Child Health. (2017). Poverty and Child Health: Views from the Frontline. www.rcpch.ac.uk/sites/default/files/2018-04/poverty20and20child20health20survey20-20views20from20the20frontline20-20final2008.05.20171.pdf.

Cicchetti, D., Rogosch, F.A., Gunnar, M.R., & Toth, S.L. (2010). The differential impacts of early physical and sexual abuse and internalizing problems on daytime cortisol rhythm in school-aged children. *Child Development*, 81, 252–269.

Clarke, T. & Costall, A. (2008). The emotional connotations of color: A qualitative investigation. *Color Research and Application*, 33, 406–410.

Cleghorn, E. (2021). *Unwell Women: A Journey through Medicine and Myth in a Man-Made World*. London: Weidenfeld & Nicholson.

Coelho, R., Viola, T.W., Walss-Bass, C., Brietzke, E., & Grassi-Oliveira, R. (2014). Childhood maltreatment and inflammatory markers: A systematic review. *Acta Psychiatrica Scandinavica*, 129, 180–192.

Collins, T.W. & Grineski, S.E. (2018). Geographic and social disparities in exposure to air neurotoxicants at U.S. public schools. *Environmental Research*, 161, 580–587.

Collins, T.W., Grineski, S.E., & Nadybal, S. (2019). Social disparities in exposure to noise at public schools in the contiguous United States. *Environmental Research*, 175, 257–265.

Combas, M., Ozturk, E., & Derin, G. (2022). Childhood trauma and dissociation in female patients with fibromyalgia. *Medicine*, 11, 1635–1640.

Commission on Social Determinants of Health. (2008). *Closing the gap in a generation – Health equity through action on the social determinants of health*. Geneva: World Health Organization.

Commodore, S., Ferguson, P.L., Neelon, B., Newman, R., & Grobman, W. (2021). Reported neighborhood traffic and the odds of asthma/asthma-like symptoms: A cross-sectional analysis of a multi-racial cohort of children. *International Journal of Environmental Research and Public Health*, 18, 243.

Coogan, P., Schon, K., Li, S., Cozier, Y., Bethea, T., & Rosenberg, L. (2020). Experiences of racism and subjective cognitive function in African American women. *Alzheimer's & Dementia (Amst)*, 12, e12067.

Cook, A., Spinazzola, J., Ford, J., Lanktree, C., *et al.* (2005). Complex trauma in children and adolescents. *Psychiatric Annals*, 35, 390–398.

Cooke, A.N. & Halberstadt, A.G. (2021). Adultification, anger bias, and adults' different perceptions of Black and White children. *Cognition and Emotion*, 35, 1416–1422.

Cooper, L.A., Roter, D.L., Carson, K.A., Beach, M.C., *et al.* (2012). The associations of clinicians' implicit attitudes about race with medical visit communication and patient ratings of interpersonal care. *American Journal of Public Health*, 102, 979–987.

Copperman, J. & Knowles, K. (2006). Developing women only and gender sensitive practices in inpatient wards: Current issues and challenges. *Journal of Adult Protection*, 8, 15–30.

Cozzarelli, C., Wilkinson, A.V., & Tagler, M.J. (2001). Attitudes toward the poor and attributions for poverty. *Journal of Social Issues*, 57, 207–227.

D'Andrea, W., Ford, J., Stolbach, B., Spinazzola, J., & Van der Kolk, B. (2012). Understanding interpersonal trauma in children: Why we need a developmentally appropriate trauma diagnosis. *American Journal of Orthopsychiatry*, 82, 187–200.

Dalia, C., Abbas, K., & Colville, G. (2013). G49 resilience, post-traumatic stress, burnout and coping in medical staff on the paediatric and neonatal intensive care unit (P/NICU) – A survey. *Archives of Disease in Childhood*, 98, A26–A27.

Dane, B. (2000). Child welfare workers: An innovative approach for interacting with secondary trauma. *Journal of Social Work Education*, 36, 27–38.

Danese, A. & McEwen, B.S. (2012). Adverse childhood experiences, allostasis, allostatic load, and age-related disease. *Physiology & Behavior*, 106, 29–39.

Danese, A., Pariante, C.M., Caspi, A., Taylor, A., & Poulton, R. (2007). Childhood maltreatment predicts adult inflammation in a life-course study. *Proceedings of the National Academy of Sciences*, 104, 1319–1324.

Danisi, C., Dustin, M., Ferreira, N., & Held, N. (2021). *Queering Asylum in Europe: Legal and Social Experiences of Seeking International Protection on Grounds of Sexual Orientation and Gender Identity*. IMISCOE Research Series. Cham: Springer International Publishing.

Davis, D.A. (2005). Are reports of childhood abuse related to the experience of chronic pain in adulthood? A meta-analytic review of the literature. *The Clinical Journal of Pain*, 21, 5, 398–405.

De Bellis, M.D., Woolley, D.P., & Hooper, S.R. (2013). Neuropsychological findings in pediatric maltreatment: Relationship of PTSD, dissociative symptoms, and abuse/neglect indices to neurocognitive outcomes. *Child Maltreatment*, 18, 171–183.

De Bellis, M.D. & Zisk, A. (2014). The biological effects of childhood trauma. *Child and Adolescent Psychiatric Clinics of North America*, 23, 185–222.

DeCasper, A. & Fifer, W. (1980). Of human bonding: Newborns prefer their mother's voices. *Science*, 208, 1174–1176.

DeCasper, A. & Spence, M. (1986). Prenatal maternal speech influences human newborn's perception of speech sounds. *Infant Behavior and Development*, 9, 133–150.

DeQuattro, K., Trupin, L., Li, J., Katz, P.P., *et al.* (2020). Relationships between adverse childhood experiences and health status in systemic lupus erythematosus. *Arthritis Care Research*, 72, 525–533.

Desai, A., Sachdeva, S., Parekh, T., & Desai, R. (2020). COVID-19 and cancer: Lessons from a pooled metaanalysis. *JCO Global Oncology*, 6, 557–559.

De Soir, E. (2012). The Management of Emotionally Disturbing Interventions in Fire and Rescue Services: Psychological Triage as a Framework for Acute Support. In R. Hughes, C. Cooper, & A. Kindler. *International Handbook of Workplace Trauma Support*. New York, NY: John Wiley & Sons.

Dettlaff, A., Rivaux, S., Baumann, D., Fluke, J., Rycraft, J., & James, J. (2011). Disentangling substantiation: The influence of race, income, and risk on the substantiation decision in child welfare. *Children and Youth Services Review*, 33, 1630–1637.

Dinsmore, A.P. (2012). A small-scale investigation of hospital experiences among people with a learning disability on Merseyside: Speaking with patients and their carers. *British Journal of Learning Disabilities*, 40, 201–212.

Dolezsar, C.M., McGrath, J.J., Herzig, A.J.M., & Miller, S.B. (2014). Perceived racial discrimination and hypertension: A comprehensive systematic review. *Health Psychology*, 33, 20–34.

Dombo, E.A. & Blome, W. (2016). Vicarious trauma in child welfare workers: A study of organizational responses. *Journal of Public Child Welfare*, 10, 505–523.

Drake, B., Jonson-Reid, M., Way, I., & Chung, S. (2003). Substantiation and recidivism. *Child Maltreatment*, 8, 4, 248–260.

Drury, V., Craigie, M., Francis, K., Aoun, S., & Hegney, D.G. (2014). Compassion satisfaction, compassion fatigue, anxiety, depression and stress in registered nurses in Australia: Phase 2 results. *Journal of Nursing Management*, 22, 519–531.

Dube, S.R., Fairweather, D., Pearson, W.S., Felitti, V.J., Anda, R.F., & Croft, J.B. (2009). Cumulative childhood stress and autoimmune disease. *Psychological Medicine*, 71, 243–250.

Duncan, G. & Magnuson, K. (2013). The Long Reach of Early Childhood Poverty. In Y.M. Yeung (ed.), *Economic Stress, Human Capital, and Families in Asia. Quality of Life in Asia* (Vol. 4). Dordrecht: Springer.

Dutheil, F. (2019). Suicide among physicians and healthcare workers: A systematic review and meta-analysis. *PLoS One*, 14, e0226361.

Dykes, G. (2011). The implications of adverse childhood experiences for the professional requirements of social work. *Social Work/Maatskaplike Werk*, 47, 521–533.

Eagle, G. & Kaminer, D. (2013). Continuous traumatic stress: Expanding the lexicon of traumatic stress. *Peace and Conflict: Journal of Peace Psychology*, 19, 2, 85.

Edmondson, A.C. (1999). Psychological safety and learning behaviour in work teams. *Administrative Science Quarterly*, 44, 350–384.

Edmondson, D. (2014). An enduring somatic threat model of posttraumatic stress disorder due to acute life-threatening medical events. *Social and Personality Psychology Compass*, 8, 118–134.

Egendorf, S.P., Mielke, H.W., Castorena-Gonzalez, J.A., Powell, E.T., & Gonzales, C.R. (2021). Soil lead (Pb) in New Orleans: A spatiotemporal and racial analysis. *International Journal of Environmental Research and Public Health*, 18, 1314.

Eiseman, L. (2006). *Color: Messages and Meanings – A Pantone Color Resource*. Gloucester, MA: Handbooks Press.

Ekkel, E.D. & de Vries, S. (2017). Nearby green space and human health: Evaluating accessibility metrics. *Landscape and Urban Planning*, 157, 214–220.

Elliot, A. & Maier, M.A. (2014). Color psychology: Effects of perceiving color on psychological functioning in humans. *Annual Review of Psychology*, 65, 95–120.

Emanuel, L. (2002). Deprivation X3: The contribution of organisational dynamics to the 'triple deprivation' of looked-after-children. *Journal of Child Psychotherapy*, 28, 163–179.

Epel, E.S., Crosswell, A.D., Mayer, S.E., Prather, A.A., *et al.* (2018). More than a feeling: A unified view of stress measurement for population science. *Frontiers in Neuroendocrinology*, 49, 146–169.

Equality and Human Rights Commission. (2018). *The lived experiences of access to healthcare for people seeking and refused asylum*. Available at: whttps://www.equalityhumanrights.com/sites/default/files/research-report-122-people-seeking-asylum-access-to-healthcare-lived-experiences.pdf.

Erikson, K.T. (1976). *Everything in its Path*. New York, NY: Simon and Schuster.

Fallot, R.D.M. & Harris, M. (2009). *Creating Cultures of Trauma-Informed Care: A Self-Assessment and Planning Protocol*. Washington, DC: Community Connections.

Fani, N., Carter, S.E., Harnett, N.G., Ressler, K.J., & Bradley, B. (2021). Association of racial discrimination with neural response to threat in Black women in the US exposed to trauma. *JAMA Psychiatry*, 78, 1005–1012.

Feldman, C.H., Malspeis, S., Leatherwood, C., Kubzansky, L., Costenbader, K.H., & Roberts, A.L. (2019). Association of childhood abuse with incident systemic lupus erythematosus in adulthood in a longitudinal cohort of women. *Journal of Rheumatology*, 46, 12, 1589–1596.

Felitti, V.J., Anda, R.F., & Nordenberg, D. (1998). Relationship of childhood abuse and household dysfunction to many of the leading causes of death in adults. The Adverse Childhood Experiences (ACE) Study. *American Journal of Preventative Medicine*, 14, 245–258.

Ferguson, L., Taylor, J., Davies, M., Shrubsole, C., Symonds, P., & Dimitroulopoulou, S. (2020). Exposure to indoor air pollution across socio-economic groups in high-income countries: A scoping review of the literature and a modelling methodology. *Environment International*, 143, 1057.

Field, T., Diego, M., & Hernandez-Reif, M. (2006). Prenatal depression effects on the fetus and newborn: A review. *Infant Behavior and Development*, 29, 445–455.

Figley, C. (1995). *Compassion Fatigue: Coping with Secondary Traumatic Stress Disorder in Those who Treat the Traumatized*. New York, NY: Brunner/Mazel.

Fisher, J. (2006). *Working with the neurobiological legacy of early trauma*. Paper presented at the Trauma Center Lecture Series, Brookline, MA.

Fisher, K., Haagen, B., & Orkin, K. (2005). Acquiring medical services for individuals with mental retardation in community-based housing facilities. *Applied Nursing Research*, 18, 155–159.

FitzGerald, C. & Hurst, S. (2017). Implicit bias in healthcare professionals: A systematic review. *BMC Medical Ethics*, 18, 19.

Fluke, J., Yuan, Y., Hedderson, J., & Curtis, P. (2003). Disproportionate representation of race and ethnicity in child maltreatment: Investigation and victimization. *Children and Youth Services Review*, 25, 359–373.

Fraiberg, S., Adelson, E., & Shapiro, V. (1975). Ghosts in the nursery: A psychoanalytic approach to the problems of impaired infant–mother relationships. *Journal of the American Academy of Child and Adolescent Psychiatry*, 14, 387–421.

Friedman, D. & Luyckx, V.A. (2019). Genetic and developmental factors in chronic kidney disease hotspots. *Seminars in Nephrology*, 34, 244–255.

Fujimura, K.E., Sitarik, A.R., Havstad, S., Lin, D.L., *et al.* (2016). Neonatal gut microbiota associates with childhood multisensitized atopy and T cell differentiation. *Nature Medicine*, 22, 1187–1191.

Fuligni, A.J., Chiang, J.J., & Tottenham, N. (2021). Sleep disturbance and the long-term impact of early adversity. *Neuroscience Biobehavioral Review*, 126, 304–313.

Funk, R.R., McDermeit, M., Godley, S.H., & Adams, L. (2003). Maltreatment issues by level of adolescent substance abuse treatment: The extent of the problem at intake and relationship to early outcomes. *Child Maltreatment*, 8, 36–45.

Garcia, C.L., Abreu, L.C., Ramos, J., Castro, C., *et al.* (2019). Influence of burnout on patient safety: Systematic review and meta-analysis. *Medicina (Kaunas, Lithuania)*, 55, 553.

Gardner-Neblett, N., Iruka, I.U., & Humphries, M. (2021). Dismantling the Black–White achievement gap paradigm: Why and how we need to focus instead on systemic change. *Journal of Education*, 203, 2.

Garrido-Hernansaiz, H., Murphy, P.J., & Alonso-Tapia, J. (2017). Predictors of resilience and posttraumatic growth among people living with HIV: A longitudinal study. *AIDS and Behavior*, 21, 3260–3270.

Gee, G.C. & Ford, C.L. (2011). Structural racism and health inequities: Old issues, new directions. *Du Bois Review*, 8, 115–132.

Gelaye, B., Kajeepeta, S., & Williams, M.A. (2016). Suicidal ideation in pregnancy: An epidemiologic review. *Archives of Women's Mental Health*, 19, 741–751.

Gensollen, T., Iyer, S.S., Kasper, D.L., & Blumberg, R.S. (2016). How colonization by microbiota in early life shapes the immune system. *Science*, 352, 539–544.

Geronimus, A.T., Hicken, M.T., Pearson, J.A., Seashols, S.J., Brown, K.L., & Cruz, T.D. (2010). Do US Black women experience stress-related accelerated biological aging? A novel theory and first population-based test of Black-White differences in telomere length. *Human Nature*, 10, 19–38.

Gibson, F. (2010). Access to justice for people with disabilities: The response of the clinic. *La Trobe Law School Legal Studies Research Paper No. 2010/3*. SSRN: https://ssrn.com/abstract=1540581.

Gilbert, P.A. & Zemore, S.E. (2016). Discrimination and drinking: A systematic review of the evidence. *Social Science & Medicine*, 161, 178–194.

Glaser, D. (2000). Child abuse and neglect and the brain – a review. *Journal of Child Psychology and Psychiatry*, 41, 97–116.

Goetz, S.B. & Taylor-Trujillo, A. (2012). A change in culture: Violence prevention in an acute behavioural health setting. *Journal of the American Psychiatric Nurses Association*, 18, 96–103.

Goldstein, M.F., Eckhardt, E.A., Joyner-Creamer, P., Berry, R., Paradise, H., & Cleland, C.M. (2010). What do deaf high school students know about HIV? *AIDS Education and Prevention*, 22, 523–537.

Goodwin, R.D., Hoven, C.W., Murison, R., & Hotopf, M. (2003). Association between childhood physical abuse and gastrointestinal disorders and migraine in adulthood. *American Journal of Public Health*, 93, 1065–1067.

Grant, J.M., Mottet, L.A., & Tanis, J. (2010). *National Transgender Discrimination Survey Report on Health and Health Care*. Washington, DC: National Center for Transgender Equality and National Gay and Lesbian Task Force.

Grasser, L.R. & Jovanovic, T. (2022). Neural impacts of stigma, racism, and discrimination. *Biological Psychiatry: Cognitive Neuroscience & Neuroimaging*, 12, 1225–1234.

Green, B.L., Saunders, P.A., Power, E., Dass-Brailsford, P., *et al.* (2016). Trauma-informed medical care: Patient response to a primary care provider communication training. *Journal of Loss and Trauma*, 21, 147–159.

Green, C.R., Mihic, A.M., & Nikkel, S.M. (2009). Executive function deficits in children with fetal alcohol spectrum disorders (FASD) measured using the Cambridge Neuropsychological Tests Automated Battery. *Journal of Child Psychology and Psychiatry*, 50, 688–697.

Greenhalgh, T., Robert, G., Macfarlane, F., Bate, P., & Kyriakidou, O. (2004). Diffusion of innovations in service organizations: Systematic review and recommendations. *Milbank Q*, 82, 581–629.

Groce, N.E., Yousafzai, A.K., & van der Maas, F. (2007). HIV/AIDS and disability: Differences in HIV/AIDS knowledge between deaf and hearing people in Nigeria. *Disability and Rehabilitation*, 29, 367–371.

Guasp, A. (2010). *Lesbian, Gay and Bisexual People Later on in Life*. London: Stonewall.

Gunnar, M.R. & Fisher, P.A. (2006). Bringing basic research on early experience and stress neurobiology to bear on preventive interventions for neglected and maltreated children. *Development and Psychopathology*, 18, 651–677.

Haider, A.H., Sexton, J., Sriram, N., Cooper, L.A., *et al.* (2011). Association of unconscious race and social class bias with vignette-based clinical assessments by medical students. *JAMA*, 306, 942–951.

Hair, N.L., Hanson, J.L., Wolfe, B.L., & Pollak, S.D. (2015). Association of child poverty, brain development, and academic achievement. *JAMA Pediatrics*, 169, 9.

Hales, T.W., Green, S.A., Bissonette, S., Warden, A., *et al.* (2019). Trauma-informed care outcome study. *Research on Social Work Practice*, 29, 529–539.

Hankivsky, O., Reid, C., & Cormier, R. (2010). Exploring the promises of intersectionality for advancing women's health research. *International Journal for Equity in Health*, 9, 5.

Hannan, E.L., Wu, Y., & Tamis-Holland, J. (2020). Sex differences in the treatment and outcomes of patients hospitalized with ST-elevation myocardial infarction. *Catheter and Cardiovascular Interventions*, 95, 196–204.

Hao, Y. & Liu, J. (2019). Sex differences in in-hospital management and outcomes of patients with acute coronary syndrome. *Circulation*, 139, 1776–1785.

Haque, A. (2010). Mental health concepts in Southeast Asia: Diagnostic considerations and treatment implications. *Psychology, Health and Medicine*, 15, 127–134.

Harris, H.R., Wieser, F., Vitonis, A.F., & Rich-Edwards, J. (2018). Early life abuse and risk of endometriosis. *Human Reproduction*, 33, 9, 1657–1668.

Harris, J. & Bamford, C. (2001). The uphill struggle: Services for deaf and hard of hearing people – issues of equality, participation and access. *Disability & Society*, 7, 969–979.

Harvey, S., Mitchell, M., Keeble, J., McNaughton Nicholls, C., & Rahim, N. (2014). *Barriers Faced by Lesbian, Gay, Bisexual and Transgender People in Accessing Domestic Abuse, Stalking, Harassment and Sexual Violence Services*. Cardiff: Welsh Government.

Hatzenbuehler, M.L., Weissman, D.G., McKetta, S., Lattanner, M.R., *et al.* (2021). Smaller hippocampal volume among black and latinx youth living in high-stigma contexts. *Journal of the American Academy of Child and Adolescent Psychiatry*, 61, 6, 809–819.

Havig, K. (2008). The health care experiences of adult survivors of child sexual abuse: A systematic review of evidence on sensitive practice. *Trauma, Violence & Abuse*, 9, 19–33.

Hawkins, P. & Shohet, R. (2012). *Supervision in the Helping Professions* (fourth edition). Milton Keynes: Open University Press.

Heard-Garris, N.J., Cale, M., Camaj, L., Hamati, M.C., & Dominguez, T.P. (2018). Transmitting trauma: A systematic review of vicarious racism and child health. *Social Science & Medicine*, 199, 230–240.

Hechanova, R. & Waelde, L. (2017). The influence of culture on disaster mental health and psychosocial support interventions in Southeast Asia. *Mental Health Religion and Culture*, 20, 31–44.

Heim, C., Newport, D., Mletzko, T., Miller, A.H., & Nemeroff, C.B. (2008). The link between childhood trauma and depression: Insights from HPA axis studies in humans. *Psycho-neuroendocrinology*, 33, 693–710.

Heitkemper, M., Cain, K., Burr, R., Jun, S.-E., & Jarrett, M. (2011). Is childhood abuse or neglect associated with symptom reports and physiological measures in women with irritable bowel syndrome? *Biological Research for Nursing*, 13, 399–408.

Helliwell, J.F. & Wang, S. (2009). 'Trust and well-being.' Paper prepared for the 3rd OECD World Forum on Statistics, Knowledge and Policy. Busan, Korea.

Henderson, J. (2013). Experiencing maternity care: The care received and perceptions of women from different ethnic groups. *BMC Pregnancy Childbirth*, 13, 1–14.

Hepper, P.G. (1991). An examination of fetal learning before and after birth. *Irish Journal of Psychology*, 12, 95–107.

Her, A.Y., Shin, E.S., Kim, Y.H., Garg, S., & Jeong, M.H. (2018). The contribution of gender and age on early and late mortality following ST-segment elevation myocardial infarction: Results from the Korean Acute Myocardial Infarction National Registry with Registries. *Journal of Geriatric Cardiology*, 15, 205–214.

Herman, J.L. (1992). *Trauma and Recovery*. New York, NY: Basic Books.

Hill, C.E. (2009). *Helping Skills: Facilitating Exploration, Insight, and Action*. Washington, DC: American Psychological Association.

Hinton, D.E., Reis, R., & de Jong, J. (2015). The 'thinking a lot' idiom of distress and PTSD: An examination of their relationship among traumatized Cambodian refugees using the 'Thinking a Lot' Questionnaire. *Medical Anthropology*, 29, 357–380.

Hlubocky, F.J., Spence, R., McGinnis, M., Taylor, L., & Kamal, A. (2020). Burnout and moral distress in oncology: Taking a deliberate ethical step forward to optimize oncologist well-being. *JCO Oncology Practice*, 16, 185–186.

Hobday, A. (2001). Timeholes: A useful metaphor when explaining unusual or bizarre behaviour in children who have moved families. *Clinical Child Psychology and Psychiatry*, 6, 41–47.

Honwana, A.M. (1997). Healing for peace: Traditional healers and post-war reconstruction in Southern Mozambique. *Peace and Conflict: Journal of Peace Psychology*, 3, 3, 293–305.

Høyvik, A.C., Willumsen, T., Lie, B., & Hilden, P.K. (2021). The torture victim and the dentist: The social and material dynamics of trauma re-experiencing triggered by dental visits. *Torture Journal*, 31, 70–83.

Huang, H., Yan, P., Shan, Z., Chen, S., *et al.* (2015). Adverse childhood experiences and risk of type 2 diabetes: A systematic review and meta-analysis. *Metabolism*, 64, 1408–1418.

Hughes, A., McMunn, A., & Bartley, M. (2015). Elevated inflammatory biomarkers during unemployment: Modification by age and country in the UK. *Journal of Epidemiology and Community Health*, 10, 113.

Hughes, K., Bellis, M.A., Hardcastle, K.A., Sethi, D., *et al.* (2017). The effect of multiple adverse childhood experiences on health: A systematic review and meta-analysis. *Lancet Public Health*, 8, 356–366.

Hunsaker, S., Chen, H.C., Maughan, D., & Heaston, S. (2015). Factors that influence the development of compassion fatigue, burnout, and compassion satisfaction in emergency department nurses. *Journal of Nursing Scholarship*, 47, 186–194.

Independent Maternity Review. (2022a). *Ockenden report – Final: Findings, conclusions, and essential actions from the independent review of maternity services at the Shrewsbury and Telford Hospital NHS Trust*. Available at: https://assets.publishing.service.gov.uk/government/uploads/system/uploads/attachment_data/file/1064302/Final-Ockenden-Report-web-accessible.pdf.

Independent Maternity Review. (2022b). *Kirkup report – Maternity and neonatal services in East Kent: 'Reading the signals' report*. Available at: www.gov.uk/government/publications/maternity-and-neonatal-services-in-east-kent-reading-the-signals-report.

Jackowski, A.P., Douglas-Palumberi, H., Jackowski, M., Win, L., *et al.* (2008). Corpus callosum in maltreated children with posttraumatic stress disorder: A diffusion tensor imaging study. *Psychiatry Research*, 162, 256–261.

Jackson, T., Provencio, A., Bentley-Kumar, K., Pearcy, C., *et al.* (2017). Discussion of: 'PTSD and surgical residents: everybody hurts sometimes'. *American Journal of Surgery*, 214, 1125–1126.

Jalil, N.A., Yunus, R.M., & Said, N.S. (2013). Students' colour perception and preference: An empirical analysis of its relationship. *Procedia-Social and Behavioral Sciences*, 90, 575–582.

Janssen, I., Krabbendam, L., & Bak, M. (2004). Childhood abuse as a risk factor for psychotic experiences. *Acta Psychiatrica Scandinavica*, 109, 38–45.

Jewkes, R., Flood, M., & Lang, J. (2015). From work with men and boys to changes of social norms and reduction of inequities in gender relations: A conceptual shift in prevention of violence against women and girls. *The Lancet*, 385, 9977, 1580–1589.

Jiang, D.M., Berlin, A., & Moody, L. (2020). Transitioning to a new normal in the post-Covid era. *Current Oncology Reports*, 22, 7, 73.

Jones, L., Bellis, M.A., Wood, S., Hughes, K., *et al.* (2012). Prevalence and risk of violence against children with disabilities: A systematic review and meta-analysis of observational studies. *The Lancet*, 380, 9845, 899–907.

Joseph Rowntree Foundation. (2020). UK Poverty 2019/20. www.jrf.org.uk/report/uk-poverty-2019-20.

Juang, K.D. & Yang, C.Y. (2014). Psychiatric comorbidity of chronic daily headache: Focus on traumatic experiences in childhood, post-traumatic stress disorder and suicidality. *Current Pain and Headache Reports*, 18, 4, 1–7.

Kadambi, M.A. & Truscott, D. (2003). An investigation of vicarious traumatization among therapists working with sex offenders. *Traumatology*, 9, 216–230.

Kakinami, L., Séguin, L., Lambert, M., Gauvin, L., Nikiema, B., & Paradis, G. (2014). Poverty's latent effect on adiposity during childhood: Evidence from a Quebec birth cohort. *Journal of Epidemiology and Community Health*, 68, 239–245.

Kapadia, D., Zhang, J., Salway, S., Nazroo, J., et al. (2022). *Ethnic Inequalities in Healthcare: A Rapid Evidence Review*. NHS Race & Health Observatory.

Karcher, N.R. & Barch, D.M. (2021). The ABCD study: Understanding the development of risk for mental and physical health outcomes. *Neuropsychopharmacology*, 46, 131–134.

Karlen, J., Ludvigsson, J., Hedmark, M., Faresjo, A., Theodorsson, E., & Faresjo, T. (2015). Early psychosocial exposures, hair cortisol levels, and disease risk. *Pediatrics*, 135, 1450–1457.

Kawamoto, K.R., Davis, M.B., & Duvernoy, C.S. (2016). Acute coronary syndromes: Differences in men and women. *Current Atherosclerosis Reports*, 18, 73.

Keesler, J.M. (2020). Promoting satisfaction and reducing fatigue: Understanding the impact of trauma-informed organizational culture on psychological wellness among direct service providers. *Journal of Applied Research in Intellectual Disabilities*, 33, 5, 939–949.

Kellerman, N.P.F. (2013). Epigenetic transmission of Holocaust trauma: Can nightmares be transmitted? *Israel Journal of Psychiatry and Related Sciences*, 50, 33–39.

Kelly, L., Runge, J., & Spencer, C. (2015). Predictors of compassion fatigue and compassion satisfaction in acute care nurses. *Journal of Nursing Scholarship*, 47, 522–528.

Kemeny, M.E., Foltz, C., Cavanagh, J.F., Cullen, M., et al. (2012). Contemplative/emotion training reduces negative emotional behavior and promotes prosocial responses. *Emotion*, 12, 338–350.

Kendall-Tackett, K.A. (2009). Psychological trauma and physical health: A psychoneuroimmunology approach to etiology of negative health effects and possible interventions. *Psychological Trauma: Theory, Research, Practice, and Policy*, 1, 1, 35–48.

Khan, A., Plummer, D., Hussain, R., & Minichiello, V. (2008). Does physician bias affect the quality of care they deliver? Evidence in the care of sexually transmitted infections. *Sexually Transmitted Infections*, 84, 150–151.

Kilpatrick, D.G., Resnick, H.S., Milanak, M.E., Miller, M.W., Keyes, K.M., & Friedman, M.J. (2013). National estimates of exposure to traumatic events and PTSD prevalence using DSM-IV and DSM-5 criteria. *Journal of Traumatic Stress*, 26, 537–547.

Kilpatrick, D.G., Saunders, B.E., & Smith, D.W. (2003). *Youth Victimization: Prevalence and Implications*. Washington, DC: U.S. Department of Justice, Office of Justice Programs, National Institute of Justice.

Kinsella, M.T. & Monk, C. (2009). Impact of maternal stress, depression and anxiety on fetal neurobehavioral development. *Clinical Obstetrics and Gynecology*, 52, 425–440.

Kirmayer, L.J. (2004). The cultural diversity of healing: Meaning, metaphor and mechanism. *British Medical Bulletin*, 16, 33–48.

Kleinman, A. (1977). Depression somatization and the new cross-cultural psychiatry. *Social Science and Medicine*, 11, 3–9.

Knight, M., Bunch, K., Tuffnell, D., Shakespeare, J., et al. (eds) on behalf of MBRRACE-UK (2018). *Saving Lives, Improving Mothers' Care – Lessons learned to inform maternity care from the UK and Ireland Confidential Enquiries into Maternal Deaths and Morbidity 2016–18*. Oxford: National Perinatal Epidemiology Unit, University of Oxford.

Knight, M., Bunch, K., Tuffnell, D., Shakespeare, J., *et al.* (eds) on behalf of MBRRACE-UK (2019). *Saving Lives, Improving Mothers' Care – Lessons learned to inform maternity care from the UK and Ireland Confidential Enquiries into Maternal Deaths and Morbidity 2015–17.* Oxford: National Perinatal Epidemiology Unit, University of Oxford.

Knight, M., Bunch, K., Tuffnell, D., Shakespeare, J., *et al.* (eds) on behalf of MBRRACE-UK (2020). *Saving Lives, Improving Mothers' Care – Lessons learned to inform maternity care from the UK and Ireland Confidential Enquiries into Maternal Deaths and Morbidity 2016–18.* Oxford: National Perinatal Epidemiology Unit, University of Oxford.

Knight, M., Bunch, K., Tuffnell, D., Shakespeare, J., *et al.* (eds) on behalf of MBRRACE-UK (2021). *Saving Lives, Improving Mothers' Care – Lessons learned to inform maternity care from the UK and Ireland Confidential Enquiries into Maternal Deaths and Morbidity 2017–19.* Oxford: National Perinatal Epidemiology Unit, University of Oxford.

Knight, M., Bunch, K., Tuffnell, D., Shakespeare, J., *et al.* (eds) on behalf of MBRRACE-UK (2022). *Saving Lives, Improving Mothers' Care Core Report – Lessons learned to inform maternity care from the UK and Ireland Confidential Enquiries into Maternal Deaths and Morbidity 2018–20.* Oxford: National Perinatal Epidemiology Unit, University of Oxford.

Kohrt, B.A. & Hruschka, D.J. (2010). Nepali concepts of psychological trauma: The role of idioms of distress, ethnopsychology and ethnophysiology in alleviating suffering and preventing stigma. *Culture, Medicine, and Psychiatry,* 34, 322–352.

Koku, P. (2010). HIV-related stigma among African immigrants living with HIV/AIDS in USA. *Sociological Research Online,* 15, 121–124.

Kouyoumdjian, F.G., Findlay, N., Schwandt, M., & Calzavara, L.M. (2013). A systematic review of the relationships between intimate partner violence and HIV/AIDS. *PLoS One,* 8, 1–25.

Kranjac, A.W., Kimbro, R.T., Denney, J.T., Osiecki, K.M., Moffett, B.S., & Lopez, K.N. (2017). Comprehensive neighborhood portraits and child asthma disparities. *Maternal & Child Health Journal,* 21, 1552–1562.

Kuderer, N.M., Choueri, T.K., & Shah, D.P. (2020). Clinical impact of Covid-19 on patients with cancer (CCC1919): A cohort study. *The Lancet,* 395, 1907–1918.

Kumagai, A.K. & Lypson, M.L. (2009). Beyond cultural competence: Critical consciousness, social justice, and multicultural education. *Academic Medicine,* 84, 782–787.

Kurtz, A. & Turner, K. (2007). An exploratory study of the needs of staff who care for offenders with a diagnosis of personality disorder. *Psychology & Psychotherapy: Theory, Research & Practice,* 80, 421–435.

Kushel, M.B., Evans, J.L., Perry, S., Robertson, M.J., & Moss, A.R. (2003). No door to lock: Victimization among homeless and marginally housed persons. *Archives of Internal Medicine,* 163, 2492–2499.

Kvam, M.H. (2004). Sexual abuse of deaf children: A retrospective analysis of the prevalence and characteristics of childhood sexual abuse among deaf adults in Norway. *Child Abuse and Neglect,* 28, 3, 241–251.

Kyle, R.G., Kukanova, M., Campbell, M., Wolfe, I., Powell, P., & Callery, P. (2011). Childhood disadvantage and emergency admission rates for common presentations in London: An exploratory analysis. *Archives of Disease in Childhood,* 96, 221–225.

Lambda Legal. (2010). *When Health Care Isn't Caring: Lambda Legal's Survey of Discrimination Against LGBT People and People with HIV.* New York, NY: Lambda Legal.

Lazinski, M.J., Shea, A.K., & Steiner, M. (2008). Effects of maternal prenatal stress on offspring development: A commentary. *Maternity and Infant Care Archives of Women's Mental Health,* 1, 363–375.

Lee, H., Andrew, M., Gebremariam, A., Lumeng, J.C., & Lee, J.M. (2014). Longitudinal associations between poverty and obesity from birth through adolescence. *American Journal of Public Health,* 104, e70–e76.

Leeners, B., Stiller, R., Block, E., Görres, G., Imthurn, B., & Rath, W. (2007). Consequences of childhood sexual abuse experiences on dental care. *Journal of Psychosomatic Research*, 62, 581–588.

Lefkowitz, D.S., Baxt, C., & Evans, J.R. (2010). Prevalence and correlates of posttraumatic stress and postpartum depression in parents of infants in the Neonatal Intensive Care Unit (NICU). *Journal of Clinical Psychology in Medical Settings*, 17, 230–237.

LeGrand, S., Muessig, K.E., McNulty, T., Soni, K., *et al.* (2016). Epic allies: Development of a gaming app to improve antiretroviral therapy adherence among young HIV-positive men who have sex with men. *JMIR Serious Games*, 4, 6–10.

Lemieux-Charles, L. & McGuire, W. (2006). What do we know about health care team effectiveness? A review of the literature. *Medical Care Research and Review*, 63, 3, 263–300.

Leserman, J. (2008). Role of depression, stress, and trauma in HIV disease progression. *Psychosomatic Medicine*, 70, 539–545.

Leung, T.I. (2021). Finding the evidence base using citation networks: Do 300 to 400 US physicians die by suicide annually? *Journal of General Internal Medicine*, 36, 4, 1129–1131.

Levine, P.A. & Kline, M. (2007). *Trauma Through a Child's Eyes: Awakening the Ordinary Miracle of Healing*. Berkeley, CA: North Atlantic Books.

Lewis, G. & Drife, J. (2004). *Confidential Enquiry into Maternal and Child Health: Improving Care for Mothers, Babies, and Children. Why Mothers Die 2000–2002. The Sixth Report of Confidential Enquiries into Maternal Deaths in the United Kingdom*. London: Royal College of Obstetricians and Gynaecologists.

Lewis, T.T., Cogburn, C.D., & Williams, D.R. (2015). Self-reported experiences of discrimination and health: Scientific advances, ongoing controversies, and emerging issues. *Annual Review of Clinical Psychology*, 11, 40–70.

Lewis, T.T. & Van Dyke, M.E. (2018). Discrimination and the health of African Americans: The potential importance of intersectionalities. *Current Directions in Psychological Science*, 27, 176–182.

Leydecker, S. (2017). Healthy patient rooms in hospitals: Emotional wellbeing naturally. *Architectural Design*, 87, 76–81.

Lieberman, A.F., Padron, E., Van Horn, P., & Harris, W.W. (2005). Angels in the nursery: The intergenerational transmission of benevolent influences. *Infant Mental Health Journal*, 26, 504–520.

Lightfoot, E. (2014). Children and youth with disabilities in the child welfare system: An overview. *Child Welfare*, 93, 23–45.

Lightfoot, E., Hill, K., & LaLiberte, T. (2011). Prevalence of children with disabilities in the child welfare system and out of home placement: An examination of administrative records. *Children and Youth Services Review*, 33, 2069–2075.

Liming, K.W. & Grube, W.A. (2018). Wellbeing outcomes for children exposed to multiple adverse experiences in early childhood: A systematic review. *Child and Adolescent Social Work Journal*, 32, 1–19.

Loftus, E.F. & Palmer, J.C. (1974). Reconstruction of auto-mobile destruction: An example of the interaction between language and memory. *Journal of Verbal Learning and Verbal Behavior*, 13, 585–589.

Lumey, L.H., Stein, A.D., & Ravelli, C.J. (1995). Timing of prenatal starvation in women and birth weight in their offspring: The Dutch famine birth cohort study. *European Journal of Obstetrics and Gynaecology and Reproductive Biology*, 61, 23–30.

Lutz, W., Leon, S.C., Martinovich, Z., Lyons, J.S., & Stiles, W.B. (2007). Therapist effects in outpatient psychotherapy: A three-level growth curve approach. *Journal of Counseling Psychology*, 54, 32–39.

Machtinger, E.L., Haberer, J.E., Wilson, T.C., & Weiss, D.S. (2012). Recent trauma is associated with antiretroviral failure and HIV transmission risk behavior among HIV-positive women and female-identified transgenders. *AIDS and Behavior*, 16, 2160–2170.

Manduca, R. & Sampson, R.J. (2019). Punishing and toxic neighborhood environments independently predict the intergenerational social mobility of black and white children. *Proceedings of the National Academy of Sciences*, 116, 16, 7772–7777.

Margellos-Anast, H., Estarziau, M., & Kaufman, G. (2006). Cardiovascular disease knowledge among culturally deaf patients in Chicago. *Preventive Medicine*, 42, 235–239.

Marmot, M. (2010). *Fair Society, Healthy Lives. The Marmot Review: Strategic Review of Health Inequalities in England Post-2010*. Marmot Review Team.

Marsella, A.J. (2011). Twelve critical issues for mental health professionals working with ethno-culturally diverse populations. *Psychology International*, 22, 7–10.

Marshall, P.J. & Fox, N.A. (2004). The BEIP Core Group. A comparison of the electroencephalogram between institutionalized and community children in Romania. *Journal of Cognitive Neuroscience*, 16, 1327–1338.

Maslach, C. (2003). *Burnout: The Cost of Caring*. Los Altos, CA: ISHK.

Mason, B. (1993). Towards positions of safe uncertainty. *Human Systems: The Journal of Systemic Consultation and Management*, 4, 189–200.

Mastrocinque, J.M., Thew, D., Cerulli, C., Raimondi, C., Pollard, R.Q., & Chin, N.P. (2015). Deaf victims' experiences with intimate partner violence: The need for integration and innovation. *Journal of Interpersonal Violence*, 10, 1077–1082.

Maty, S.C., Lynch, J.W., Raghunathan, T.E., & Kaplan, G.A. (2008). Childhood socioeconomic position, gender, adult body mass index, and incidence of type 2 diabetes mellitus over 34 years in the Alameda County Study. *American Journal of Public Health*, 98, 1486–1494.

May, P.A., Chambers, C.D., & Kalberg, W.O. (2018). Prevalence of fetal alcohol spectrum disorders in 4 US communities. *Journal of the American Medical Association*, 319, 474–478.

McCann, I.L. & Pearlman, L.A. (1990). Vicarious traumatization: A framework for understanding the psychological effects of working with victims. *Journal of Traumatic Stress*, 3, 131–149.

McCarthy, R., Mukherjee, R.A.S., Fleming, K.M., Green, J., Clayton-Smith, J., Price, A.D., Allely, C.S., Cook, P.A. (2021). Prevalence of fetal alcohol spectrum disorder in Greater Manchester, UK: An active case ascertainment study. *Alcohol Clin Exp Res*. 45, 2271-2281.

McCormick, R. (2017). Does access to green space impact the mental well-being of children? A systematic review. *Journal of Pediatric Nursing*, 37, 3–7.

McDonald, J. (2020). 'It's fine; I'm fine': Considerations for trauma-informed healthcare practices. *Journal of Aggression, Maltreatment & Trauma*, 29, 4, 385–399.

McElvaney, R. & Tatlow-Golden, M. (2016). A traumatised and traumatising system: Professionals' experience in meeting the mental health needs of young people in the care and youth justice systems in Ireland. *Children and Youth Services Review*, 65, 62–69.

McEwen, B.S. & Akil, H. (2020). Revisiting the stress concept: Implications for affective disorders. *Journal of Neuroscience*, 40, 12–21.

McFadden, P., Neill, R.D., Mallett, J., Manthorpe, J., *et al.* (2022). Mental well-being and quality of working life in UK social workers before and during the COVID-19 pandemic: A propensity score matching study. *British Journal of Social Work*, 52, 2814–2833.

McLaughlin, K.A., Breslau, J., Green, J.G., Lakoma, M.D., *et al.* (2011). Childhood socio-economic status and the onset, persistence, and severity of DSM-IV mental disorders in a US national sample. *Social Science and Medicine*, 73, 7, 1088–1096.

McManus, B.M., Richardson, Z., Schenkman, M., & Murphy, N.J. (2020). Child characteristics and early intervention referral and receipt of services: A retrospective cohort study. *BMC Pediatrics*, 20, 1, 84.

Meaney, M.J. & Szyf, M. (2005). Environmental programming of stress responses through DNA methylation: Life at the interface between a dynamic environment and a fixed genome. *Dialogues in Clinical Neuroscience*, 7, 103–123.

Mehta, L.S., Beckie, T.M., & DeVon, H.A. (2016). Acute myocardial infarction in women: A scientific statement from the American Heart Association. *Circulation*, 133, 916–947.

Mehta, R. & Zhu, R.J. (2009). Blue or red? Exploring the effect of color on cognitive task performances. *Science*, 323, 1226–1229.

Mendes, A.P., Zhang, L., Prietsch, S.O., Franco, O.S., *et al.* (2011). Factors associated with asthma severity in children: A case-control study. *Journal of Asthma*, 48, 235–240.

Mesquita, B. & Walker, R. (2003). Cultural differences in emotions: A context for interpreting emotional experiences. *Behaviour Research and Therapy*, 41, 777–793.

Meyer, J.P., Stanley, D.J., Herscovitch, L., & Topolnytsky, L. (2002). Affective, continuance, and normative commitment to the organization: A meta-analysis of antecedents, correlates, and consequences. *Journal of Vocational Behavior*, 61, 20–52.

Michopoulos, V., Powers, A., Gillespie, C.F., Ressler, K.J., & Jovanovic, T. (2017). Inflammation in fear- and anxiety-based disorders: PTSD, GAD, and beyond. *Neuropsychopharmacology*, 42, 254–260.

Minnes, P. & Steiner, K. (2009). Parent views on enhancing the quality of health care for their children with fragile X syndrome, autism or Down syndrome. *Child: Care, Health and Development*, 35, 250–256.

Miró, E., Martínez, M.P., & Sánchez, A.I. (2020). Clinical manifestations of trauma exposure in fibromyalgia: The role of anxiety in the association between posttraumatic stress symptoms and fibromyalgia status. *Journal of Trauma and Stress*, 33, 1082–1092.

Mohr, D.C., Hart, S.L., & Julian, L. (2004). Association between stressful life events and exacerbation in multiple sclerosis: A meta-analysis. *British Medical Journal*, 328, 731–742.

Monk, C., Spicer, J., & Champagne, F.A. (2012). Linking prenatal maternal adversity to developmental outcomes in infants: The role of epigenetic pathways. *Development and Psychopathology*, 24, 1361–1376.

Morris, D., Webb, E., Dionelis, C., Parmar, E., & Wallang, P. (2020). Adverse Childhood Experiences (ACEs) and their relationship to BMI in a developmental disorder adolescent population. *Abuse*, 1, 2.

Morrissey, T.W., Hutchison, L., & Winsler, A. (2014). Family income, school attendance, and academic achievement in elementary school. *Developmental Psychology*, 50, 741–753.

Motta, R.W. (2012). Secondary trauma in children and school personnel. *Journal of Applied School Psychology*, 28, 256–269.

Mudrick, N.R., Breslin, M.L., Yee, S., & Liang, M. (2010). Accessibility of Primary Health Care Provider Settings for People with Disabilities: Information from Health Plan Audits [Slides]. Presented at the annual meeting of the American Public Health Association, Denver, CO, 8 November.

Mullen, C., Grineski, S., Collins, T., Xing, W., & Whitaker, R. (2020). Patterns of distributive environmental inequity under different PM2.5 air pollution scenarios for Salt Lake County public schools. *Environmental Research*, 186, 109543.

Näring, G.W.B. & Van Lankveld, W.G.J.M. (2007). Somatoform dissociation and traumatic experiences in patients with rheumatoid arthritis and fibromyalgia. *Clinical and Experimental Rheumatology*, 25, 872–877.

Neigh, G.N., Gillespie, C.F., & Nemeroff, C.B. (2009). The neurobiological toll of child abuse and neglect. *Trauma, Violence, & Abuse*, 10, 389–410.

NHS Digital. (2021). National Child Measurement Programme, England 2020/21 School Year. Available at: https://digital.nhs.uk/data-and-information/publications/statistical/national-child-measurement-programme/2020-21-school-year.

NHS England. (2015). About the survey. GP Patient Survey. Available at: https://gp-patient. co.uk/about.

NHS England. (2021). *A Good Practice Guide to Support Implementation of Trauma Informed Care in the Perinatal Period*. Available at: www.england.nhs.uk/publication/a-good-practice-guide-to-support-implementation-of-trauma-informed-care-in-the-perinatal-period.

Nichter, M. (2010). Idioms of distress revisited. *Culture, Medicine and Psychiatry*, 34, 401–416.

Niedzwiedz, C.L., Green, M.J., & Benzeval, M. (2021). Mental health and health behaviours before and during the initial phase of the COVID-19 lockdown: Longitudinal analyses of the UK household longitudinal study. *Journal of Epidemiology and Community Health*, 75, 224–231.

Niimura, J., Nakanishi, M., Okumura, Y., Kawano, M., & Nishida, A. (2019). Effectiveness of 1-day trauma-informed care training programme on attitudes in psychiatric hospitals: A pre-post study. *International Journal of Mental Health Nursing*, 28, 980–988.

Nijenhuis, E.R.S., Van Dyck, R., Ter Kuile, M.M., Mourits, M.J.E., Spinhoven, P., & Van der Hart, O. (2003). Evidence for associations among somatoform dissociation, psychological dissociation and reported trauma in patients with chronic pelvic pain. *Journal of Psychosomatic Obstetrics and Gynaecology*, 24, 87–98.

Noll, J.G., Trickett, P., Susman, E.J., & Putnam, F.W. (2006). Sleep disturbances and childhood sexual abuse. *Journal of Pediatric Psychology*, 31, 469–480.

Nomura, Y., Rompala, G., Pritchett, L., Aushev, V., Chen, J., & Hurd, Y.L. (2021). Natural disaster stress during pregnancy is linked to reprogramming of the placenta transcriptome in relation to anxiety and stress hormones in young offspring. *Molecular Psychiatry*, 26, 6520–6530.

Norful, A.A., Rosenfeld, A., Schroeder, K., Travers, J.L., & Aliyu, S. (2021). Primary drivers and psychological manifestations of stress in frontline healthcare workforce during the initial COVID-19 outbreak in the United States. *General Hospital Psychiatry*, 69, 20–26.

Ntinda, R. (2009). Customary Practices and Children with Albinism in Namibia: A Constitutional Challenge? In O.C. Ruppel (ed.), *Children's Rights in Namibia* (pp.243–254). Windhoek, Namibia: Macmillan Education.

Oberlander, T.F., Weinberg, J., Papsdorf, M., Grunau, R., Misri, S., & Devlin, A.M. (2008). Prenatal exposure to maternal depression, neonatal methylation of human glucocorticoid receptor gene (NR3C1) and infant cortisol stress responses. *Epigenetics*, 3, 97–106.

Ogden, P. & Fisher, J. (2014). *Sensorimotor Psychotherapy: Interventions for Trauma and Attachment*. New York, NY: W.W. Norton.

Orton, S., Jones, L.L., Cooper, S., Lewis, S., & Coleman, T. (2014). Predictors of children's secondhand smoke exposure at home: A systematic review and narrative synthesis of the evidence. *PLoS ONE*, 9, e11269.

Ozeke, O., Ozeke, V., Coskun, O., & Budakoglu, I.I. (2019). Second victims in health care: Current perspectives. *Advances in Medical Education and Practice*, 10, 593–603. Palfrey, N., Reay, R.E., Aplin, V., Cubis, J.C., *et al.* (2019). Achieving service change through the implementation of a trauma-informed care training program within a mental health service. *Community Mental Health*, 55, 467–475.

Panagioti, M., Geraghty, K., Johnson, J., Zhou, A., *et al.* (2018). Association between physician burnout and patient safety, professionalism, and patient satisfaction: A systematic review and meta-analysis. *JAMA Internal Medicine*, 178, 10, 1317–1331.

Papadopoulos, R. (2007). Refugees, trauma and adversity-activated development. *European Journal of Psychotherapy and Counselling*, 9, 301–312.

Pascoe, E.A. & Smart Richman, L. (2009). Perceived discrimination and health: A meta-analytic review. *Psychology Bulletin*, 135, 531–554.

Patrick, E.T. & Bryan, Y. (2005). Research strategies for optimizing pregnancy outcomes in minority populations. *American Journal of Obstetrics and Gynaecology*, 192, S64–70.

Pereira, P.C. & Fortes, P.A. (2010). Communication and information barriers to health assistance for deaf patients. *American Annals of the Deaf*, 155, 31–37.

Perez, L., Jones, J., Englert, D., & Sachau, D. (2010). Secondary traumatic stress and burnout among law enforcement investigators exposed to disturbing media images. *Journal of Police and Criminal Psychology*, 25, 113–124.

Perry, B.D. (1997). Incubated in Terror: Neurodevelopmental Factors in the 'Cycle of Violence'. In J. Osofsky (ed.), *Children in a Violent Society* (pp.124–148). New York, NY: Guilford Press.

Perry, B.D. (2009). Examining child maltreatment through a neurodevelopmental lens: Clinical application of the neurosequential model of therapeutics. *Journal of Loss and Trauma*, 14, 240–255.

Pistorius, K.D. (2006). The Personal Impact on Female Therapists from Working with Sexually Abused Children. All Theses and Dissertations. Paper 394. Brigham Young University, Provo, Utah.

Pollard, R.Q. & Barnett, S. (2009). Health-related vocabulary knowledge among deaf adults. *Rehabilitation Psychology*, 54, 182–185.

Pollock, L. (2004). *Experiences of Maternity Services: Muslim Women's Perspectives*. London: The Maternity Alliance.

Porges, S.W. (2007). The polyvagal perspective. *Biological Psychology*, 74, 2, 116–143.

Porter, J.L. & Williams, L.M. (2011). Auditory status and experiences of abuse among college students. *Violence and Victims*, 26, 6, 788–798.

Poulton, R., Moffitt, T.E., & Silva, P.A. (2015). The Dunedin Multidisciplinary Health and Development Study: Overview of the first 40 years, with an eye to the future. *Social Psychiatry and Psychiatric Epidemiology*, 50, 679–693.

Prasad, K., McLoughlin, C., Stillman, M., Poplau, S., *et al.* (2021). Prevalence and correlates of stress and burnout among U.S. healthcare workers during the COVID-19 pandemic: A national cross-sectional survey study. *EClinicalMedicine*, 16, 35, 100879.

Priebe, S. & McCabe, R. (2006). The therapeutic relationship in psychiatric settings. *Acta Psychiatrica Scandinavica*, 113, 69–72.

Public Health England. (2018). *National Dental Epidemiology Programme for England: Oral health survey of five-year-old children 2017: A report on the inequalities found in prevalence and severity of dental decay*. London: Public Health England.

Puolakka, E., Pahkala, K., Laitinen, T.T., Magnussen, C. G., *et al.* (2016). Childhood socioeconomic status in predicting metabolic syndrome and glucose abnormalities in adulthood: The Cardiovascular Risk in Young Finns Study. *Diabetes Care*, 39, 12, 2311–2317.

Purtle, J. (2020). Systematic review of evaluations of trauma-informed organizational interventions that include staff trainings. *Trauma, Violence, & Abuse*, 21, 4, 725–740.

Puthussery, S. (2016). Perinatal outcomes among migrant mothers in the United Kingdom: Is it a matter of biology, behaviour, policy, social determinants or access to health care? *Best Practice and Research in Clinical Obstetrics and Gynaecology*, 32, 39–49.

Quinn, K., Frueh, B.C., Scheidell, J., Schatz, D., Scanlon, F., & Khan, M.R. (2019). Internalizing and externalizing factors on the pathway from adverse experiences in childhood to non-medical prescription opioid use in adulthood. *Drug and Alcohol Dependency*, 197, 212–219.

Quosh, C. & Gergen, K.J. (2008). Constructing Trauma and its Treatment: Knowledge, Power and Resistance. In K.J. Gergen, T. Sugiman, W. Wagner, & Y. Yamada (eds), *Meaning in Action Constructions, Narratives, and Representations* (pp.97–111). New York, NY: Springer.

Rae, B.E. & Rees, S. (2015). The perceptions of homeless people regarding their healthcare needs and experiences of receiving health care. *Journal of Advanced Nursing*, 71, 2096–2107.

Raharja, A., Tamara, A., & Kok, L.T. (2021). Association between ethnicity and severe COVID-19 disease: A systematic review and meta-analysis. *Journal of Racial and Ethnic Health Disparities*, 8, 6, 1563–1572.

Randolph, M. & Reddy, D. (2006). Sexual abuse and sexual functioning in a chronic pelvic pain sample. *Journal of Child Sexual Abuse*, 15, 61–78.

Rasmussen, C. & Bisanz, J. (2009). Executive functioning in children with fetal alcohol spectrum disorders: Profiles and age-related differences. *Child Neuropsychology*, 15, 201–215.

Reith, T.P. (2018). Burnout in United States healthcare professionals: A narrative review. *Cureus*, 10, 12, e3681.

Remen, R.N. (1996). *Kitchen Table Wisdom: Stories that Heal*. New York, NY: Riverhead Books.

Restauri, N. & Sheridan, A.D. (2020). Burnout and posttraumatic stress disorder in the coronavirus disease 2019 (COVID-19) pandemic: Intersection, impact, and interventions. *Journal of the American College of Radiology: JACR*, 17, 7, 921–926.

Rey, J.H. (1994). *Universals of Psychoanalysis in the Treatment of Psychotic and Borderline States*. London: Free Association Books.

Rhodes-Kropf, J., Carmody, S.S., & Seltzer, D. (2005). 'This is just too awful; I just can't believe I experienced that…': Medical students' reactions to their 'most memorable' patient death. *Academic Medicine*, 80, 634–640.

Rivaux, S.L., James, J., Wittenstrom, K., Baumann, D., *et al.* (2008). The intersection of race, poverty, and risk: Understanding the decision to provide services to clients and to remove children. *Child Welfare*, 87, 151–168.

Rod, N.H., Bengtsson, J., Budtz-Jørgensen, E., Clipet-Jensen, C., *et al.* (2020). Trajectories of childhood adversity and mortality in early adulthood: A population-based cohort study. *The Lancet*, 396, 10249, 489–497.

Rosen, M.A., DiazGranados, D., Dietz, A.S., Benishek, L.E., *et al.* (2018). Teamwork in healthcare: Key discoveries enabling safer, high-quality care. *American Psychology*, 73, 433–450.

Rosenthal, L., Earnshaw, V.A., Moore, J.M., Ferguson, D.N., & Lewis, T.T. (2018). Intergenerational consequences: Women's experiences of discrimination in pregnancy predict infant social-emotional development at six months and one year. *Journal of Developmental and Behavioral Pediatrics*, 39, 228–237.

Ross, C., Dimitrova, S., Howard, L.M., Dewy, M., *et al.* (2015). Human trafficking and health: A cross-sectional survey of NHS professionals' contact with victims of human trafficking. *BMJ Open*, 5, e008682.

Ross, C.A. (2005). Childhood sexual abuse and psychosomatic symptoms in irritable bowel syndrome. *Journal of Child Sexual Abuse*, 14, 1, 27–38.

Rothschild, B. (2000). *The Body Remembers: The Psychophysiology of Trauma and Trauma Treatment*. New York, NY: Norton.

Royal College of Paediatrics and Child Health. (2022). Child health inequalities driven by child poverty in the UK – position statement. www.rcpch.ac.uk/resources/child-health-inequalities-position-statement.

Rutter, M., O'Connor, T.G., & English and Romanian Adoptees (ERA) Study Team. (2004). Are there biological programming effects for psychological development? Findings from a study of Romanian adoptees. *Developmental Psychology*, 40, 1, 81–94.

Sachs-Ericsson, N., Kendall-Tackett, K., & Hernandez, A. (2007). Childhood abuse, chronic pain and depression in the National Comorbidity Survey. *Child Abuse & Neglect*, 3, 5, 531–547.

Salyers, M.P., Bonfils, K.A., Luther, L., Firmin, R.L., *et al.* (2017). The relationship between professional burnout and quality and safety in healthcare: A meta-analysis. *Journal of General Internal Medicine*, 32, 475–482.

Sarkar, P., Bergman, K., Fisk, N.M., & Glover, V. (2006). Maternal anxiety at amniocentesis and plasma cortisol. *Prenatal Diagnosis*, 26, 505–509.

Scanzano, A. & Cosentino, M. (2015). Adrenergic regulation of innate immunity: A review. *Frontiers in Pharmacology*, 6, 171.

Schaufeli, W.B. & Bakker, A.B. (2004). Job demands, job resources, and their relationship with burnout and engagement: A multi-sample study. *Journal of Organizational Behavior*, 25, 293–315.

Scheier, D.B. (2009). Barriers to health care for people with hearing loss: A review of the literature. *The Journal of the New York State Nurses' Association*, 40, 4–10.

Schernhammer, E. (2005). Taking their own lives: The high rate of physician suicide. *New England Journal of Medicine*, 352, 24, 2473–2476.

Schild, S. & Dalenberg, C.J. (2012). Trauma exposure and traumatic symptoms in deaf adults. *Psychological Trauma: Theory, Research, Practice, and Policy*, 4, 117–127.

Schmidt, K.L., Merrill, S.M., Gill, R., Miller, G.E., Gadermann, A.M., & Kobor, M.S. (2021). Society to cell: How child poverty gets 'under the skin' to influence child development and lifelong health. *Developmental Review*, 61, 100983.

Schore, A. (2009a). Relational trauma and the developing right brain. *Annals of the New York Academy of Sciences*, 1159, 189–203.

Schore, A. (2009b). Right Brain Affect Regulation: An Essential Mechanism of Development, Trauma, Dissociation, and Psychotherapy. In D. Fosha, D.J. Siegel, & M. Solomon (eds), *The Healing Power of Emotions: Affective Neuroscience, Development and Clinical Practice* (pp.112–144). New York, NY: W.W. Norton and Company.

Schrag, D. *et al.* (2020). Oncology practice during the COVID19 Pandemic. *JAMA*, 323, 20, 2005–2006.

Schrepf, A., Naliboff, B., Williams, D.A., Stephens-Shields, A.J., *et al.* (2018). MAPP Research Network. Adverse childhood experiences and symptoms of urologic chronic pelvic pain syndrome: A multidisciplinary approach to the study of chronic pelvic pain research network study. *Annals of Behavioral Medicine*, 13, 52, 865–877.

Schulman, K.A. (1999). The effect of race and sex on physicians' recommendations for cardiac catheterization. *New England Journal of Medicine*, 340, 618–626.

Schulz, A.J., Williams, D.R., Israel, B.A., & Lempert, L.B. (2002). Racial and spatial relations as fundamental determinants of health in Detroit. *Milbank Q*, 80, 677–707.

Schuster, M. & Dwyer, P.A. (2020). Post-traumatic stress disorder in nurses: An integrative review. *Journal of Clinical Nursing*, 29, 2769–2787.

Schwaiger, M., Grinberg, M., Moser, D., Zang, J.C., *et al.* (2016). Altered stress-induced regulation of genes in monocytes in adults with a history of childhood adversity. *Neuropsychopharmacology*, 10, 2530–2540.

Segelov, E., Underhill, C., & Prenen, H. (2020). Practical considerations for treating patients with cancer in the Covid-19 pandemic. *JCO Oncology Practice*, 16, 8, 467–482.

Semiz, M., Kavakcı, O., & Peksen, H. (2014). Post-traumatic stress disorder, alexithymia and somatoform dissociation in patients with fibromyalgia. *Turkish Journal of Physical Medicine*, 60, 245–251.

Shalev, A.Y., Peri, T., Brandes, D., Freedman, S., Orr, S.P., & Pitman, R.K. (2000). Auditory startle response in trauma survivors with posttraumatic stress disorder: A prospective study. *American Journal of Psychiatry*, 157, 255–261.

Shanafelt, T.D., Hasan, O., Dyrbye, L.N., Sinsky, C., *et al.* (2015). Changes in burnout and satisfaction with work-life balance in physicians and the general US working population between 2011 and 2014. *Mayo Clinic Proceedings*, 90, 1600–1613.

Sharifi, M., Asadi-Pooya, A.A., & Mousavi-Roknabadi, R.S. (2020). Burnout among healthcare providers of COVID-19: A systematic review of epidemiology and recommendations. *Archives of Academic Emergency Medicine*, 9, 1, e7.

Shavers, V.L., Fagan, P., Jones, D., Klein, W.M., Boyington, J., & Moten, C. (2012). The state of research on racial/ethnic discrimination in the receipt of health care. *American Journal of Public Health*, 102, 953–966.

Shen, L. (2019). Early-life exposure to severe famine is associated with higher methylation level in the IGF2 gene and higher total cholesterol in late adulthood: The Genomic Research of the Chinese Famine (GRECF) study. *Clinical Epigenetics*, 11, 88.

Shevlin, M., Dorahy, M.J., & Adamson, G. (2007). Trauma and psychosis: An analysis of the National Comorbidity Survey. *American Journal of Psychiatry*, 164, 166–169.

Shires, D.A. & Jaffee, K. (2015). Factors associated with health care discrimination experiences among a National Sample of female-to-male transgender individuals. *Health and Social Work*, 40, 134–141.

Shohet, R. & Shohet, J. (2019). *In Love With Supervision: Creating Transformative Conversations*. Monmouth: PCCS Books.

Shotter, J. (1993). *Cultural Politics of Everyday Life*. Milton Keynes: Open University Press.

Siegel, D.J. (2012). *The Developing Mind: How Relationships and the Brain Interact to Shape Who We Are*. London and New York, NY: The Guilford Press.

SignHealth. (2013). *Research into the Health of Deaf People*. Available at: https://signhealth.org.uk/wp-content/uploads/2019/07/SignHealth-Deaf-Health-Survey-Report-1.pdf.

Sinclair, I., Baker, C., Lee, J., & Gibbs, I. (2007). *The Pursuit of Permanence: A Study of the English Childcare System*. London: Jessica Kingsley Publishers.

Singer, L.T., Nelson, S., Short, E., Min, M.O., *et al.* (2008). Prenatal cocaine exposure: Drug and environmental effects at 9 years. *Journal of Pediatrics*, 153, 105–111.

Slopen, N., Lewis, T.T., & Williams, D.R. (2016). Discrimination and sleep: A systematic review. *Sleep Medicine*, 18, 88–95.

Smedley, B.D., Stith, A.Y., & Nelson, A.R. (eds) (2003). *Unequal Treatment: Confronting Racial and Ethnic Disparities in Health Care*. Institute of Medicine (US) Committee on Understanding and Eliminating Racial and Ethnic Disparities in Health Care. Washington, DC: National Academies Press.

Smeijers, A.S. & Pfau, R. (2009). Towards a treatment for treatment: On communication between general practitioners and their deaf patients. *The Sign Language Translator and Interpreter*, 3, 1–14.

Smith, J. (2021). *Nurturing Maternity Staff: How to Tackle Trauma, Stress and Burnout to Create a Positive Working Culture in the NHS*. London: Pinter and Martin.

Smith, R.P. (2017). Burnout in obstetricians and gynecologists. *Obstetrics and Gynecology Clinics of North America*, 44, 297–310.

Soares, A.L.G., Howe, L.D., Matijasevich, A., Wehrmeister, F.C., Menezes, A.M., & Gonçalves, H. (2016). Adverse childhood experiences: Prevalence and related factors in adolescents of a Brazilian birth cohort. *Child Abuse Neglect*, 51, 21–30.

Spencer, N.J., Blackburn, C.M., & Read, J.M. (2015). Disabling chronic conditions in childhood and socioeconomic disadvantage: A systematic review and meta-analyses of observational studies. *BMJ Open*, 5, e007062.

Stamm, B.H. (1999). *Secondary Traumatic Stress: Self-Care Issues for Clinicians, Researchers, and Educators*. Lutherville, MD: Sidran Press.

Stelnicki, A.M., Carleton, R.N., & Reichert, C. (2020). *Mental Disorder Symptoms among Nurses in Canada*. Ottawa, ON: Canadian Federation of Nurses Unions.

Stepanikova, I. & Cook, K.S. (2008). Effects of poverty and lack of insurance on perceptions of racial and ethnic bias in health care. *Health Services Research*, 43, 915–930.

Straus, L. (2009). Somali women's experience of childbirth in the UK: Perspectives from Somali health workers. *Midwifery*, 25, 181–186.

Studer Group. (2015). Healing Physician Burnout Survey. Available at: www.huronlearninglab.com/resources/articles-and-industry-updates/articles-and-whitepapers/studer-group-releases-results-of-physician-burnout.

Substance Abuse and Mental Health Services Administration. (2014). *SAMHSA's concept of trauma and guidance for a trauma-informed approach*. Rockville: Department of Health and Human Services.

Sue, D.W. (2010). *Microaggressions in Everyday Life: Race, Gender, and Sexual Orientation*. Hoboken, NJ: John Wiley & Sons.

Sullivan, P. & Knutson, J. (2000). Maltreatment and disabilities: A population-based epidemiological study. *Child Abuse & Neglect*, 24, 1257–1273.

Summerfield, D. (2004). Cross-Cultural Perspectives on the Medicalization of Human Suffering. In G.M. Rosen (ed.), *Posttraumatic Stress Disorder: Issues and Controversies* (pp.233–245). Chichester: John Wiley.

Sundin, E. & Baguley, T. (2015). Prevalence of childhood abuse among people who are homeless in Western countries: A systematic review and meta-analysis. *Social Psychiatry and Psychiatric Epidemiology*, 50, 183–194.

Szalma, J.L. & Hancock, P.A. (2011). Noise effects on human performance: A meta-analytic synthesis. *Psychological Bulletin*, 137, 682–707.

Sze, S., Pan, D., & Nevill, C.R. (2020). Ethnicity and clinical outcomes in COVID-19: A systematic review and meta-analysis. *EClinicalMedicine*, 29, 100630.

Talge, N.M., Neal, C., & Glover, V. (2007). Antenatal maternal stress and long-term effects on child neurodevelopment: How and why? *Journal of Child Psychology and Psychiatry*, 48, 245–261.

Tamayo-Sarver, J.H., Hinze, S.W., Cydulka, R.K., & Baker, D.W. (2003). Racial and ethnic disparities in emergency department analgesic prescription. *American Journal of Public Health*, 1, 93, 2067–2073.

Taylor, J., Bradbury-Jones, C., & Lund, P. (2019). Witchcraft-related abuse and murder of children with albinism in sub-saharan Africa: A conceptual review. *Child Abuse Review*, 28, 13–26.

Teicher, M.H., Samson, J.A., Anderson, C.M., & Ohashi, K. (2016). The effects of childhood maltreatment on brain structure, function and connectivity. *Nature*, 17, 652–666.

Tervalon, M. & Murray-García, J. (1998). Cultural humility versus cultural competence: A critical distinction in defining physician training outcomes in multicultural education. *Journal of Health Care for the Poor and Underserved*, 9, 117–125.

Thames, A.D., Irwin, M.R., Breen, E.C., & Cole, S.W. (2019). Experienced discrimination and racial differences in leukocyte gene expression. *Psychoneuroendocrinology*, 106, 277–283.

Thayer, J.F. & Lane, R.D. (2009). Claude Bernard and the heart–brain connection: Further elaboration of a model of neurovisceral integration. *Neuroscience and Biobehavioral Review*, 33, 81–88.

The Food Foundation. (2021). *The Broken Plate 2021: The State of the Nation's Food System*. Available at: foodfoundation.org.uk/publication/broken-plate-2021.

Thiara, R.K., Hague, G., & Mullender, A. (2011). Losing out on both counts: Disabled women and domestic violence. *Disability and Society*, 26, 757–771.

Thomas, J. (2016). Adverse childhood experiences among MSW students. *Journal of Teaching in Social Work*, 36, 235–255.

Tidmarsh, L.V., Harrison, R., Ravindran, D., Matthews, S.L., & Finlay, K.A. (2022). The influence of adverse childhood experiences in pain management: Mechanisms, processes, and trauma-informed care. *Frontiers in Pain Research*, 3, 923866. doi: 10.3389/fpain.2022.923866.

Tietjen, G.E., Brandes, J.L., Peterlin, B.L., Eloff, A., *et al.* (2010). Childhood maltreatment and migraine (part I). Prevalence and adult revictimization: A multicenter headache clinic survey. *Headache*, 50, 1, 20–31.

Tingle, C. & Vora, S. (2018). *Break the Barriers: Girls' Experiences of Menstruation in the UK.* London: Plan International UK.

Tottenham, N., Hare, T.A., Quinn, B.T., McCarry, T.W., Nurse, M., *et al.* (2010). Prolonged institutional rearing is associated with atypically large amygdala volume and difficulties in emotion regulation. *Developmental Science*, 13, 46–61.

Treisman, K. (2016). *Working with Relational and Developmental Trauma in Children and Adolescents.* London: Routledge.

Treisman, K. (2017a). *A Therapeutic Treasure Box for Working with Children and Adolescents with Developmental Trauma: Creative Techniques and Activities.* London: Jessica Kingsley Publishers.

Treisman, K. (2017b). *A Therapeutic Treasure Deck of Cards: Grounding, Soothing, Coping, and Regulating.* London: Jessica Kingsley Publishers.

Treisman, K. (2019). *Presley the Pug Relaxation Activity Book.* London: Jessica Kingsley Publishers.

Treisman, K. (2020). *The Parenting Patchwork Treasure Deck: A Creative Tool for Assessments, Interventions, and Strengthening Relationships with Parents, Carers, and Children.* London: Jessica Kingsley Publishers.

Treisman, K. (2021). *A Treasure Box for Creating Trauma-Informed Organizations: A Ready-to-Use Resource for Trauma, Adversity, and Culturally Informed, Infused, and Responsive Systems.* London: Jessica Kingsley Publishers.

Treisman, K. (2022). *The Trauma Treasure Deck of Cards: A Creative Tool for Assessments, Interventions, and Learning for Work with Adversity and Stress.* London: Jessica Kingsley Publishers.

Ueda, M., Martins, R., & Hendrie, P.C. (2020). Managing cancer care during the Covid-19 pandemic: Agility and collaboration toward a common goal. *Journal of the National Comprehensive Cancer Network*, 1–4.

Ulrich, R.S., Zimring, C., Zhu, X., DuBose, J., *et al.* (2008). A review of the research literature on evidence-based healthcare design. *HERD: Health Environments Research and Design Journal*, 1, 61–125.

United Nations. (2000). *Annex II: The definition of trafficking in persons and the mandate for the Global Report.* Available at: www.unodc.org/documents/data-and-analysis/glotip/Annex_II_-_Definition_and_mandate.pdf.

Upshur, C.C., Bacigalupe, G., & Luckmann, R. (2010). 'They don't want anything to do with you': Patient views of primary care management of chronic pain. *Pain Medicine*, 11, 1791–1798.

Upshur, C.C., Luckmann, R.S., & Savageau, J.A. (2006). Primary care provider concerns about management of chronic pain in community clinic populations. *Journal of General Internal Medicine*, 21, 652–655.

Ussher, J.M. (2013). Diagnosing difficult women and pathologising femininity: Gender bias in psychiatric nosology. *Feminism & Psychology*, 23, 63–69.

van Daalen., K.R., Kaiser, J., & Kebede, S. (2022). Racial discrimination and adverse pregnancy outcomes: A systematic review and meta-analysis. *BMJ Global Health*, 7, e009227.

Van der Kolk, B. (2005). Developmental trauma disorder: Toward a rational diagnosis for children with complex trauma histories. *Psychiatric Annals*, 35, 401–408.

Van der Kolk, B. (2014). *The Body Keeps the Score: Brain, Mind, and Body in the Healing of Trauma*. New York, NY: Viking Penguin.

Van Mol, M.M., Kompanje, E.J., Benoit, D.D., Bakker J., & Nijkamp, M.D. (2015). The prevalence of compassion fatigue and burnout among healthcare professionals in intensive care units: A systematic review. *PLoS One*, 10, 618.

van Ryn, M. & Burke, J. (2000). The effect of patient race and socio-economic status on physicians' perceptions of patients. *Social Science and Medicine*, 50, 813–828.

Vohra, J., Marmot, M.G., Bauld, L., & Hiatt, R.A. (2016). Socioeconomic position in childhood and cancer in adulthood: A rapid-review. *Journal of Epidemiology and Community Health*, 70, 6, 629–634.

Ward, R.L., Nichols, A.D., & Freedman, R.I. (2010). Uncovering health care inequalities among adults with intellectual and developmental disabilities. *Health and Social Work*, 35, 280–290.

Warner, E. & Koomar, J. (2009). Arousal Regulation in Traumatised Children: Sensorimotor Interventions. International Trauma Conference: Boston.

Warrington, C., Ackerley, E., Becket, H., Walker, M., *et al.* (2016). *Making Noise: Children's Voices for Positive Change After Sexual Abuse*. Luton: University of Bedfordshire/Office of Children's Commissioner.

Webber, E.K., Bird, C.M., deRoon-Cassini, T.A., Weis, C.N., *et al.* (2010). Hospital experiences of older people with intellectual disability: Responses of group home staff and family members. *Journal of Intellectual Development Disability*, 35, 155–164.

Wei, J., Mehta, P.K., & Grey, E. (2017). Sex-based differences in quality of care and outcomes in a health system using a standardized STEMI protocol. *American Heart Journal*, 191, 30–36.

Weissbecker, I., Roshania, R., Cavallera, V., Mallow, M., *et al.* (2018). Integrating psychosocial support at Ebola treatment units in Sierra Leone and Liberia. Webber, E.K., Bird, C.M., deRoon-Cassini T.A., Weis, C.N., Huggins, A.A., Fitzgerald, J.M., Miskovich, T., Bennett K., Krukowski, J., Torres, L., Larson, C.L. (2022). Racial Discrimination and Resting-State Functional Connectivity of Salience Network Nodes in Trauma-Exposed Black Adults in the United States. *JAMA Netw Open*. 4-5. *Intervention*, 16, 69–79.

Wen, C.K., Hudak, P.L., & Hwang, S.W. (2007). Homeless people's perceptions of welcomeness and unwelcomeness in healthcare encounters. *Journal of General Internal Medicine*, 22, 1011–1017.

Wheeler, D.C., Raman, S., Jones, R.M., Schootman, M., & Nelson, E.J. (2019). Bayesian deprivation index models for explaining variation in elevated blood lead levels among children in Maryland. *Spatio-Temporal Epidemiology*, 30, 100286.

Wilkinson, R. & Pickett, K. (2010). *The Spirit Level: Why Equality is Better for Everyone*. London: Penguin.

Willard-Grace, R., Knox, M., Huang, B., Hammer, H., Kivlahan, C., & Grumbach, K. (2019). Burnout and health care workforce turnover. *Annals of Family Medicine*, 17, 1, 36–41.

Williams, D.R. & Collins, C. (2001). Racial residential segregation: A fundamental cause of racial disparities in health. *Public Health Reports*, 116, 5, 404–416.

Williams, D.R., Lawrence, J.A., & Davis, B.A. (2019). Racism and health: Evidence and needed research. *Annual Review of Public Health*, 1, 40, 105–125.

Williams, E.S., Rathert, C., & Buttigieg, S.C. (2020). The personal and professional consequences of physician burnout: A systematic review of the literature. *Medical Care Research
and Review*, 77, 5, 371–386.

Willumsen, T. (2004). The impact of childhood sexual abuse on dental fear. *Community
Dental Oral Epidemiology*, 32, 73–79.

Wood, L.C.N. (2020). Child modern slavery, trafficking and health: A practical review of
factors contributing to children's vulnerability and the potential impacts of severe
exploitation on health. *BMJ Paediatrics Open*, 4, 1, e000327.

World Health Organization. (2013). *Review of Social Determinants and the Health Divide in the
WHO European Region: Final Report*. Copenhagen: World Health Organization.

Wu, N.S., Schairer, L.C., Dellor, E., & Grella, C. (2010). Childhood trauma and health outcomes in adults with comorbid substance abuse and mental health disorders. *Addictive
Behaviors*, 35, 68–71.

Wu, R., Zhu, H., Wu, M.Y., Wang, G.H., & Jiang, C.L. (2022). Childhood trauma and suicide:
The mediating effect of stress and sleep. *International Journal of Environmental Research
and Public Health*, 19, 14, 8493.

Wullink, M., Veldhuijzen, W., Lantman-de Valk, H.M.J., Metsemakers, J.F.M., & Dinant,
G-J. (2009). Doctor-patient communication with people with intellectual disability: A
qualitative study. *BMC Family Practice*, 10, 82.

Yavne, Y., Amital, D., & Watad, A. (2018). A systematic review of precipitating physical and
psychological traumatic events in the development of fibromyalgia. *Seminars in Arthritis
and Rheumatism*, 48, 121–133.

Yehuda, R., Mulherin Engel, S., Brand, S.R., Seckl, J., Marcus, S.M. & Berkowitz, G.S. (2005).
Transgenerational effects of posttraumatic stress disorder in babies of mothers exposed
to the World Trade Center attacks during pregnancy. *Journal of Clinical Endocrinology
and Metabolism*, 90, 4115–4118.

Zarse, E.M., Neff, M.R., Yoder, R., Hulvershorn, L., *et al.* (2019). The adverse childhood
experiences questionnaire: Two decades of research on childhood trauma as a primary
cause of adult mental illness, addiction, and medical diseases. *Cogent Medicine*, 6, 1–5.

Subject Index

Author Index